Shoulder Surgery Made Easy!

The Singapore Shoulder & Elbow Society Guide to Arthroscopic and Open Shoulder Procedures

Denny T.T. Lie

Singapore General Hospital, Singapore

World Scientific

NEW JERSEY • LONDON • SINGAPORE • BEIJING • SHANGHAI • HONG KONG • TAIPEI • CHENNAI • TOKYO

Published by

World Scientific Publishing Co. Pte. Ltd.
5 Toh Tuck Link, Singapore 596224
USA office: 27 Warren Street, Suite 401-402, Hackensack, NJ 07601
UK office: 57 Shelton Street, Covent Garden, London WC2H 9HE

Library of Congress Cataloging-in-Publication Data
Names: Lie, Denny T.T. (Denny Tjiauw Tjoen), author.
Title: Shoulder surgery made easy! : the Singapore Shoulder & Elbow Society
guide to arthroscopic and open shoulder procedures / Denny T.T. Lie.
Description: Hackensack, NJ : World Scientific, [2023] | Includes bibliographical references and index.
Identifiers: LCCN 2021049380 | ISBN 9789811249839 (hardcover) |
ISBN 9789811249846 (ebook : for institutions) | ISBN 9789811249853 (ebook : for individuals)
Subjects: MESH: Shoulder--surgery | Shoulder Joint--surgery | Arthroscopy--methods
Classification: LCC RD557.5 | NLM WE 810 | DDC 617.5/72059--dc23/eng/20211101
LC record available at https://lccn.loc.gov/2021049380

British Library Cataloguing-in-Publication Data
A catalogue record for this book is available from the British Library.

For any available supplementary material, please visit
https://www.worldscientific.com/worldscibooks/10.1142/12657#t=suppl

Desk Editors: Soundararajan Raghuraman/Joy Quek

Typeset by Stallion Press
Email: enquiries@stallionpress.com

This book is dedicated to my wife Juliana, who lovingly and patiently supported me as I wrote this book during the challenging months of the COVID pandemic; and to my daughters Hannah and Rachel, who are my source of joy and my inspiration.

I am grateful to Professor Christian Gerber and Professor Jon JP Warner, my teachers and mentors when I first embarked on my journey into the shoulder world. Thank you!

https://doi.org/10.1142/9789811249846_fmatter

Foreword

It is with great honour that I introduce this textbook by my friend Professor Denny T.T. Lie.

Denny is a consummate professional physician and teacher. He recognised the need for a surgical guide for residents, fellows and early in career surgeons to standardise the process of surgical procedures. Rather than just help his own students, he decided to help everyone worldwide by putting together a guide book for shoulder arthroscopy. This text should be utilised by all surgeons in training as a baseline to prepare for preoperative, intra-operative, and post-operative care. This text will improve care and education worldwide.

I congratulate Professor Lie for this excellent contribution to medical education.

Professor Felix Savoie III
President of the American Academy of Orthopaedic Surgeons (AAOS)
Past President, American Shoulder and Elbow Society (ASES)
Past President, Arthroscopy Association of North America (AANA)

https://doi.org/10.1142/9789811249846_fmatter

About the Author

Denny T.T. Lie has been practising shoulder and sports surgery at the Singapore General Hospital since 2004, when he returned from his fellowship training at both Balgrist Hospital, Zurich, Switzerland and Massachusetts General Hospital, Boston, USA. To date, he has performed more than 2,000 shoulder procedures and authored about 100 publications. He is the current President of Singapore Orthopaedic Association, Vice President of the ASEAN Orthopaedic Association and incoming President of the Asian Shoulder & Elbow Association. He founded the Singapore Shoulder & Elbow Society (SSES) in 2018. He is passionate about teaching and is currently the Program Director of SingHealth Orthopaedic Residency. He enjoys and is equally passionate about biomechanics research. This is his first book.

https://doi.org/10.1142/9789811249846_fmatter

List of Contributors

Dr Lim Chee Yeong Department of Diagnostic Radiology, Singapore General Hospital, Singapore

Dr Dennis Ng Zhaowen The Orthopaedic Centre, Singapore

Dr Geoffrey Liew Haw Chieh Department of Anaesthesiology, Singapore General Hospital, Singapore

Dr Bryan Wang Dehao Shoulder Elbow Orthopaedic Group, Singapore

Dr Mak Wai Keong Department of Orthopaedic Surgery, Sengkang General Hospital, Singapore

Dr Lai Mun Chun Department of Orthopaedic Surgery, Tan Tock Seng Hospital, Singapore

Dr Andrew Chou Chia Chen Department of Orthopaedic Surgery, Singapore General Hospital, Singapore

Dr Abby Choke Department of Hand & Reconstructive Microsurgery, Singapore General Hospital, Singapore

Dr Bryan Loh Huai Gu Department of Orthopaedic Surgery, Singapore General Hospital, Singapore

Dr Lim Mui Hong Synergy Orthopaedic Group Pte Ltd, Singapore

Dr Thomas Kuo Department of Orthopaedic Surgery, Changi General Hospital, Singapore

Dr Zhu Meng Department of Orthopaedic Surgery, Changi General Hospital, Singapore

Dr Don Thong Siang Koh Department of Orthopaedic Surgery, Singapore General Hospital, Singapore

Dr Goh Keng Meng Jeremy Department of Orthopaedic Surgery, Singapore General Hospital, Singapore

Dr Punn Kuhataparuks MOH Holdings Pte Ltd, Singapore

Dr Cheow Xunqi Department of Orthopaedic Surgery, Sengkang General Hospital, Singapore

Dr Lee Jian Hui, Merrill Department of Orthopaedic Surgery, Singapore General Hospital, Singapore

Dr Tay Eileen The Orthopaedic Practice and Surgery, Singapore

Dr Gerald Joseph Zeng Sheng Xiang Department of Orthopaedic Surgery, Singapore General Hospital, Singapore

Dr Ong Hang Shyan Desmond Shoulder Elbow Orthopedic Group, Singapore

Dr Hamid Rahmatullah Bin Abd Razak Department of Orthopaedic Surgery, Sengkang General Hospital, Singapore

Dr Wong Merng Koon Department of Orthopaedic Surgery, Sengkang General Hospital, Singapore

Dr Edwin Tan Tze Sheng Livingstone Health, Mt Elizabeth Hospital, Singapore

Dr Puah Ken Lee Department of Orthopaedic Surgery, Singapore General Hospital, Singapore

Dr Ruben Manohara Shoulder Elbow Orthopaedic Group, Singapore

https://doi.org/10.1142/9789811249846_fmatter

Acknowledgements

I thank the following:

- Dr Punn Kuhataparuks for his excellent medical illustrations.
- Dr Shahid Khan and Dr Eric Cher for their help in Chapter 1.
- Ms Chern Lim for taking photos of the instruments in Chapter 3.

https://doi.org/10.1142/9789811249846_fmatter

Contents

https://doi.org/10.1142/9789811249846_fmatter

Introduction

Denny T.T. Lie

A Unique Shoulder Book!

This book serves as a template and a guide, with proven surgical techniques developed by the authors over the past 15 years at the Singapore General Hospital. Each surgical technique has proven published results and thus provides an assurance to the readers that these techniques are reproducible.

This is the first book published by Singapore shoulder surgeons and is the effort of Denny Lie, with contributions from his colleagues in the Singapore Shoulder & Elbow Society. *A book by Singapore surgeons for the region and the world!*

Do Orthopaedic Residents Need Another Book?

This book was written for orthopaedic residents and general orthopaedic surgeons who are interested in shoulder surgery. It is written in a simple form, with relevant salient points for successful surgery, illustrated with hundreds of surgical pictures and schematic diagrams.

The first chapter of this book is dedicated to a diagnostic approach to shoulder problems, often a confusing problem that is not well studied. The various physical examination techniques are then shown and illustrated. Imaging and other surgical preparations are also discussed. More than 20 surgical techniques are described in detail, each chapter beginning with an introduction to the problem, followed by the succinct points in imaging, diagnosis and approach; then the surgical technique(s) which the author(s) found useful, post-operative care and ending off with the clinical results of this technique.

It is hoped that the reader will enjoy reading this book and would find it useful for his/her surgical practice.

Deo Gratias!

https://doi.org/10.1142/9789811249846_0001

Chapter 1

History-Taking and Physical Examination of the Shoulder

Denny T.T. Lie

Summary of Chapter

1. History-taking and symptomology of shoulder pathologies
2. Physical examination
3. Approach based on symptoms, differential diagnoses
4. The dominant symptom, overlapping symptoms
5. Age dependent diagnoses

1. History-Taking and Symptomology of Shoulder Pathologies

1.1 *The Preliminary Questions*

- **Age:** It is a key factor as there is certain age predilection to some pathologies. For example, in young patients (20–40 years old), anterior labral and SLAP tears are more common, while middle aged patients (40–60 years of age) have more cases of tendinosis, small tears, capsulitis, ACJ and biceps pathology. It is in the age group >60 years, that the diversity of diagnoses appears; from large to massive tears, to arthritis and capsulitis. Though not exclusive, certain diagnoses tend to occur in certain age groups (see Section 5).

- **Gender** and **hand dominance**.
- **Trauma:** It is an important preliminary question. The mechanism of injury and severity needs to be understood. In all age groups, obvious bony fractures and shoulder dislocations need to be excluded. High energy falls tend to cause large tears, as opposed to low energy repetitive injuries which tend to cause small tears.
- **Occupation:** Certain occupations like professional athletes, military and police forces are more physically demanding and require stable and strong upper limbs. Others like the airline industry are time-sensitive and patients in these industries cannot take prolonged leave; hence it affects choice of treatment and timing of surgery.
- **Sports involvement:** More than a cursory question, the patient's specific involvement in the specific sports needs to be understood and his/her aspiration to return to the specific level of sports needs to be appreciated. For example, for a young patient to return to swimming, the swimming style (front crawl or breast stroke) is important. In rugby, the specific position the patient plays, is just as important.
- **Previous shoulder surgery:** It may cause capsulitis and will affect any future surgeries. Further, revision surgeries have an increased risk of infection.

1.2 *The Cardinal Questions*

Shoulder pathologies present with overlapping symptoms and it is difficult, if not impossible, to diagnose a condition on the basis of the symptoms alone. It is thus proposed that these five cardinal symptoms are asked and the interviewing physician needs to weigh which of these symptom(s) are ***dominant****, and affect the patient most (Fig. 1).*

- **Pain:** Pain is the most common presenting symptom in most orthopaedic conditions and this is certainly true in the spectrum of shoulder pathologies. The presenting pain can range from **mild to excruciating** in severity, tends to be initiated by movement and **effort-related**, that is, made worse with increased exertion and use of the shoulder. It is often described as **sharp** but often may be **throbbing in nature**. Patients often complain it is worse at night and they are unable to sleep on the affected side. Though the various pathologies may not be diagnosed just by the location or site of pain, localising the area of pain would prove useful in categorising the possible differential diagnoses. The pain could be **anterior, postero-lateral**, over the acromio-clavicular joint, or **generalised deep**.

- **Stiffness:** Many shoulder pathologies present with some limitation to range of motion, whether due to pain or a real physical limitation. It could be mild; a gradually increasing tightness as the shoulder is moved preventing full range of motion, which is termed **terminal tightness**. In its most severe form, patients complain of a **physical block** in the early to mid-range of motion.
- **Weakness:** In most shoulder conditions the weakness is **mild** and does not affect the ability of the patient to actively move the shoulder nor does it affect the patent's activity of daily living (ADL). However, when compared to the contralateral side, the patient may notice the weakness ranges from a sense of **hesitation** to **outright weakness**. In the most severe form, the patient's arm cannot be actively lifted, even with shrugging of the shoulder, and the needs to be passively lifted. The patient may not be able to maintain the arm in the lifted (abducted) position, resulting in the **drop arm sign**.
- **Instability:** The symptoms presented by patients with recurrent dislocations are usually mild and do not affect their ADL. However, when they may have a sense of **apprehension**, an uncomfortable feeling of impending dislocation when the arm is in the overhead position. This is common among overhead athletes, like netball players and rock climbers. This apprehension leads them to hesitate and robs them of the confidence they need. In more severe cases of chronic shoulder instability, patients complain of their shoulders feeling "**loose**" and may subluxate easily at the mildest provocation.
- **Numbness and referred pain:** Numbness is not a common symptom of the shoulder pathology itself. Occasionally patients may present with numbness around the regimental badge are of the deltoids, resulting from axillary nerve injury after a shoulder dislocation. Patients may present with severe numbing pain radiating down the ulnar side

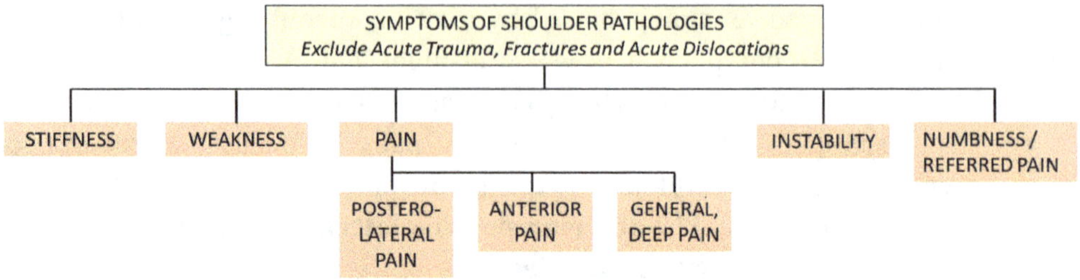

Fig. 1: The five main/cardinal symptoms of shoulder pathologies.

of the arm, which can be due to scapula-thoracic dissociations. Scapula pathologies may also present with sharp penetrating pain, often with numbness radiating down the arm. The majority of causes of numbness is radiculopathy, cervicogenic in origin and the cervical spine needs to be examined and investigated. Peripheral neuropathy may have numbness originating from or radiating to the shoulder region.

1.3 *The Other Questions*

- Allergy (including to contrast);
- Co-morbidities;
- Pain medications;
- Peri-operative anaesthesia consideration;
- Pregnancy (if applicable);
- Physiotherapy potential pre and post-surgery;
- Social support.

2. Physical Examination, Flow of Examination

2.1 *Inspection and Palpation*

- Begin with proper exposure of the patient, within limits of modesty and what is acceptable to the patient.
- Look for obvious wasting of the deltoids and squaring of the shoulders, wasting and hollowing of the supraspinatus and infraspinatus

fossae. Observe for any surgical scars, obvious lumps and swellings including prominence of the acromio-clavicular joint. Look out for the Popeye deformity.

- Palpate the entire shoulder girdle:
  (a) Begin with the sternoclavicular joint (SCJ). Prominent and tender SCJ is usually due to arthritis, and occasionally due to pyogenic bacterial infection and rarely, TB infection.
  (b) Palpate the entire clavicle, feeling for acute fractures and old deformities.
  (c) The acromio-clavicular joint (ACJ) is then palpated at the lateral end of the clavicle; feel for tenderness, swelling and deformity due to arthritis and subluxation. Occasionally, a fluctuant cystic swelling may be palpated over the ACJ, this is the Geyser's sign, a cystic swelling seen in massive cuff tear and secondary arthritis of the glenohumeral joint.
  (d) Inferior to the ACJ, palpate the long head of the biceps tendon (LHBT). Tenderness and occasionally a sense of fullness may be felt in tendinosis.
  (e) Next, palpate the entire lateral edge of the acromion and attachment of the deltoid muscle. Occasionally tenderness may be elicited in patients with cuff tears but this is not a hard sign.
  (f) Posteriorly it may be necessary in some patients to palpate the borders of the scapula. Patients with deep penetrating aching pain may have periscapular tendinosis and tenderness can be elicited in the medial scapula border especially at the supero-medial corner.

2.2 *Examination of the Cardinal Questions*

Building on the approach of the five cardinal symptoms, examination follows this pattern and helps to construct a mental diagnostic picture. Instead of the "Look-Feel-Move-Special Tests" approach, the special tests are divided and placed under the columns that reflect the predominant symptom. All the tests are routinely done but as the tests are performed, it is incumbent on the examiner to ask again if the symptom was the

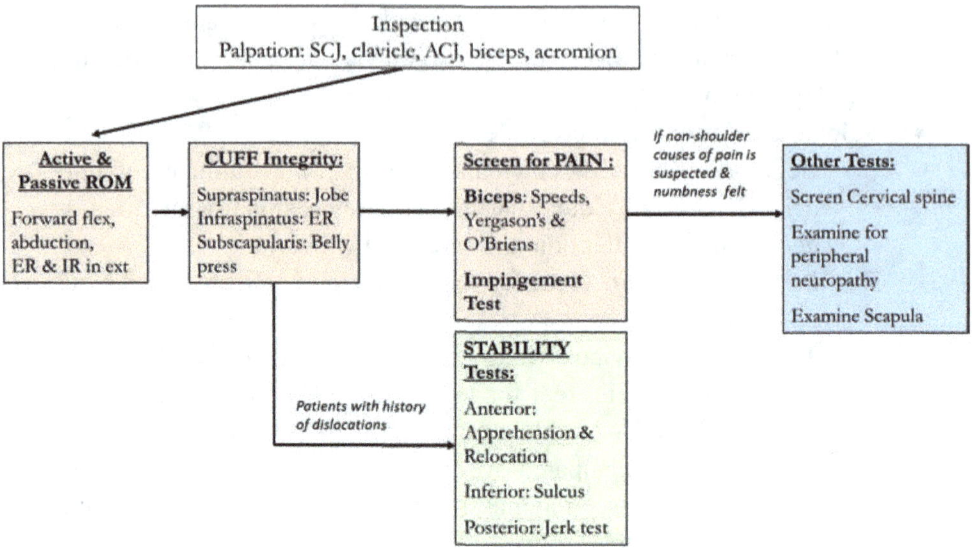

Fig. 2: Flow of examination, each group of test follows the five cardinal symptom approach.

dominant one, and accordingly if the sign being elicited is likewise, the main sign. Section 2.3 below is a table showing how each test is performed and the known sensitivity and specificity (Fig. 2).

2.3 *Common Tests of Shoulder Pathologies [1–5]*

Cuff Pathology — Tests of Supraspinatus Integrity		
Jobes test (Empty can) *Sen: 81%* *Spe: 89%*	• Position the shoulder in internal rotation with the thumb pointing down, at 30° abduction in the plane of the scapula. • Apply a downward force at the distal forearm to test for the supraspinatus strength.	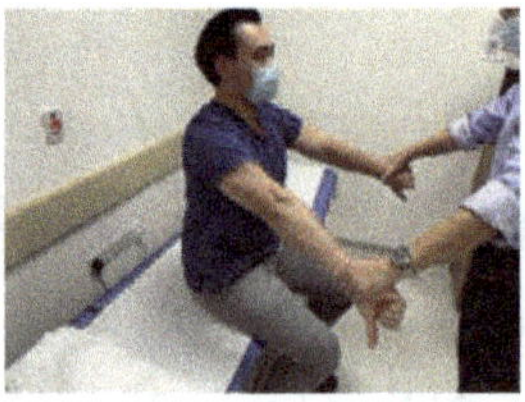

(*Continued*)

Drop test	• Passively abduct the shoulder to 180° and instruct the patient to slowly lower the arm. • Inability to slowly lower the arm between 90° and 0° abduction indicates a supraspinatus pathology.	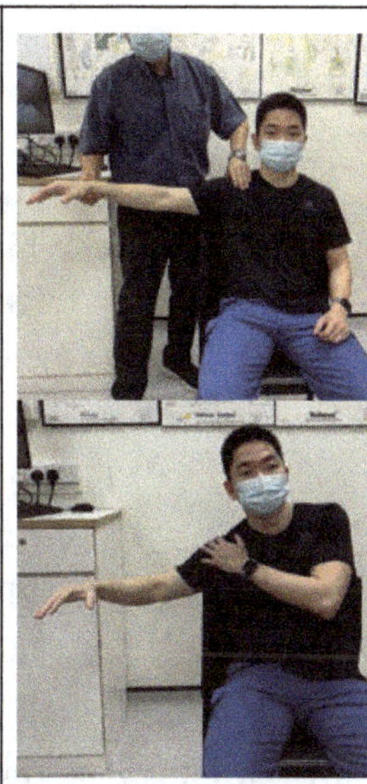
Cuff Pathology — Tests of Infraspinatus Integrity		
Resisted external rotation test *Sen: 76%* *Spe: 57%*	• Position the patient with arm in neutral rotation and elbow flexed to 90°. • Strength of infraspinatus is tested with patient exerting an ER force while the examiner apply a medially directed force. This test examines the integrity of the infraspinatus and teres minor.	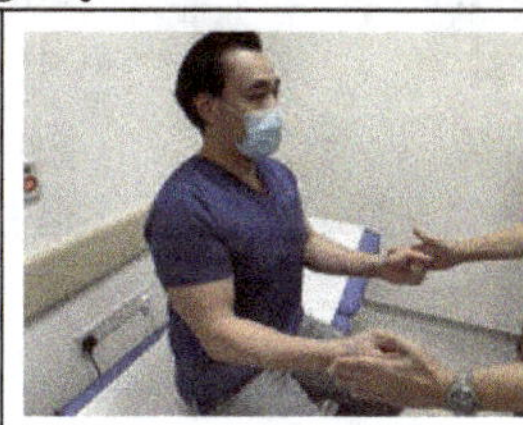

(*Continued*)

(*Continued*)

External rotation lag sign	• Position the patient with elbow 90° flexed, shoulder 20° elevated in the plane of scapula and max ER. • While holding the elbow, release the wrist and inability to maintain the position suggest an infraspinatus tear. This test examines the integrity of the infraspinatus and supraspinatus.	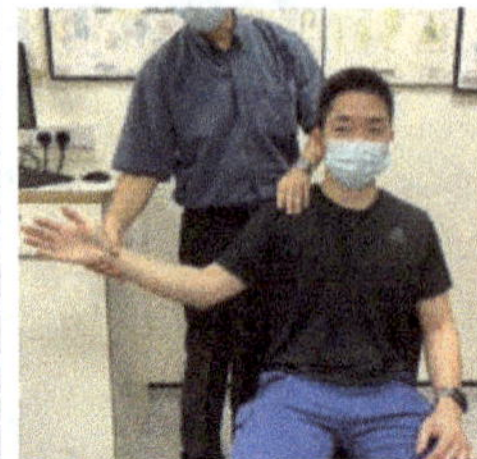 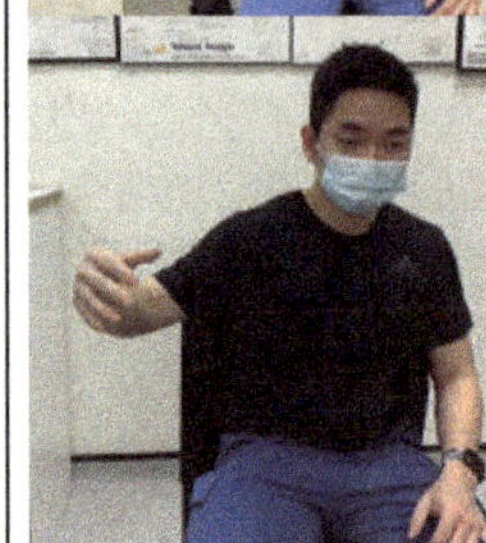
Cuff Pathology — Tests of Subscapularis Integrity		
Belly press test *Sen: 86%* *Spe: 91%*	• Position the patient seated with arm at 45°, full internal rotation and palm towards the belly. • Inability to maintain the elbow and wrist straight while pressing the belly indicates a subscapularis weakness. Passive belly off test • Bring the patient's arm into full IR and place the palm onto the belly. • Inability to keep the elbow and wrist straight upon release of the examiner's hand suggest weakness of the subscapularis.	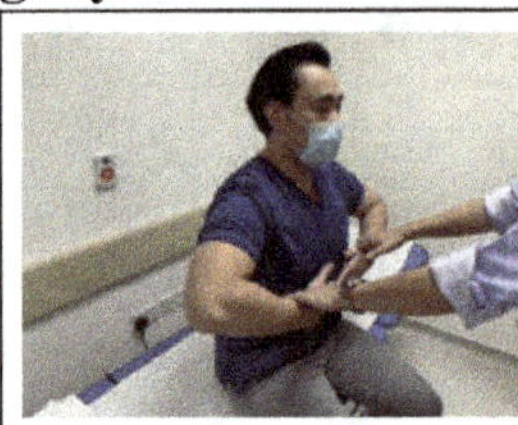

(*Continued*)

Napoleon test *Sen: 41%* *Spe: 80%*	The patient is asked to place the hand on the belly. The test is graded as • negative (or normal) if the patient can push the hand against the belly with the wrist straight; • positive, if the wrist was flexed to 90° to push against the belly; • Intermediate, if the wrist is flexed from 30° to 60° to do the belly press.	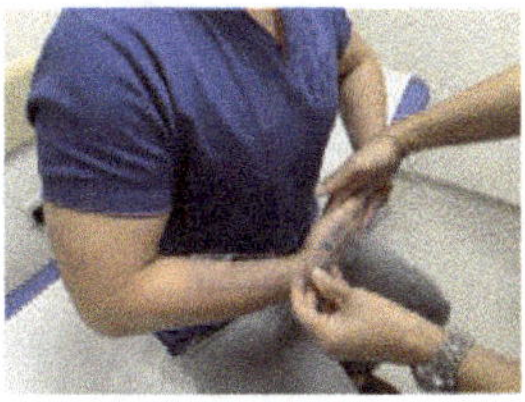
Gerber's lift-off test *Sen: 69%* *Spe: 84%*	• Position the patient with his hand behind the lower back with shoulder fully internal rotated. • Inability to lift the dorsum of the hand off the back suggest weakness of the subscapularis. Passive lift off test: • Bring the patient's hand backwards away from the lower back. • Inability to maintain the position suggest weakness of the subscapularis.	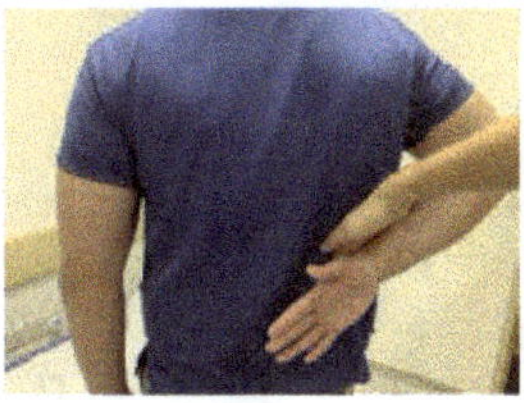

(*Continued*)

(*Continued*)

Bear hug test *Sen: 60%* *Spe: 92%*	Place the palm of the involved arm on the opposite shoulder while keeping the elbow anterior to the body, maintain position against resistance. A positive test is indicated by inability to maintain the hand position against the shoulder.	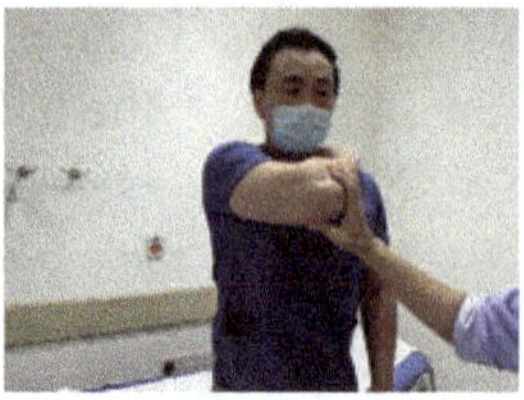
Cuff Pathology — Tests of Teres Minor Integrity		
Hornblower sign	• Position the patient with his arm at 90° abduction and elbow 90° flexed. • Instruct the patient to exert an external rotation force of the forearm against the examiner's resistance. Inability to maintain the external rotation suggest weakness of the teres minor.	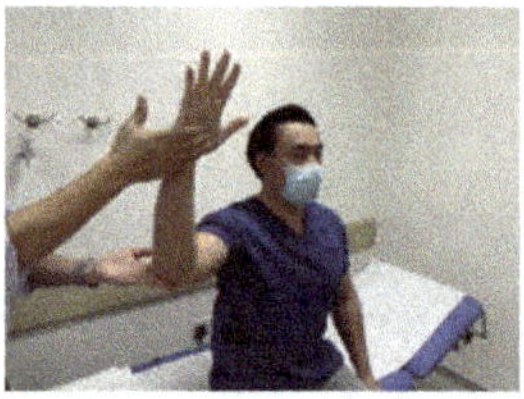
Tests for Subacromial Impingement		
Painful arc *Sen: 53%* *Spe: 76%*	• Abduct the arm in the scapular plane. • Pain between 60 and 120° of abduction due to impingement of supraspinatus or/and subacromial bursa under the acromion.	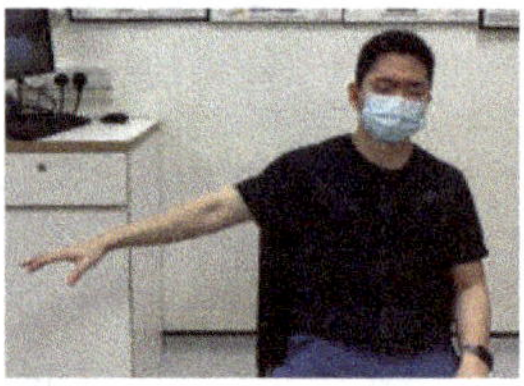
Hawkin–Kennedy test *Sen: 80%* *Spe: 56%*	• Forward flex the shoulder and elbow to 90°. • Internal rotate the shoulder causing supraspinatus and GT impingement under the CC ligament and coracoid process.	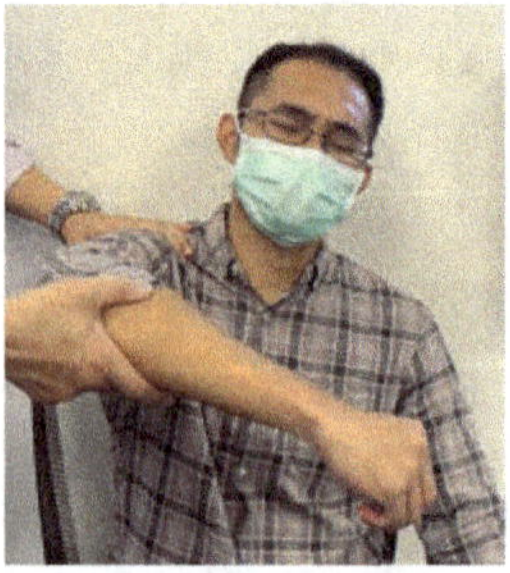

(*Continued*)

Neer's Sign *Sen: 72%* *Spe: 60%*	• Stabilise the scapular with one hand. • Passively flex the arm while internally rotated.	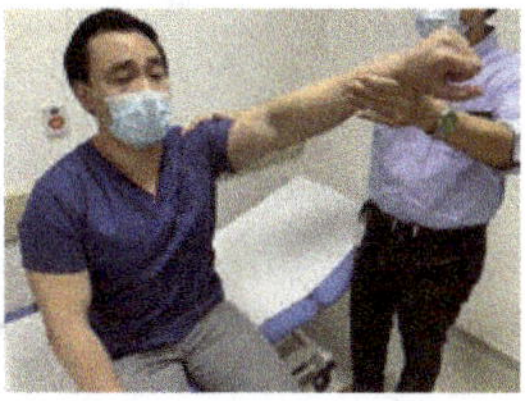
Test for ACJ Pathology		
Cross body adduction *Sen: 57%* *Spe: 96%*	• Position the patient with 90° elbow flexion and 90° shoulder flexion. • Cross adduction with hand resting on top of opposite shoulder elicits pain, indicating ACJ pathology.	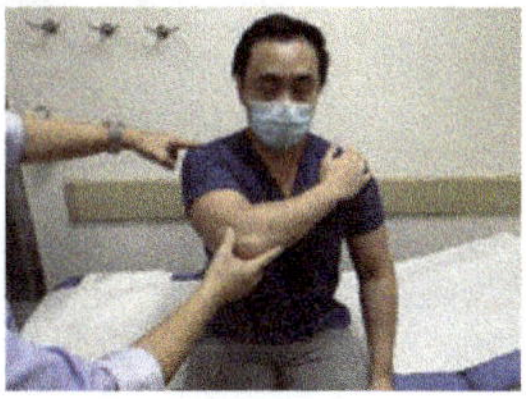
Tests for Biceps and SLAP Pathologies		
Speeds test *Sen: 20%* *Spe: 78%*	• Position the shoulder in flexion, external rotation and forearm in supination. • A downward force is applied over the forearm while the patient resists it. • Pain localised in the bicipital tendon.	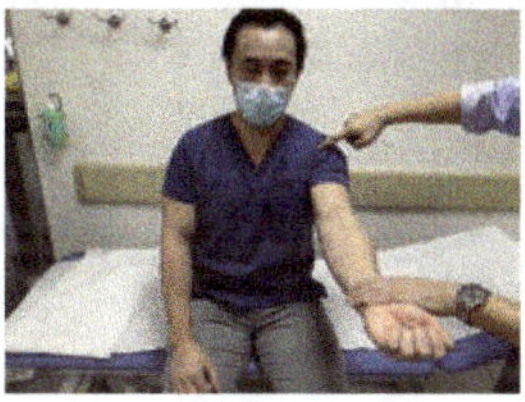
Yergason's test	• Position the affected arm in neutral position, with the elbow at 90° flexion and palm facing the ground. • Pain is localised to the bicipital groove when patient externally rotates and supinates the arm.	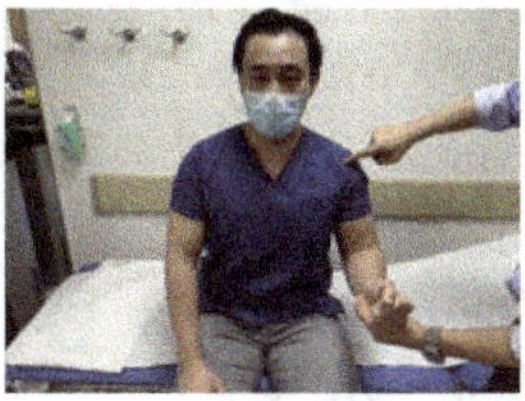

(*Continued*)

(*Continued*)

<table>
<tr><td>O'Brien active compression
Sen: 34%
Spe: 75%</td><td>• Position the shoulder in 90° flexion, 10° adduction, full internal rotation and elbow in pronation.
• Apply a distal force as the patient exerts an upward force.
• Repeat the resisted upward force with the arm in supination.
• A positive test is when pain is felt on pushing up with the arm in pronation, and relieved when the arm is in supination.</td><td>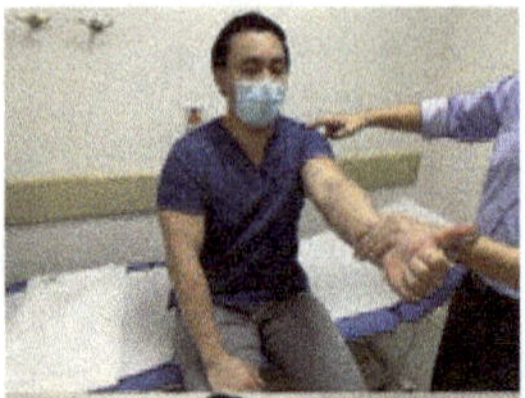
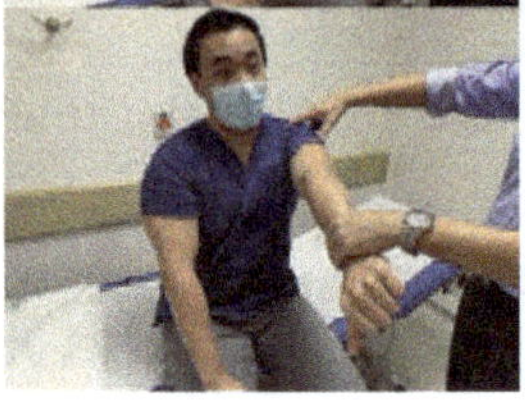</td></tr>
<tr><td>Crank Compression rotation test</td><td>• Position the patient either supine or seated, with arm in 160° elevation, elbow in 90° flexion.
• Apply a compression force along the humeral axis.
• Moving the humerus into internal and external rotation causes pain.</td><td>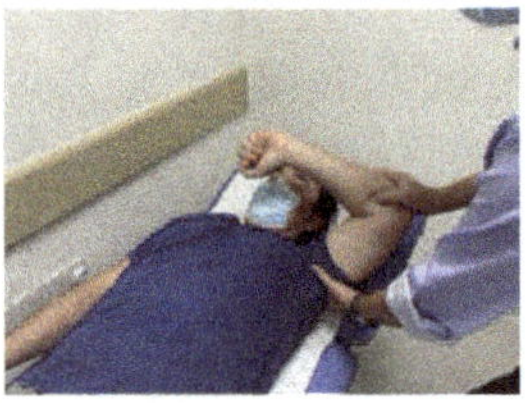</td></tr>
<tr><td colspan="3">**Tests of Anterior Stability and Pathology**</td></tr>
<tr><td>Anterior apprehension (by position)
Sen: 65.6%
Spe: 95.4%</td><td>• Position the patient either in supine or seated with shoulder in 90° abduction and elbow in 90° flexion.
• Moving the arm from neutral to 90° will result in discomfort and apprehension.</td><td>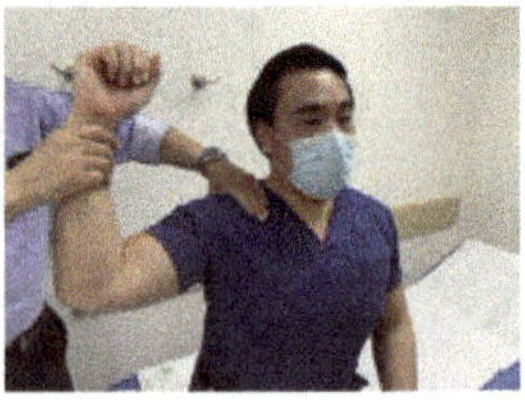</td></tr>
</table>

(*Continued*)

Apprehension and relocation test	• Perform the anterior apprehension test and exert an antero-inferior directed force from the back. • Patient's discomfort is reduced upon application of a posteriorly directed force on the shoulder to reduce any instability.	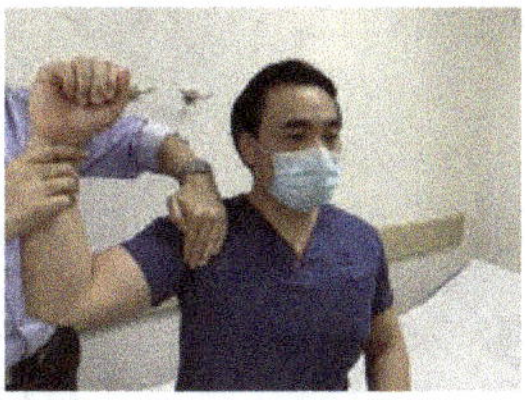
Anterior load and shift test	• Position the patient seated with scapular stabilised to the thorax using one hand. • Place the other hand across the humeral head and apply a load and shift force in an anteromedial direction. • Movement of more than half the humeral head distance is considered abnormal.	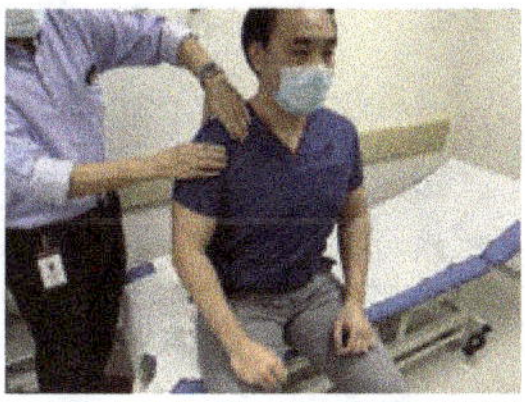
Tests of Inferior Stability and Pathology		
Inferior sulcus sign	• Position the patient seated and apply a downward force on the elbow. • Inferior GH instability will result in visible dimpling at the lateral edge of the acromion.	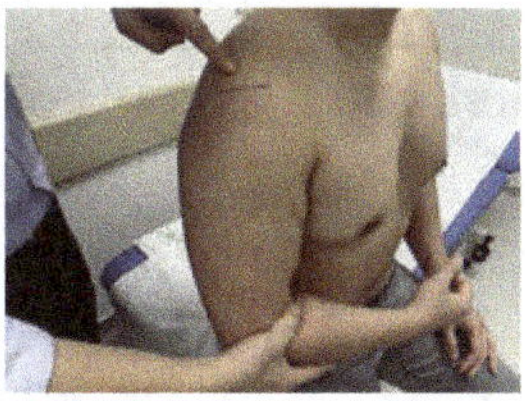

(*Continued*)

(*Continued*)

Kim's test	• Position the patient seated with arm in either 90° abduction or 45° upwards. • In 90° abduction: Hold the elbow and apply a strong axial loading force. • In 45° upwards: Hold the arm and apply a downwards and backwards force. • Pain during the test will indicate an inferior labral lesion.	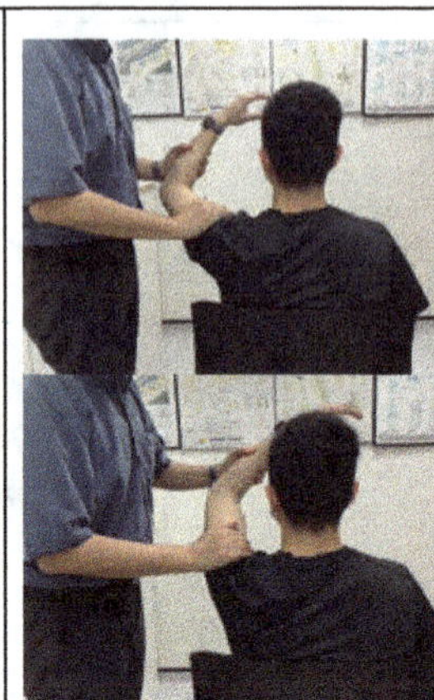
Tests of Posterior Stability and Pathology		
Posterior apprehension test	• Position the patient either in supine or seated with shoulder in IR and 90° flexion, elbow in 90° flexion. • Application of an anterior to posterior pressure will result in discomfort and apprehension.	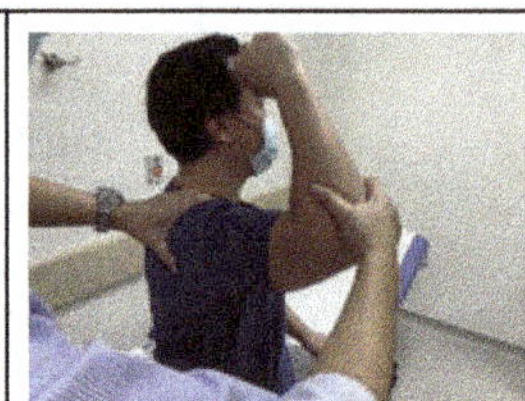
Jerk test	• Position the patient seated upright with arm in 90° abduction and IR. Stabilise the scapular with one hand. • While applying a proximally directed axial force over the elbow, move the arm horizontally across the body. • A clunk is felt when the subluxed humeral head is suddenly reduced back into position.	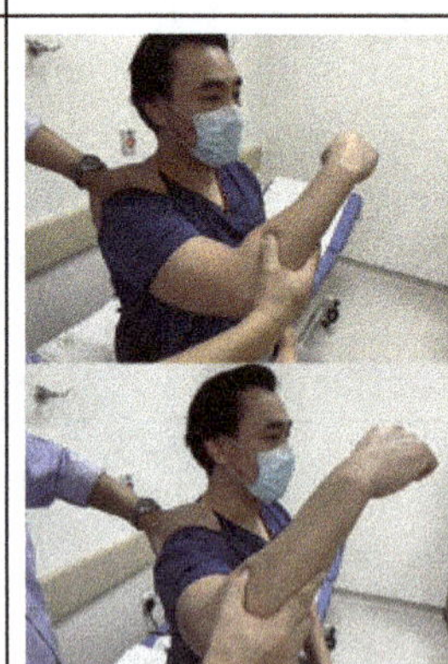

(*Continued*)

Other Tests Used		
Shrug test for arthritis/frozen shoulder *Sen: 91%* *Spe: 57%*	• The patient is instructed to abduct both arms to 90° in the plane of the body and to maintain this position for short time. • A positive test is indicated by elevation of the whole scapula to lift the arm to 90°.	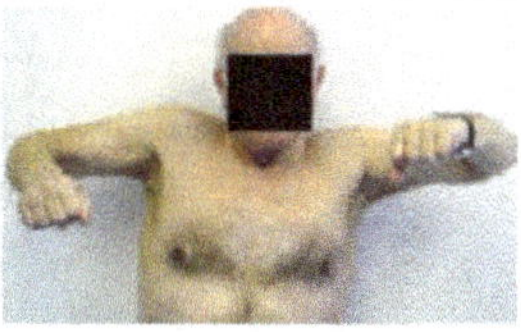
Winging of the scapula	• The patient is made to do a push-up against the wall, with the arm at the chest level • Prominence of the medial border of the scapula is a positive sign.	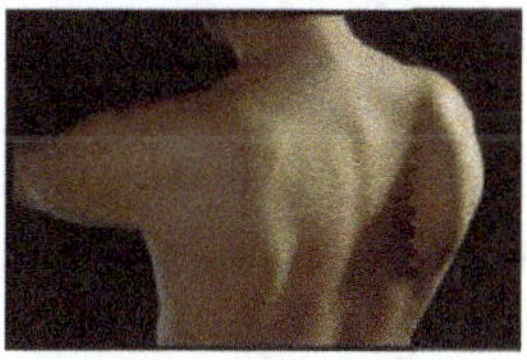
Scapula retraction test	• The examiner stabilises the medial border of the scapula as the arm is elevated. The patient may initially have difficulty flexing forward or experience subacromial pain. • Relief of impingement symptoms or ease of forward flexion is a positive test.	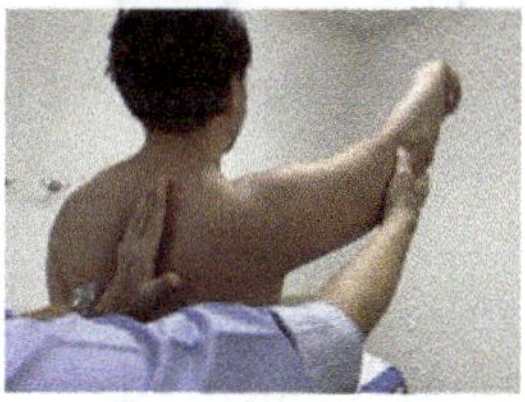

(*Continued*)

(*Continued*)

Scapula retraction test with resistance	• The examiner performs a traditional "empty can" test. • The examiner stabilises the medial border of the scapula and repeats the test. • If the impingement symptoms are relieved, the test is positive.	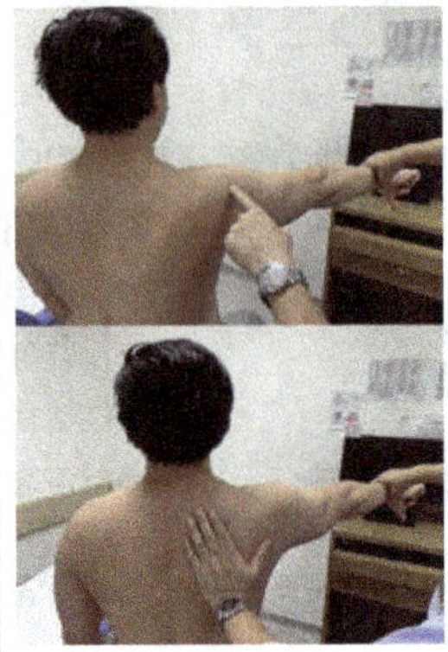

2.4 *Building a Mental Diagnostic Picture*

A composite mental picture can now be put together combining symptoms and signs as elicited above. It must be borne in mind that shoulder symptoms and signs tend to overlap but the examiner must determine which symptoms **predominate** and affect the patient most, and hence which sign are the most **significant**.

After the relevant history is taken, the examination steps are followed in routine, as shown in red arrows (Fig. 3). Hence after inspection and palpation, ROM and cuff integrity are routinely examined. In elderly patients, it is necessary to screen for the conditions that cause pain like impingement syndromes, biceps pathology and arthritis. In young patients with a history of dislocation, this is not needed; instead examination for instability is done. In special cases, it may be necessary to examine for numbness and referred pain, from cervical spine or scapula.

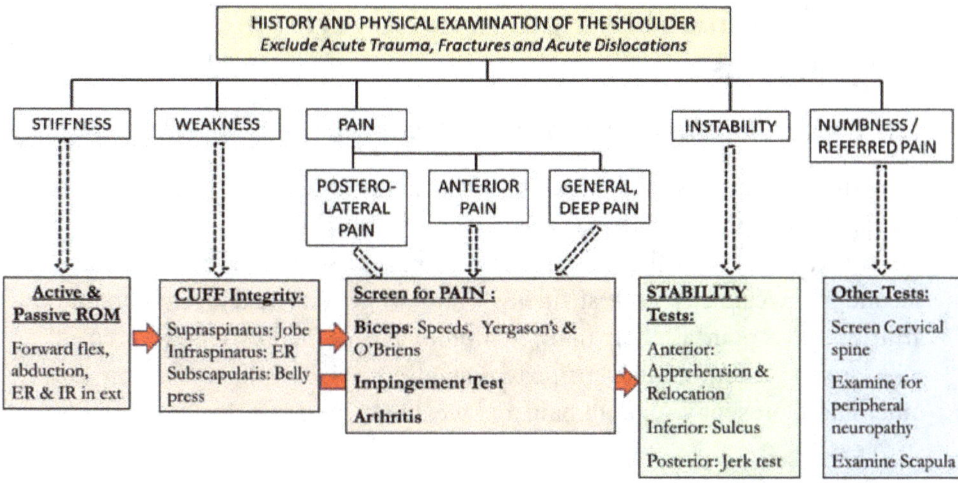

Fig. 3: Integrating symptoms and signs, each cardinal symptom has its related physical signs. But the routine of physical examination must be observed. The examiner needs to decide the dominant symptom and most significant sign.

3. An Approach Based on Symptoms, Differential Diagnosis

Each predominant cardinal symptom if supported by its corresponding significant sign, often leads to a working diagnosis. The flow chart is shown below (Fig. 4). It must be reiterated that there can be overlapping symptoms and symptom-diagnosis relationship is not reciprocal nor exclusive.

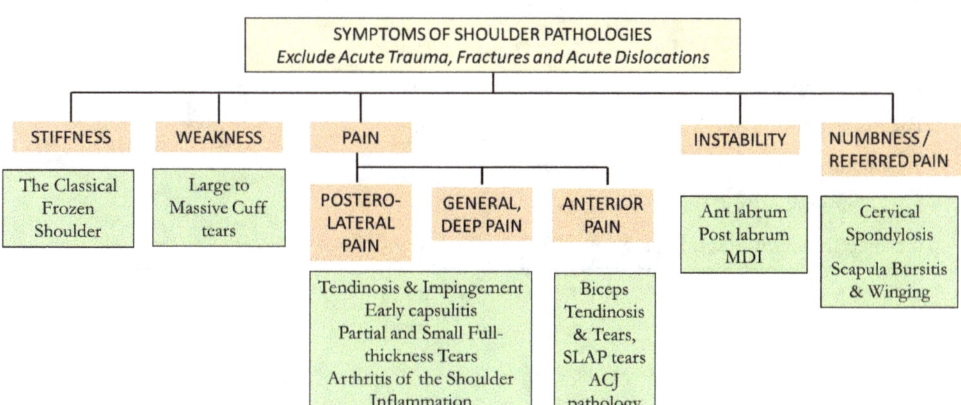

Fig. 4: Each cardinal symptom with its relevant sign often is associated with a working diagnosis. This approach helps to simplify the approach to shoulder pathologies. But symptom-diagnosis relationship is never exclusive.

4. The Dominant Symptom and Overlapping Symptoms

4.1 *Understanding Overlapping Symptoms*

Each diagnosis lends itself to a dominant main or cardinal symptom and secondary symptoms. These are shown above. Thus, cuff tendinosis, small full thickness and partial tears present primarily with pain but may have secondary weakness and stiffness. Similarly, ACJ and glenohumeral arthritis have pain as their main symptom but secondarily, may present with some weakness and stiffness that affect ADL. Large tears on the other hand, present with both pain and weakness, and may have secondary stiffness.

Adhesive capsulitis classically presents with severe stiffness but may have secondary pain and hence weakness. Any chronic instability arising from labral tears present primarily with instability, but may cause pain in SLAP lesions, and some degree of weakness (Table 1 and Fig. 5).

Table 1. Showing the main symptom of common shoulder diagnoses and secondary symptoms.

	Cardinal Symptoms that Dominate			
Shoulder Pathologies	**Pain**	**Weakness**	**Stiffness**	**Instability**
Cuff tendinosis	+++	+	+/–	–
Small and partial cuff tears	+++	+	+	–
Large to massive cuff tears	++	+++	+/–	+/–
Adhesive capsulitis	+	+	+++	–
Biceps tendinosis and SLAP	++	+/–	–	–
ACJ pathology	+++	+/–	–	–
Glenohumeral arthritis	+++	++	+	–
Chronic instability/labral tears	+/–	+/–	–	+++

4.2 *Cardinal (Primary) and Secondary Symptoms*

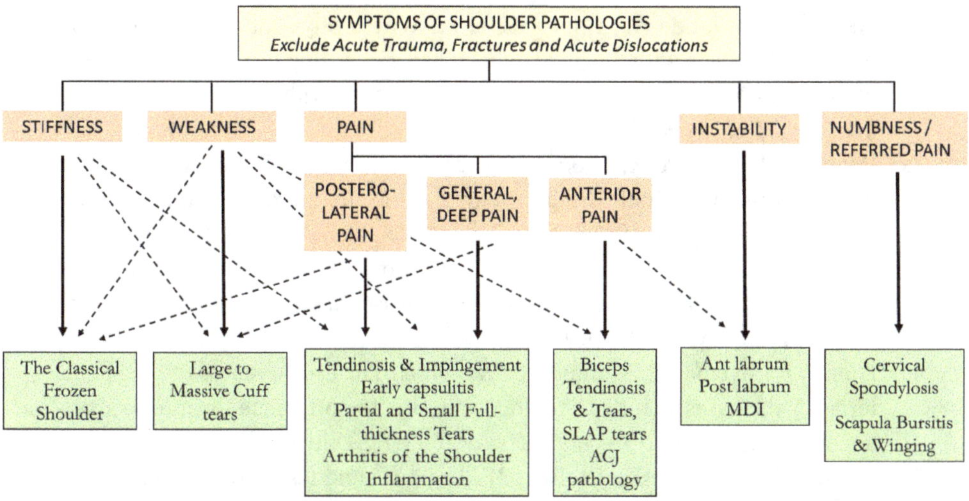

Fig. 5: Bold arrows show how the common pathologies are caused by the main (cardinal) symptoms and broken arrows show the secondary symptoms. Symptoms overlap and diagnosis-symptom relationships are never exclusive.

5. Age Differentiation of Diagnoses

Another possibility is to stratify the various diagnoses to age predilection. Once again, these categorisations are not fixed and certainly not exclusive. There is a tendency however, for certain diagnoses to be seen in certain age groups and this association can prove useful in clinical diagnosis (Table 2).

Table 2. Various diagnoses categorised under age groups.

Young (20–40 years)	Middle-aged (40–60 years)	Elderly (>60 years)
Biceps pathology including SLAP tears	Biceps tendinosis and tears	Cuff tendinosis
Labral tears causing shoulder instabilities	Adhesive capsulitis	Cuff tears (usually large to massive)
Cuff tendinosis	Cuff tendinosis	ACJ arthritis
Scapula bursitis/winging	Cuff tears (usually partial, small or medium sized)	Glenohumeral arthritis including cuff arthropathy
	Scapula bursitis	Referred pain
	Referred pain	

Note: Though not exclusive nor fixed, nevertheless the tendency for certain conditions to occur at certain ages helps in clinical diagnosis.

References

1. Hegedus EJ, Goode AP, Cook CE, *et al*. Which physical examination tests provide clinicians with the most value when examining the shoulder? Update of a systematic review with meta-analysis of individual tests. *Br J Sports Med* 2012;46(14):964–978.
2. Beaudreuil J, Nizard R, Thomas T, *et al*. Contribution of clinical tests to the diagnosis of rotator cuff disease: a systematic literature review. *Joint Bone Spine* 2009;76(1):15–19.
3. Hawkins RJ, Bokor DJ. Clinical evaluation of shoulder problems. In: Rockwood CA Jr, Matsen FA (eds.), *The Shoulder*, 2nd edn. Saunders, Philadelphia, PA, 1998, pp. 164–197.
4. Dinnes J, Loveman E, McIntyre L, Waugh N. The effectiveness of diagnostic tests for the assessment of shoulder pain due to soft tissue disorders: a systematic review. *Health Technol Assess* 2003;7(29):iii,1–166.
5. Barth JR1, Burkhart SS, De Beer JF. The bear-hug test: a new and sensitive test for diagnosing a subscapularis tear. *Arthroscopy* 2006;22(10): 1076–1084.

https://doi.org/10.1142/9789811249846_0002

Chapter 2

Imaging of the Shoulder

Lim Chee Yeong

Summary of Chapter

1. Introduction

Medical imaging serves as an integral link between bedside clinical assessment and subsequent therapeutic management. When utilised appropriately, imaging aids in diagnosis of contributory pathologies and classify the severity of diseases. Direct visualisation of structural abnormalities in the shoulder using radiological images improves clinician-patient communications by augmenting diagnostic confidence of the clinician and provides means for clear explanation of underlying injuries to patients. Accurate assessment of disease severity leads to accurate prognostication, enabling shared decision making between both parties to select the most appropriate management plan. In more complex cases, information from images are used to plan surgical approaches thereby optimising surgical outcomes. Finally, imaging may be used as an adjunct in therapy as well by image-guided intervention procedures.

Over the last two decades, the number and complexity of various imaging modalities available have proliferated tremendously. As medical practice moves towards value-based approach, focus on diagnostic imaging has also shifted towards selection of the most appropriate investigation for specific patient conditions [1]. In this chapter, we will review the most commonly used imaging modalities in workup of shoulder sports injuries and discuss their appropriate usages.

2. X-ray (Fig. 1)

Projection radiography, or X-ray for short, utilises differential attenuation of ionising radiation though different tissue material to generate images on radiographic films or modern-day solid-state detectors (digital radiography). It is a ubiquitous, readily available, low cost and high yield imaging modality used in almost all patients who present with shoulder pain. X-rays serve as a first line screening tool for joint alignment, fractures, neoplasm, infection, arthritis or other metabolic conditions. Disadvantages include limitations to the degree of densities demonstrated (especially poor for soft tissue), summative projection of tissue within a single projection and use of ionising radiation.

Since X-rays are not a cross sectional imaging modality, it is important to at least obtain two orthogonal views when assessing any appendicular skeleton. A standard set of shoulder radiographs for trauma should include at least three views: anterior–posterior (AP) views in internal and external rotation and an axillary or scapula-Y view [2]. External and internal rotation allows for full visualisation of the humeral head, allowing for better assessment of greater tuberosity and Hill-Sach injury respectively. Axillary or scapula-Y views are essential in workup of traumatic shoulder injuries as acromioclavicular and glenohumeral dislocations can be misclassified on AP views.

If patient is unable to abduct the shoulder for the axillary view due to pain, an apical oblique (modified trauma axial) view should be considered, where the X-ray tube is instead angled 45 degrees caudally from the vertical [3]. For atraumatic shoulder pain, the conventional AP view may be replaced by an AP oblique Grashey [4]. This is a true AP view of the

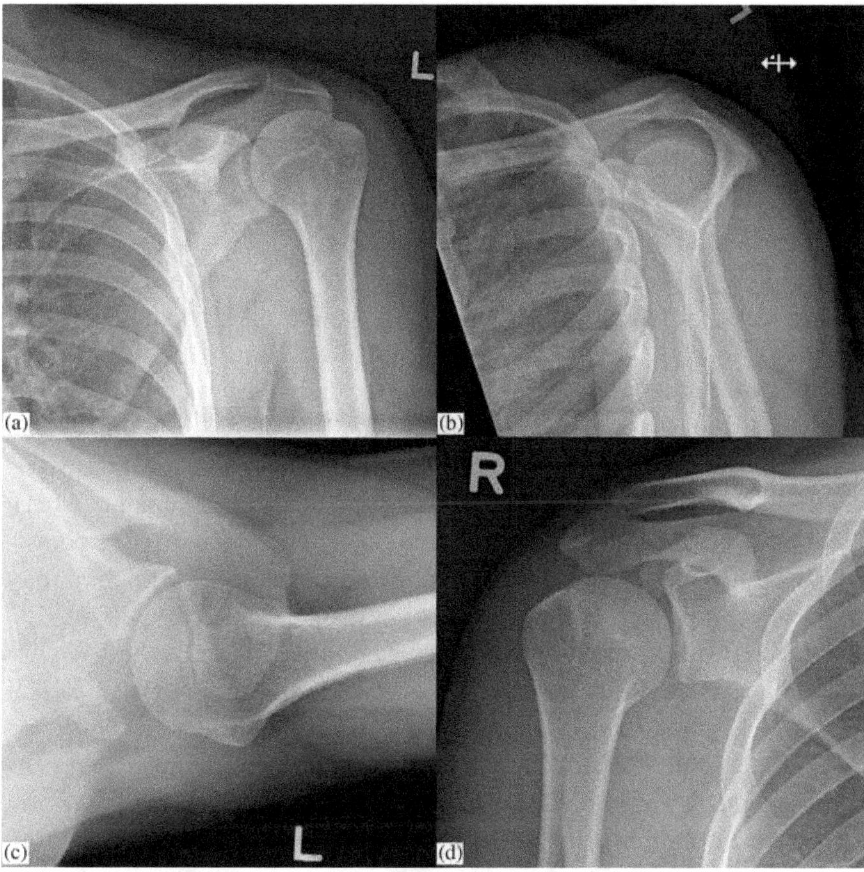

Fig. 1: Standard X-ray of the shoulder in (a) anteroposterior, (b) scapula-Y, (c) axillary and (d) Grashey projections. Note the lack of overlap between humerus and glenoid in (d) Grashey projection compared to (a) anterposterior projection.

shoulder joint that is free from the overlap between the humerus and glenoid, allowing better evaluation of the glenohumeral cartilage space, joint congruity and humeral head subluxation.

3. Computed Tomography (Fig. 2)

Computed tomography (CT) is a cross sectional imaging modality comprising of a gantry with rotating X-ray beam and multiple detectors in various arrays rotating continuously around a patient. After data is acquired, computer algorithms are used to generate 2D (1-3 mm) thin slice images which are then formatted into multiple imaging planes or 3D models. Modern dual energy CT scanners also allow additional functions such metal artifact reduction, urate crystal (gout) and marrow oedema detection [5].

CT scan is widely available and allows for very fast cross-sectional imaging. Pertaining to orthopaedic practice, it is commonly used to acquire high resolution multiplanar images of bone fractures as part of pre-surgical planning, for example in fixation of complex proximal humerus fractures. Volumetric data acquisition allows for life-like 3D virtual models to be reconstructed, currently the gold standard for assessing glenoid bone loss in shoulder instability management [6]. It is also useful in post-surgical assessment given the relatively low level of metallic imaging artifacts in comparison to magnetic resonance imaging (MRI). By administering iodine-based intravenous contrast during scan acquisition, any surrounding soft tissue inflammation or abscess formation may be elicited.

There are, however, several disadvantages of CT. CT scanners require much higher levels of ionising radiation administered to the patient compared to projection radiography. Furthermore, while the ability to expand grey scale is much higher than projection radiograph, high contrast visualisation of soft tissue structures such as tendons, cartilage and labrum is vastly inferior to ultrasound and MRI. On the other hand, CT shoulder arthrography remains a suitable alternative for assessment of labral pathologies in patients contraindicated to MRI. In CT arthrography, intra-articular injection of iodine based contrast into the glenohumeral joint to outline labral deficiencies is shown to be comparable to accuracy to MR arthrography [7].

4. Ultrasound (Fig. 3)

Ultrasound imaging, or ultrasonography, is a non-ionising modality that makes use of high frequency sound waves in ranges inaudible to humans (>20,000 Hz). An ultrasound probe both generates ultrasonic signals and measures echoes reflecting off different tissue material, which are then used to generate images. It is inexpensive, safe, widely available and portable, while providing high resolution assessment of soft tissue

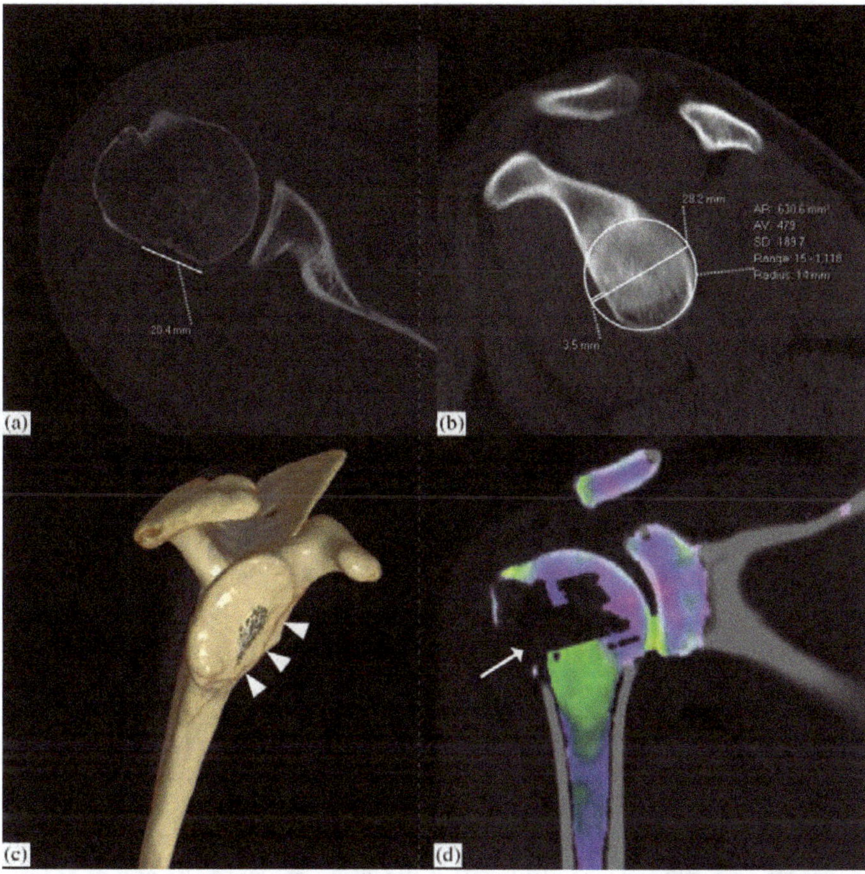

Fig. 2: (a) Axial and (b) sagittal CT images in bone window of the same patient after prior episode of anteroinferior glenohumeral dislocation. Measurement in (a) demonstrated Hill-Sach lesion at the posterior aspect of humeral head. Glenoid bone loss in (b) is measured using best fit circle Pico method. (c) 3D CT reconstruction of different patient demonstrates glenoid bone loss (arrowheads) en face. (d) Colour overlay coronal CT image of another patient using dual energy CT data, demonstrating marrow oedema (in green) adjacent to acute humerus surgical neck fracture (arrow). The fracture itself is better shown on other reformats within the CT study (not included).

structures. However, the modality demands technical expertise from users, so the degree of diagnostic accuracy is highly operator dependent.

Superficial structures such as shoulder rotator cuff tendons are convenient to assess via ultrasound given the availability of an unobstructed acoustic window for scanning. Instead of axial, coronal and sagittal planes commonly used to CT and MRI, ultrasound imaging nomenclature consists of longitudinal and transverse images, in relation to the long axis of the imaged structure. The operator needs to be wary of anisotropy artifacts when scanning curved structures like rotator cuff tendons that may mimic pathologies. This may be compensated by ensuring the probe is as parallel to the assessed component of the tendon as possible.

Sensitivity and specificity of ultrasound for diagnosis of full thickness rotator cuff tears is high and comparable to MRI, approaching 0.9 [8]. However, evidence for diagnosis of partial thickness tear and tendinosis is more heterogeneous and likely more challenging [9]. MRI is also poor in assessing the width, retraction and degree of muscle atrophy [10]. Studies in newer experimental ultrasound modes like pressure or shear wave elastography are still underway, aiming to improve assessment of tendon quality and muscular atrophy in cuff tears [11,12]. Since a full thickness tear is usually the threshold for surgical management and ultrasound is much more cost-effective than MRI, it is currently recommended as the first line investigation for rotator cuff tendinopathy work up [4]. In the context of shoulder impingement syndromes, ultrasound also provides opportunity for direct visualisation of relationships between the acromion, humeral head, and intervening soft tissues in dynamic manoeuvres to pinpoint exact causes [13].

As ultrasound machines get smaller and cheaper, point of care ultrasound and ultrasound guided injections are becoming more prevalent in the sports and orthopaedic clinics. It is therefore crucial to be aware of two essential limitations to ultrasound in the shoulder workup. Firstly, ultrasonography remains a high operator dependant tool, demanding rigorous training and experience for an operator to be competent. Secondly, ultrasound provides high diagnostic accuracy in very limited, albeit commonly injured, component of the shoulder — the rotator cuff tendons. It is not useful in assessment of instability, bone and articular pathologies. In other words, it is great tool only in limited situations and in the right hands.

5. Magnetic Resonance Imaging (Fig. 4)

MRI uses high field strength magnets (1.5–3 Tesla), field gradients and radio waves to manipulate hydrogen atoms in the body, thereby generating

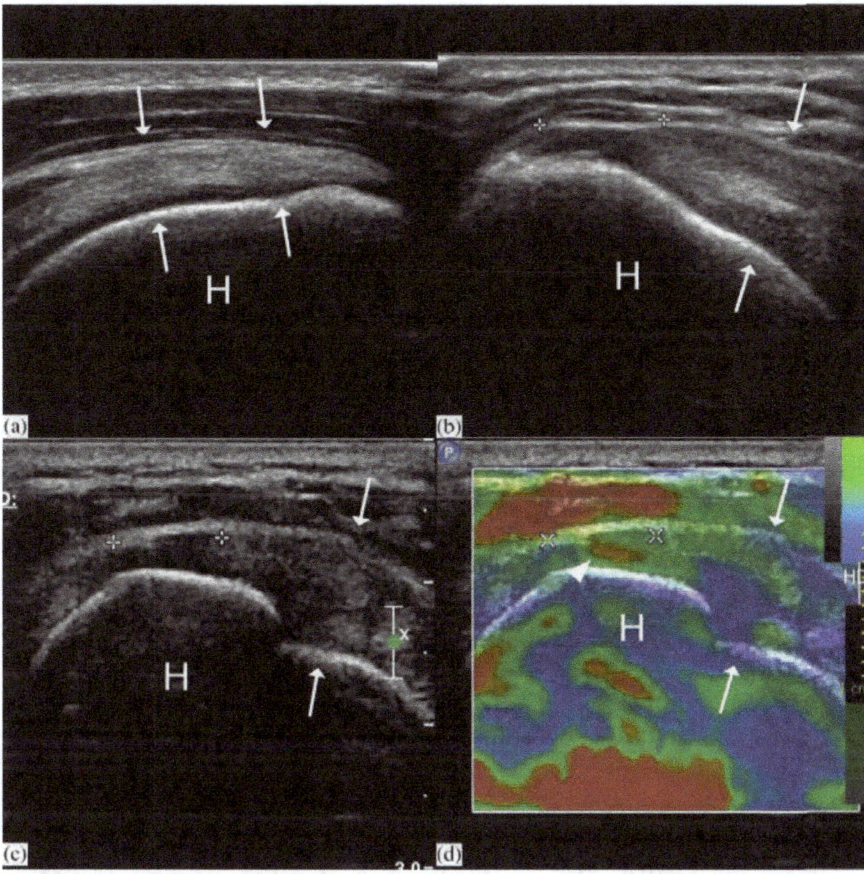

Fig. 3: (a) B-mode ultrasound image in longitudinal plane of normal supraspinatus tendon (arrows). "H" detonates humeral head. (b) Longitudinal B-mode, (c) transverse B-mode and (d) transverse B-mode with stress elastography colour overlay of different patient showing a supraspinatus tendon tear (hypoechoic area within calliper markings). Arrows denote the supraspinatus tendon, "H" denotes the humeral head. In (d), the arrowhead points to red area of softening within the supraspinatus tendon when the tendon tear is located.

localising and tissue specific signals which allow complex computer programs to generate cross sectional images. Acquisition parameters are varied to obtain either 2D or volumetric 3D images with different contrast weightage — typically T1-weighted, T2-weighted, proton density or intermediate-weighted, with or within fat suppression.

The main advantage of MRI is that it allows for the highest level of contrast between different soft tissue types compared to other imaging modalities. This provides a huge advantage in shoulder imaging where multiple structures are potentially injured. When coupled with a high-quality shoulder surface coil, high resolution images with small voxel size and high signal to noise ratio may be obtained for accurate assessment of the smallest structural abnormalities in the shoulder.

For rotator cuff tendinopathy, MRI provides the highest specificity and accuracy in diagnosis of partial and full thickness tears, with slightly lower sensitivity in detection of partial thickness tears (0.8) [14]. It is more sensitive for detection of partial tears and tendinosis compared to ultrasound and may be a secondary investigation in patients with negative ultrasound findings. It also allows for accurate assessment of tear shape, tendon retraction and muscular atrophy [15]. These additional information allows the clinician to assess severity of disease and provide reasonable prognostic projections pre-operatively [16].

MRI is the main tool for assessing labral and capsular injuries in shoulder instability, either through high resolution 3T conventional MRI or MRI arthrography [4]. In MRI arthrography, gadolinium-based contrast is injected into the glenohumeral joint under ultrasound or fluoroscopy guidance before the MRI scan. The distention of the joint allows for better visualisation of any labral injuries as contrast seeps into the tears. When MRI arthrography is available, it appears to add accuracy to diagnosis of labral injuries [17,18]. This is likely more significant in patients with chronic symptoms that is suspected to be subtle based clinical assessment. Patients with acute symptoms or severe injuries tend to have intrinsic image contrast in the form of effusion or soft-tissue changes that allow diagnosis without joint distention [19]. In patients with glenoid bone loss, 3D MRI may also be used in place of CT, sparing young patients from unnecessary ionising radiation dose [20].

In contrast to ultrasound, MRI is the jack of all trades and master of many. Other than rotator cuff and labral injuries, it is able to assess the glenohumeral and sternoclavicular joint, cartilage, bones, surrounding muscles and ligaments. Main limitations are high cost and clinical contraindications to MRI. Patients with non-compatible cardiac implants or claustrophobia and are unable to tolerate prolonged scan time will not be able to undergo this investigation. Furthermore, MRI is highly susceptible

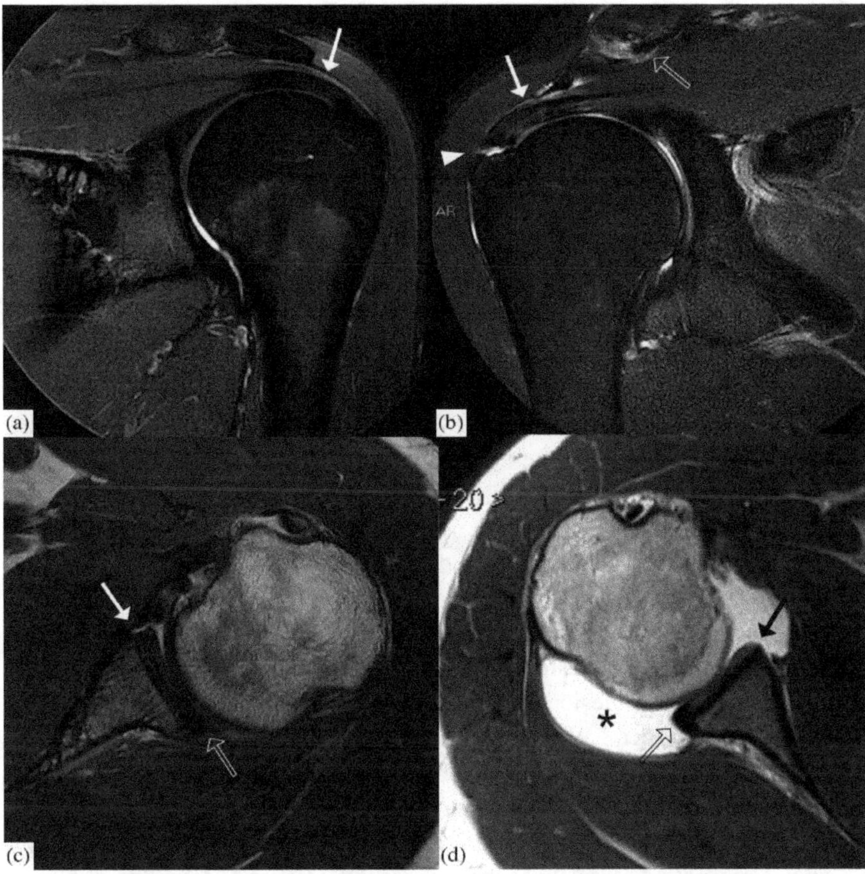

Fig. 4: (a) Coronal T2 weighted fat suppressed image of normal supraspinatus tendon (arrow). (b) Coronal T2 weighted fat suppressed image of supraspinatus tendon with tendinosis (arrow) and focal footprint tear (arrowhead). Block arrow points to concomitant acromioclavicular osteoarthritis. (c) and (d) are both axial PD weighted images of shoulder in different patients where arrows point to deficient anterior labra (Bankart lesion) and block arrows point to intact posterior labra for comparison. (c) is a conventional MRI but done in high magnet field strength (3T) to increase image quality while (d) is a MR arthrogram where the glenohumeral joint is distended with contrast (*) to increased accuracy of labral pathology detection despite lower field strength (1.5T).

to various imaging artifacts such as metallic susceptibility from orthopaedic implants or magic angle artifacts [21]. The former may limit usage in post-surgical workup unless advanced scanners with modern artifact reduction protocol are used [22].

References

1. American College of Radiology. ACR Appropriateness Criteria®. American College of Radiology [Internet]. 31 May 2020. Available from: https://acsearch.acr.org/list.
2. Amini B, Beckmann NM, Beaman FD, Wessell DE, Bernard SA, Cassidy RC, *et al.* ACR Appropriateness Criteria® Shoulder Pain — Traumatic American College of Radiology [Internet]. 31 May 2020. Available from: https://acsearch.acr.org/docs/69433/Narrative/.
3. Neep M, Aziz A. Radiography of the acutely injured shoulder. *Radiography* 2011;17(3):188–192.
4. Small KM, Adler RS, Shah SH, Roberts CC, Bencardino JT, Appel M, *et al.* ACR Appropriateness Criteria® Shoulder Pain — Atraumatic. American College of Radiology [Internet]. 31 May 2020. Available from: https://acsearch.acr.org/docs/3101482/Narrative/.
5. Rajiah P, Sundaram M, Subhas N. Dual-Energy CT in Musculoskeletal Imaging: What is the Role Beyond Gout? *Am J Roentgenol* 2019;213(3): 493–505.
6. Di Giacomo G, Itoi E, Burkhart SS. Evolving concept of bipolar bone loss and the Hill-Sachs lesion: From "engaging/non-engaging" lesion to "on-track/off-track" lesion. *Arthroscopy* 2014;30(1):90–98.
7. Jarraya M, Roemer FW, Gale HI, Landreau P, D'Hooghe P, Guermazi A. MR-arthrography and CT-arthrography in sports-related glenolabral injuries: A matched descriptive illustration. *Insights into Imaging* 2016;7(2):167–177.
8. Roy J-S, Braën C, Leblond J, Desmeules F, Dionne CE, MacDermid JC, *et al.* Diagnostic accuracy of ultrasonography, MRI and MR arthrography in the characterisation of rotator cuff disorders: A systematic review and meta-analysis. *Br J Sports Med* 2015;49(20):1316–1328.
9. Smith T, Back T, Toms A, Hing C. Diagnostic accuracy of ultrasound for rotator cuff tears in adults: A systematic review and meta-analysis. *Clin Radiol* 2011;66(11):1036–1048.
10. Okoroha KR, Fidai MS, Tramer JS, Davis KD, Kolowich PA. Diagnostic accuracy of ultrasound for rotator cuff tears. *Ultrasonography* 2019;38(3):215.
11. Hatta T, Giambini H, Uehara K, Okamoto S, Chen S, Sperling JW, *et al.* Quantitative assessment of rotator cuff muscle elasticity: Reliability and feasibility of shear wave elastography. *J Biomech* 2015;48(14):3853–3858.
12. Hou SW, Merkle AN, Babb JS, McCabe R, Gyftopoulos S, Adler RS. Shear wave ultrasound elastographic evaluation of the rotator cuff tendon. *J Ultrasound Med* 2017;36(1):95–106.

13. Bureau NJ, Beauchamp M, Cardinal E, Brassard P. Dynamic sonography evaluation of shoulder impingement syndrome. *Am J Roentgenol* 2006; 187(1):216–220.
14. Smith TO, Daniell H, Geere J-A, Toms AP, Hing CB. The diagnostic accuracy of MRI for the detection of partial-and full-thickness rotator cuff tears in adults. *Magn Reson Imaging* 2012;30(3):336–346.
15. Morag Y, Jacobson JA, Miller B, De Maeseneer M, Girish G, Jamadar D. MR imaging of rotator cuff injury: What the clinician needs to know. *Radiographics* 2006;26(4):1045–1065.
16. Kijowski R, Thurlow P, Blankenbaker D, Liu F, McGuine T, Li G, *et al.* Preoperative MRI Shoulder Findings Associated with Clinical Outcome 1 Year after Rotator Cuff Repair. *Radiology* 2019;291(3):722–729.
17. Magee T. 3-T MRI of the shoulder: Is MR arthrography necessary? *Am J Roentgenol* 2009;192(1):86–92.
18. Major NM, Browne J, Domzalski T, Cothran RL, Helms CA. Evaluation of the glenoid labrum with 3-T MRI: Is intraarticular contrast necessary? *Am J Roentgenol* 2011;196(5):1139–1144.
19. De Coninck T, Ngai SS, Tafur M, Chung CB. Imaging the glenoid labrum and labral tears. *Radiographics* 2016;36(6):1628–1647.
20. Vopat BG, Cai W, Torriani M, Vopat ML, Hemma M, Harris GJ, *et al.* Measurement of glenoid bone loss with 3-dimensional magnetic resonance imaging: A matched computed tomography analysis. *Arthroscopy* 2018;34(12):3141–3147.
21. Singh DR, Chin MS, Peh WC (eds.), *Artifacts in Musculoskeletal MR Imaging. Seminars in Musculoskeletal Radiology*. Thieme Medical Publishers, 2014.
22. Jungmann PM, Agten CA, Pfirrmann CW, Sutter R. Advances in MRI around metal. *J Magn Reson Imaging* 2017;46(4):972–991.

https://doi.org/10.1142/9789811249846_0003

Chapter 3

Patient Positioning, Anaesthesia and OT Preparations

Denny T.T. Lie, Geoffrey Liew and Dennis Ng

Summary of Chapter

1. Patient positioning: Beach chair vs lateral decubitus
2. Anaesthesia
3. The arthroscope and camera stack
4. Surgical arthroscopic instruments
5. Other OT preparations

1. Patient Positioning: Beach Chair vs Lateral Decubitus

Patient positioning is important in shoulder surgery to provide the best possible access to the shoulder, whilst maintaining safety of the patient. Either the beach-chair position or lateral decubitus is used, though there are several variations. The arm in the beach chair is then supported in an arm-holder or passively supported at the side of the patient.

1.1 *The Beach Chair Position (Fig. 1)*

The patient is seated propped up, and orientation to the arthroscopic views are thus anatomical. Some of the advantages and disadvantages include:

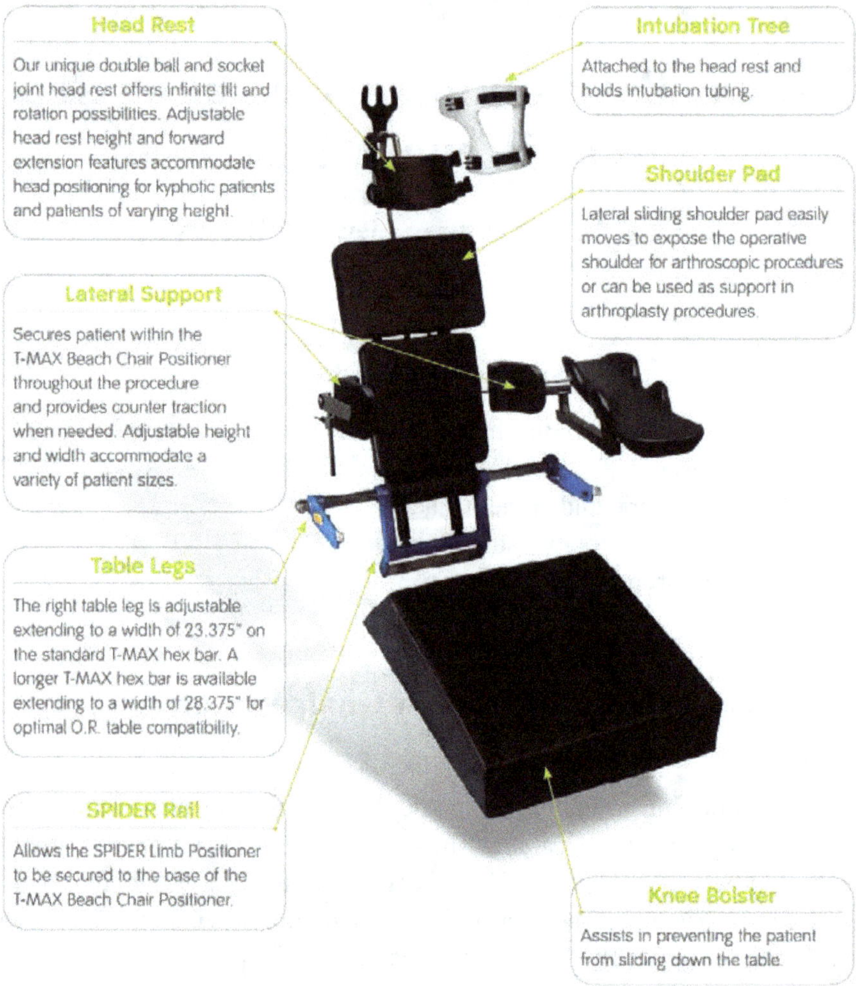

Fig. 1: T-Max Beach Chair (Smith & Nephew).

(a) Advantages:

- Unimpeded access to front and back of shoulder.
- Ability to convert from arthroscopy to open surgery.
- Complete freedom of the arm to move across entire ROM.
- Views and perspective to structures are anatomical.
- Structures and capsule are not under tension and hence amenable to plication and tightening procedures.

(b) Disadvantages:

- Surgery to the posterior labrum is challenging and views thereof not easy.
- There are some anaesthetic concerns when the patient is being propped up.
- Retracted cuff tears may be more challenging and require the arm to be supported in abduction.

(c) Components and set-up of the beach chair are as follows:

- *Head support*: The head of the patient must be securely supported (Fig. 2) yet permitted to adjust (Fig. 3) and so take into account different body habitus of the patient and possible cervical deformities. Airway access must remain unimpeded. The masks used should also be easy to use and be disposable.
- *Truncal support*: There are side supports (Fig. 4) to ensure even large patients do not run the risk of falling over. Further, the upper

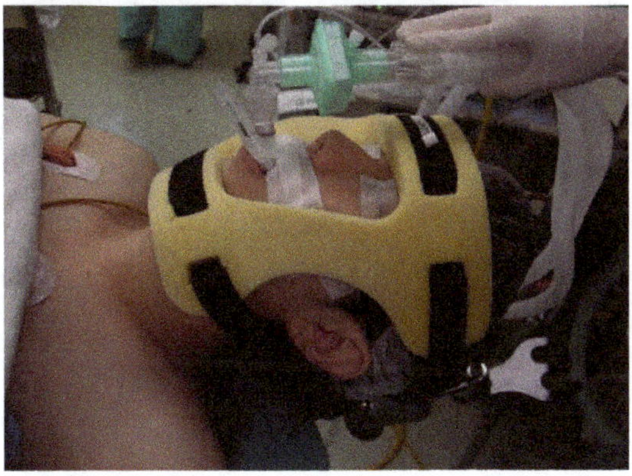

Fig. 2: Patient's head is secured with a face mask.

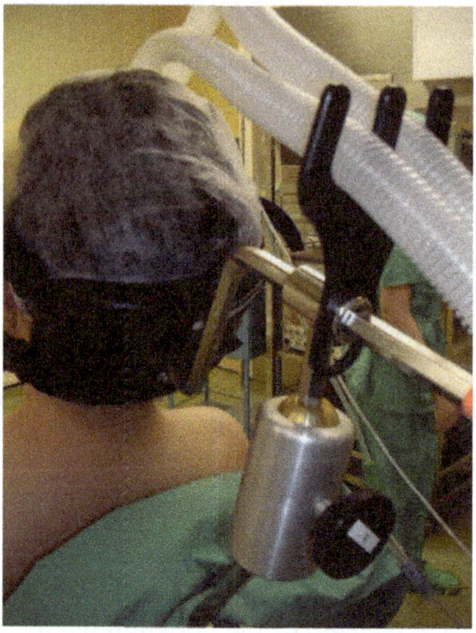

Fig. 3: The headrest is adjustable.

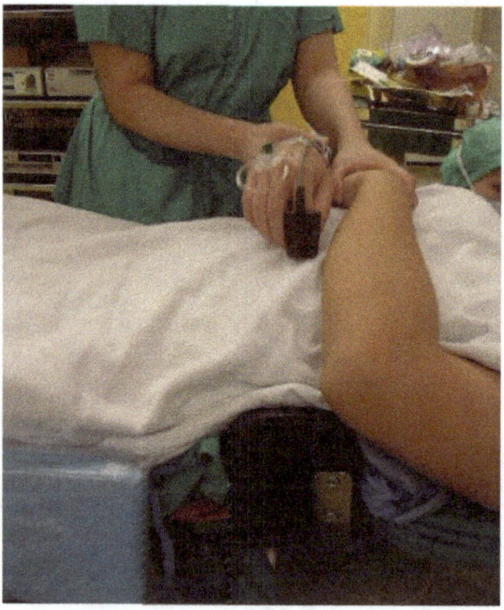

Fig. 4: Side supports stabilise the patient.

truncal support should be able to slide, either to provide additional support or to provide even greater access to the posterior aspects of the shoulder.

- *Arm support*: The contralateral arm is usually supported in an arm-holder whilst the ipsilateral arm is either passively supported on a table or in a hydraulic arm-holder. The key is not to restrict the mobility of the arm.
- *Leg support*: The legs of the patient are propped up by a large cushion or several pillows, and strapped firmly (Fig. 5).
- The patient can be put under anaesthesia either on a separate trolley or on the table fitted with a beach chair. As the airways are being secured, priority is to secure the truncal side supports, then the face-mask is applied (but not tied firmly yet), and the leg supports placed in position and straps applied. The patient is then propped up slowly, usually a hydraulic mechanism helps support the weight of the patient. **Tip: it is recommended to prop up to 30° first, repeat the blood pressure and if stable, then to continue propping up to the final 70°–80°.**

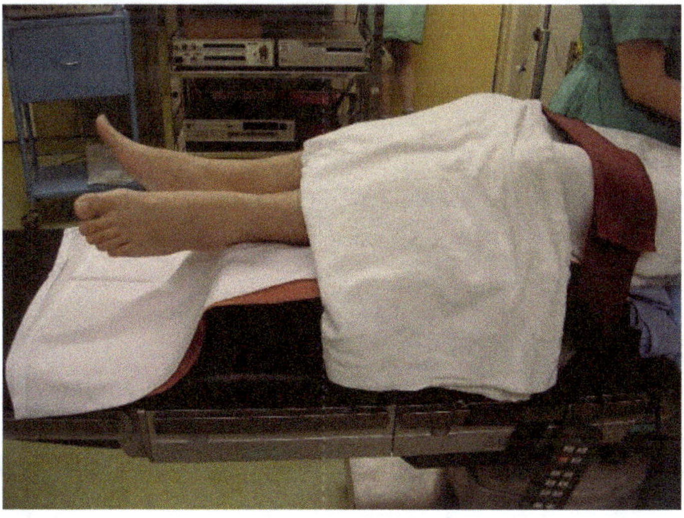

Fig. 5: The patient's legs are raised on a cushion to prevent sliding down.

1.2 *The Lateral Decubitus Position*

(a) Advantages:

- Excellent access all around the shoulder.
- Clear access to the posterior structures of the shoulder.
- Retracted structures are already reduced to some extent as the arm is brought to abduction.

(b) Disadvantages:

- Limited movement of the arm.
- Structures and capsule are already under some tension and thus tightening procedures would be limited.
- Needs some getting used to with regards to orientation of the structures.

(c) Setting up the Lateral Decubitus position:

- Most operating tables can be used.
- Patient stabilisation devices such as a beanbag.
- Padding to avoid pressure injuries. Axillary roll under the axilla. Knee is slightly bent and fibula head of lower leg padded to prevent injury to common peroneal nerve.
- Arm is placed in a sling and traction is applied (Fig. 6).
- Tilt patient approximately 20° posterior to orient glenoid parallel to floor.
- Keep head of patient clear of anaesthesia so surgeon can access anterior portals.
- Suspend arm with about 10 lbs of weight.
- Approximately 70° of abduction (30°–70° depending on preference).
- Approximately 15° of forward flexion (Fig. 7).

1.3 *Arm Holder (Fig. 8)*

Surgeons familiar with the beach chair position enjoy the liberty of the arm being free to be moved. They can thus access various corners of the shoulder with the minimum number of portals. However, if assistant

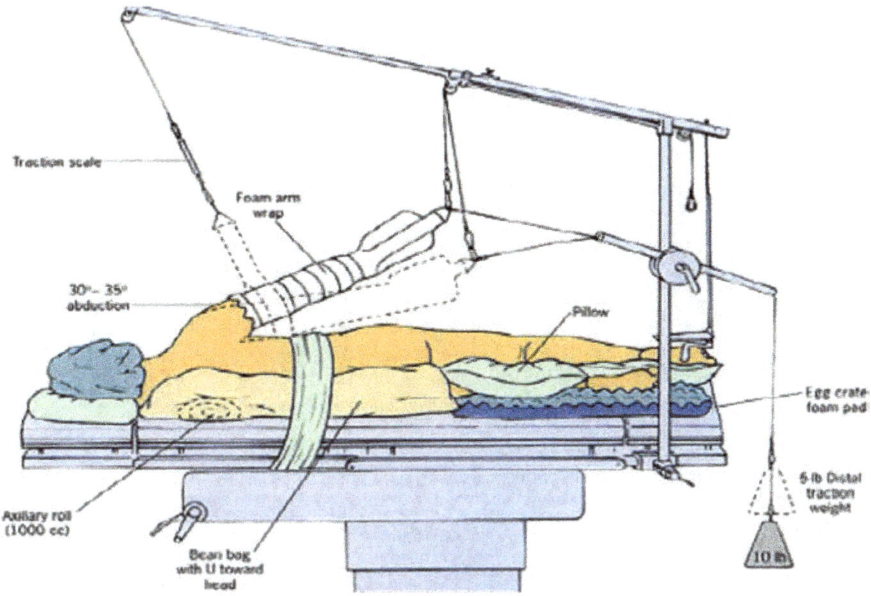

Fig. 6: The Lateral decubitus position. The arm is placed under traction and all bony prominences are well padded [7].

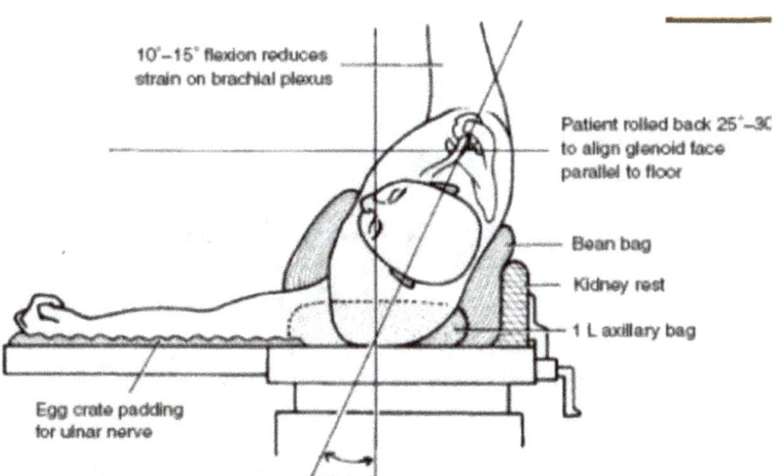

Fig. 7: The Lateral decubitus position. The patient is tilted 20° posterior so that the glenoid surface is parallel to the floor.

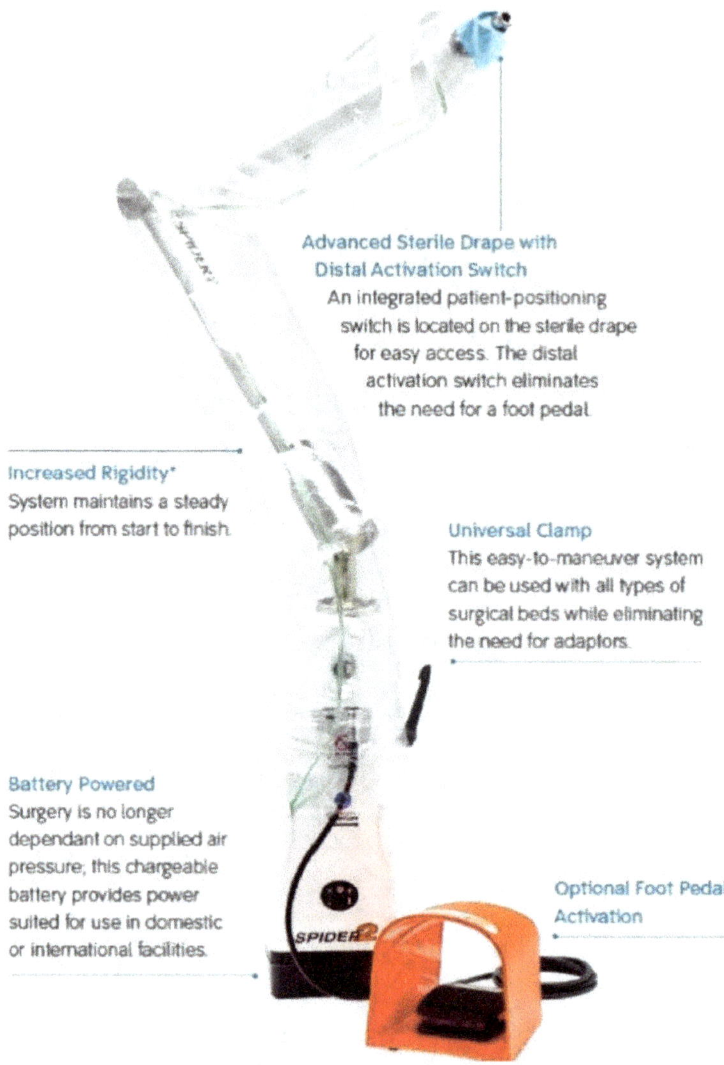

Fig. 8: Spider2 arm holder (Smith & Nephew).

support is limited, there is often a need for the arm to be supported, to be moved to a desired position and more importantly, to be held firmly in that position. The Tenet arm-holder is used in our institution. A hydraulic system enables the mechanical arm to support the load of the patient's arm. A foot pedal releases the hydraulic mechanism lock, enabling the arm to be re-positioned before locking it again by releasing the foot pedal. Some preparation is needed to wrap the arm in sterile holders and takes some getting used to.

Details of setting up of the arm holder is not given here and surgeons are advised to speak to their local Smith & Nephew representative for further details.

2. Anaesthesia: General Anaesthesia, Blocks and Local Anaesthetic

2.1 *Pre-op Anaesthesia Considerations*

Patients presenting for shoulder surgery can range from the fit and robust young adults with sports-related injuries requiring a stabilisation procedure, to the frail elderly individuals with pre-existing co-morbidities such as diabetes mellitus and rheumatoid arthritis requiring decompression surgery or arthroplasty. Rheumatoid arthritis is a multisystem disorder with potential articular (e.g. atlanto-axial instability) and extra-articular (e.g. pulmonary) involvements. These effects might pose great challenges to the anaesthetists in the conduct of anaesthesia, airway management, and surgical positioning of patients.

Therefore, a full preoperative anaesthetic assessment is imperative in the pre-optimisation as well as in choosing the appropriate anaesthetic technique. Careful patient selection and pre-operative psychological preparation are also vital if awake techniques are considered, as some patients might find it intolerable despite having excellent regional block because of the close proximity of the patient's face to the surgical site and instruments, and the claustrophobia under the surgical drapes.

2.2 *Considerations for GA During Shoulder Surgery*

Shoulder surgery can be performed under general anaesthesia (GA), regional anaesthesia (with or without sedation), or a combination of both. The choice of anaesthetic technique is generally guided by factors such as the type of shoulder surgery, surgical duration, patient's fitness and preference, surgeon's familiarity and preference, institutional practice and anaesthetic expertise. GA or GA supplemented by regional anaesthesia is the usual practice in our institution.

Adequate intravenous access is often required as blood loss can be considerable, particularly in arthroscopic surgery. In the conduct of GA, the patient's airway is secured with an endotracheal tube or a supraglottic airway. Endotracheal tube provides a more secure airway in the beach-chair position. Conversely, supraglottic airway is favoured by some for being less stimulating with head movement due to surgical traction, nonetheless troubleshooting the airway device in a beach-chair position with the patient's face under surgical drapes can be difficult. Patient's head and neck are secured in a headrest and padded facemask, and care should be undertaken to ensure no excessive stretching of the brachial plexus by surgical tractions. The legs are raised with several pillows or a large pad under the knees, to reduce stretch on the hamstrings and to improve venous return. All bony prominences should be well padded and supported including the non-surgical arm. A warm air blanket system should be applied to maintain normothermia.

Patients in the sitting beach chair position are more predisposed to hypotension, with cerebral ischaemia known to occur. This can be mitigated in susceptible patients by more gradual head elevation, fluid preloading and vasopressors. The non-invasive blood pressure should ideally be maintained close to baseline values to ensure adequate cerebral perfusion, considering the hydrostatic pressure difference between the cuffed arm and the brain in an upright position. Cerebral oximetry monitoring has also been utilised to try and achieve adequate cerebral perfusion, although evidence for its use is inconclusive to date [1].

Shoulder surgery is associated with excruciating post-operative pain. In the absence of regional anaesthetic blockade, an intra-operative multimodal regime should include a strong opioid, parenteral paracetamol and intravenous non-steroidal inflammatory drugs (NSAID) such as parecoxib unless contraindicated.

2.3 *Interscalene Block*

Interscalene block (ISB) is the most commonly performed brachial plexus block for shoulder surgery. It anaesthetises C5 to C7 nerve roots as well as the superficial cervical plexus. The traditional nerve stimulation block technique has largely been supplanted by the use of ultrasound. Ultrasound guided block allows visualisation of relevant anatomical structures, the needle-tip position, the spread of local anaesthetic (LA), which is associated with less needle passes, less LA volumes and better post-operative pain relief.

To perform the ultrasound guided ISB, the patient is placed supine with head turned away from the block site. After skin asepsis, the high frequency linear array probe is placed transversely parallel and above the clavicle with the beam directed caudally to the first rib to obtain the supraclavicular brachial plexus view. The subclavian artery is identified, and the brachial plexus trunks with its "bunch of grapes" appearance lying lateral and superficial to the artery. Then trace the brachial plexus by scanning superiorly. At the level of C6, the trunks of the brachial plexus should give way to the roots (C5, C6, and C7), which lie in the interscalene groove between the two scalene muscles (Fig. 9). An in-plane approach directing from lateral to medial using a 50 mm ultrasound short-bevelled needle is preferred. Colour doppler is applied to identify any vessels to avoid along

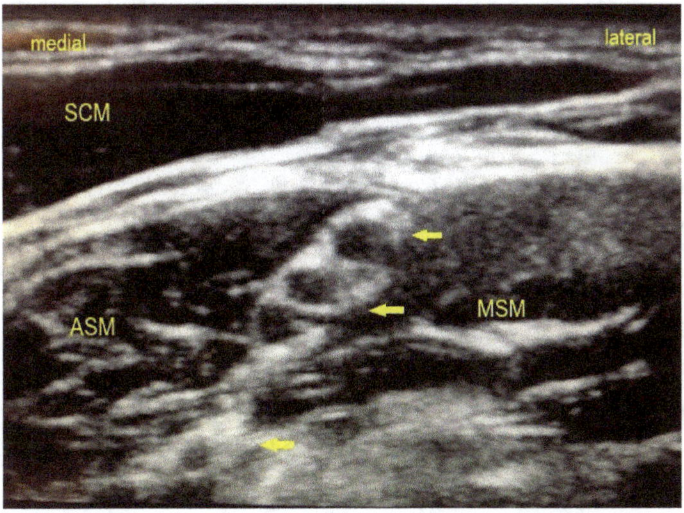

Fig. 9: Sono-anatomy of the interscalene brachial plexus. SCM: sternocleidomastoid muscle. ASM: anterior scalene muscle. MSM: middle scalene muscle. Arrows: C5, bifid C6, C7 roots in the interscalene groove.

the needle trajectory. Phrenic nerve can be observed superficial to the anterior scalene muscle away from C5 root by scanning up and down. The needle tip is placed adjacent to the nerve root C6 then C5 to deposit the LA, occasionally having to go between C5 and C6. After negative aspiration, LA can be injected slowly while observing the spread. Typically, up to 10 ml of 0.5% Ropivacaine or Levobupivacaine should suffice for regional analgesia when combined with GA, whereas a higher volume of 15 mL might be needed for the awake regional anaesthesia technique.

The phrenic nerve is almost always blocked with the traditional landmark block technique with larger volumes of LA, resulting in ipsilateral diaphragmatic paresis. The incidence is lower with LA volume reduction and ultrasound guidance [2]. Most patients can tolerate the unilateral reduced diaphragmatic activity; however, this might cause problems in patients with obesity or poor lung reserves. Other side effects can also be caused by LA spread to the surrounding structures, such as Horner's syndrome from block of the sympathetic trunk, and voice hoarseness from recurrent laryngeal nerve block. Both are self-limiting which resolve after the block wears off. Pneumothorax can still occur but is less likely than supraclavicular block.

2.4 *Alternative Blocks and Infiltration*

2.4.1 *Superior trunk block*

To perform the block, the ultrasound probe is tracked distally from the interscalene view where the C5 and C6 roots fuse to form the superior trunk, until the suprascapular nerve branches off the superior trunk. Using an in-plane approach, the ultrasound needle is advanced from lateral to medial, LA is deposited inferior and then superior to the trunk. It has been shown that superior trunk block can provide effective anaesthesia while preserving the diaphragmatic function (phrenic nerve sparing) when compared with ISB [3]. Hence it is a good alternative to ISB in shoulder surgery.

2.4.2 *Supraclavicular brachial plexus block*

Supraclavicular block has traditionally not been regarded as the block of choice for shoulder surgery because of the concerns that the proximal branches might be missed. Nevertheless, it has been shown to produce effective shoulder anaesthesia comparable to that of ISB. There is a reduced incidence of adverse effects such as voice hoarseness and Horner's syndrome. However, the incidence of phrenic nerve palsy is similar to ISB [4]. It also produces a denser motor block which might negatively affect patient satisfaction and early rehabilitation.

2.5 *Post-op Pain Management*

The post-operative pain is significant, which can remain severe for 48 hours after surgery. Early mobilisation with physical therapy on the first post-operative day is necessary for better functional outcome, but pain can be a hinderance to early rehabilitation. Furthermore, in spite of excellent analgesia provided by the regional blockade, some patients will complain of excruciating pain after block resolution. Hence it is important to initiate a multimodal analgesic treatment before the block regresses. Analgesic options such as oral paracetamol, oral NSAID (unless contraindicated), and a strong oral opioid (morphine or oxycodone) should be provided.

3. The Arthroscope and Camera Stack

3.1 *The Ideal Arthroscopy Instruments and Camera System*

There are many camera systems in the market, and the choice of camera systems should be driven by practicalities of the market where one practises. There are some criteria which can guide one in choosing the camera and visualisation systems. These factors include:

- Clarity of pictures and videos. Some systems display a subtle flicker and others have a bluish hue in background. Images should be sharp with vibrant colours. Focus should not be lost with minimal bleeding.
- The entire system should be easy to set up by the OT nurses.
- The scopes should be resistant to scratches and durable against RF burns.

- The scopes and light cables should be able to undergo autoclaving instead of using sheaths, as sheaths are known to have perforations which breach sterility barriers [5].
- Camera systems should be integrated with shaver, fluid pump and the RF machine.
- The entire system should be housed in a trolley stack and should be portable.

3.2 *Image Capture, Processing and Transmission*

It is essential in any camera system that images and videos can be captured with clarity and fidelity. Some systems have confusing ways of storing and copying videos onto personal storage devices and this is discouraging. Another problem commonly faced is that videos tend to be stored in a codex not familiar to most computer operating systems, and converting them is not easy; though this is less of a problem these days.

3.3 *The Mitek PureVue System*

The Mitek Lock family of scopes (Fig. 10) works with the PureVue system (Fig. 11), which is a single-chip camera system that provides real-time 1080 pixel HD videos. Image clarity is enhanced via 4K camera control system on a 32" display (Fig. 12). The entire system is also linked with the FMS VUE II Fluid Management and Tissue Debridement system, as well as the VAPR VUE Radiofrequency Electrode System.

4. Surgical Arthroscopic Instruments

Every industrial vendor has its own unique instruments. Mitek instruments come in a set which are versatile enough to cover most arthroscopic shoulder surgeries (Fig. 13). We have chosen to separate them into functional sets, this is to enable faster turn-around times between surgeries while waiting for the instruments to be autoclaved.

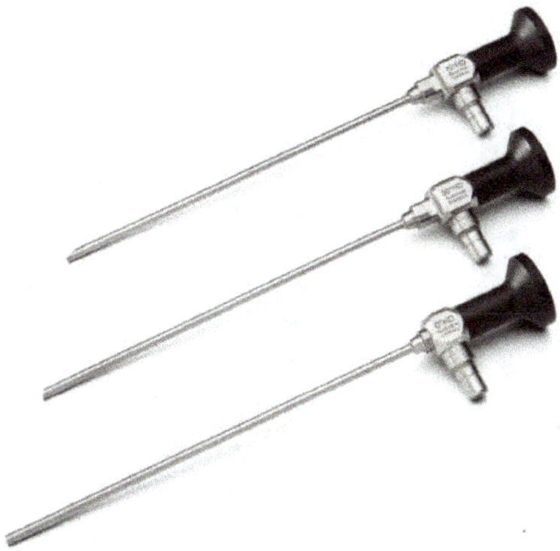

Fig. 10: Mitek Lock family of scopes.

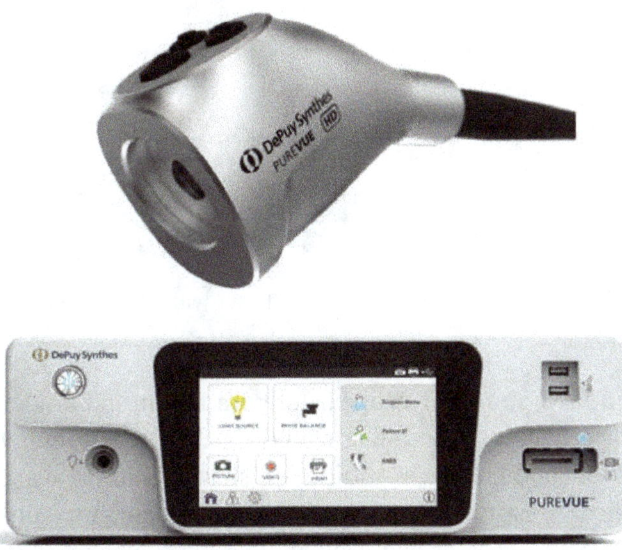

Fig. 11: PUREVUE Camera and CCS.

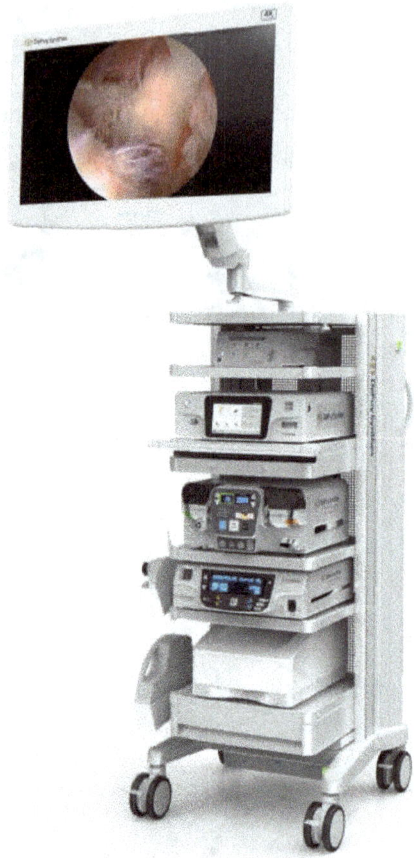

Fig. 12: PUREVUE Tower with 4K Monitor.

1. **Standard shoulder scopes:** Camera trocar and holder, probe, tissue grasper, suture manipulator, knot-pusher, suture cutter, arthroscopic scissors and punch, in addition to shavers and RF wand.
2. **Labral repairs:** Awl and drill for specific anchor, suture passers like Ideal Suture passer and Acupass (Smith & Nephew), suture retrievers like bird beak, crochet hook (Table 1).
3. **Cuff repair:** Awl and drill for specific anchor, antegrade suture passers like Express Sew III, suture retrievers like bird beak retrievers or cleaver hooks (Table 2).

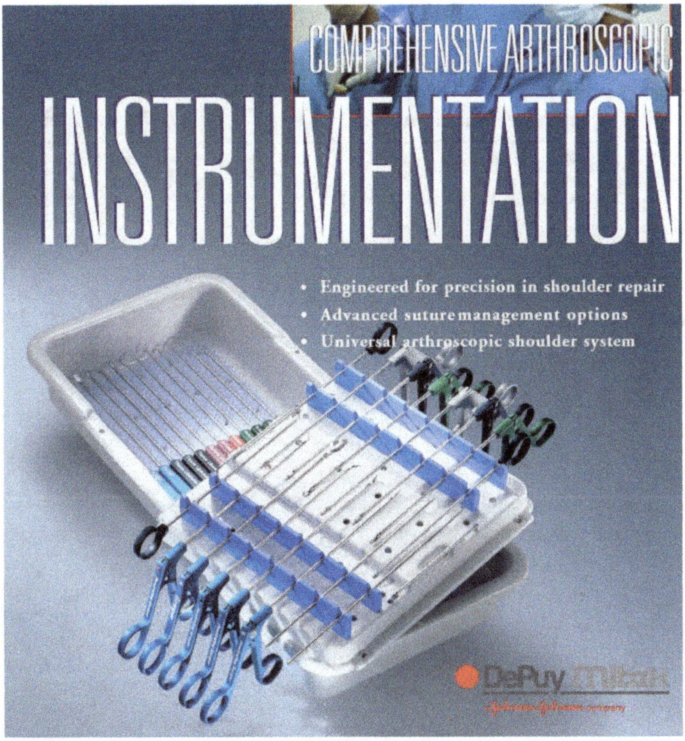

Fig. 13: Mitek instruments.

Table 1: Table showing the standard and common instruments used in labral repairs.

Standard Instruments for Labral Repairs		
Name	**Purpose, Notes on Use**	**Illustrations**
Cannula inserters	• Orange (5.5 mm) for suture management in the antero-superior portal. • Yellow (8.5 mm) main working cannula in antero-inferior portal. Cannula insertors can be used to dilate the portals prior to inserting the cannulas.	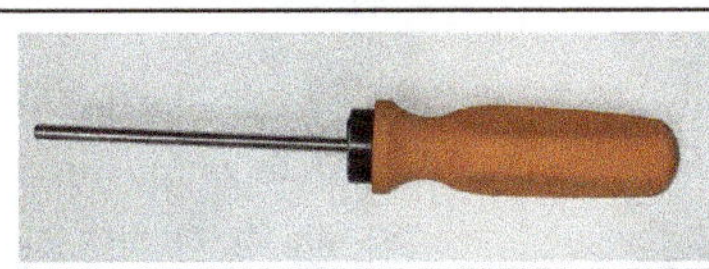 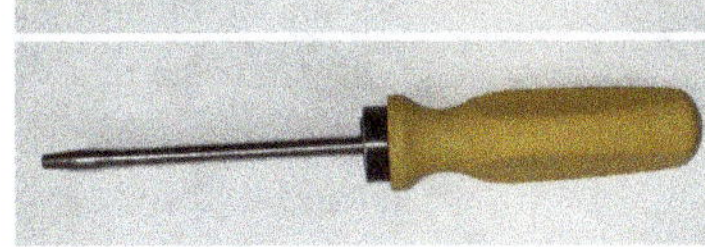

(*Continued*)

Table 1: (*Continued*)

Standard Instruments for Labral Repairs		
Name	**Purpose, Notes on Use**	**Illustrations**
Liberators	Liberators with the blade directed upwards (as shown) or downwards, are used to free and mobilise the adherent labrum, prior to repair.	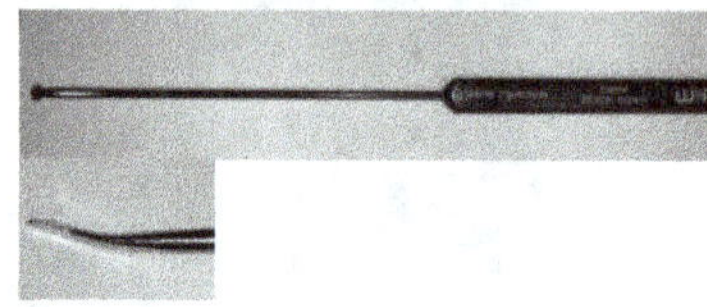
Rasp	Rasps with roughened surface facing down (as shown) or facing up, are used to roughen the glenoid edge for better labral healing.	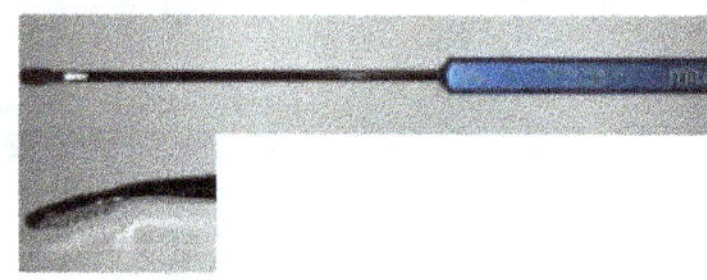
Drill guides	• Gryphon anchor drill guide (fishmouth opening) • Gryphon anchor drill guide (sawtooth opening) • Gryphon Proknot drill guide Gryphon drill guides come with four mouth openings, these two are most commonly used, the fish mouth and saw tooth openings.	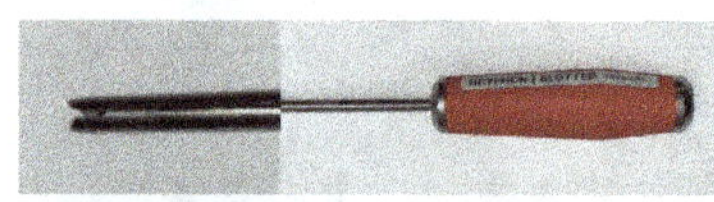 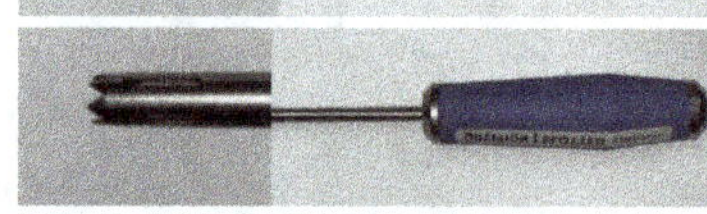 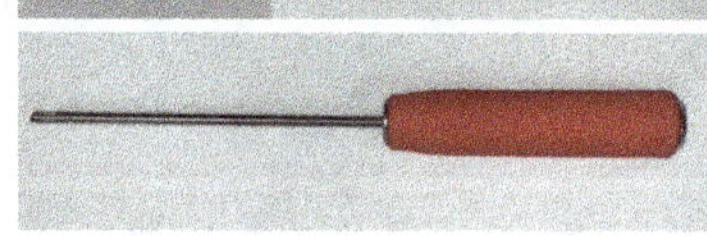
Tissue grasper	Tissue graspers have different teeth serrations, and are used to mobilize the liberated labral, as well as to tent up ligaments and capsule.	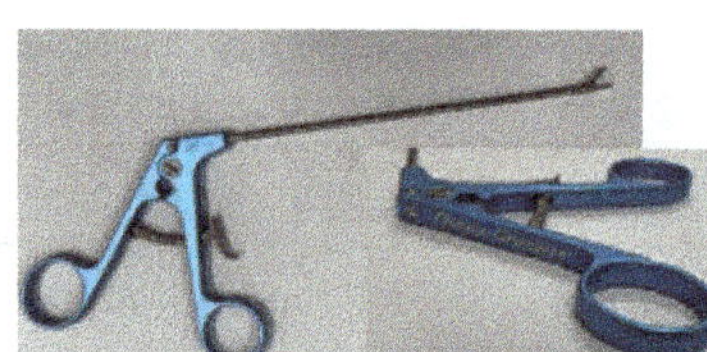
Suture retrievers	Suture retrievers are important to separate sutures into different portals, to ensure sutures exit within the same soft tissue portal (opening) prior to tying sutures and for general suture management.	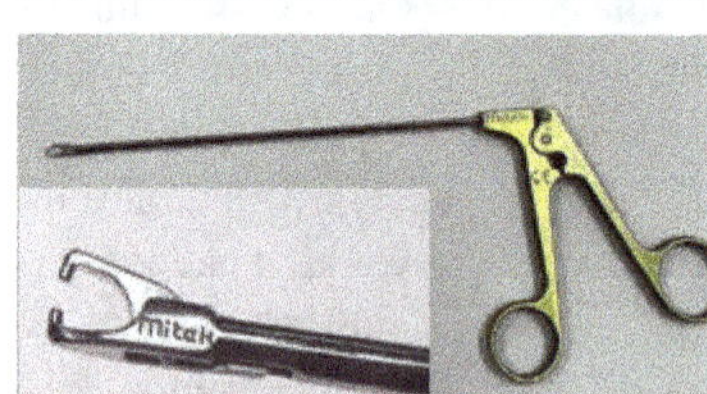

Table 1: (*Continued*)

Standard Instruments for Labral Repairs		
Name	**Purpose, Notes on Use**	**Illustrations**
Suture passers	The IDEAL suture shuttle has a sharp penetrating tip, there are variations of tip directions. Suture passing is done using a CHIA wire.	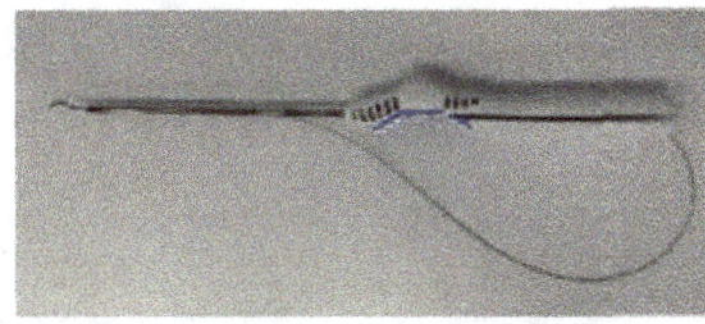
Penetrating grasper	Also called the bird beak retriever, this grasper is useful to retrogradely retrieve sutures. Hence it is useful in both labral and cuff repairs.	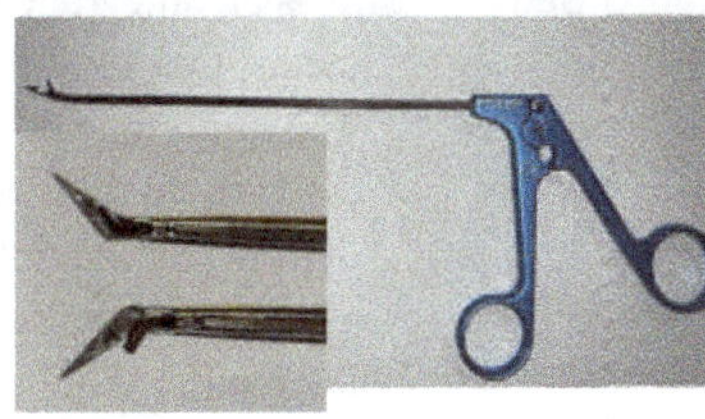
Crochet hook	This functions as a suture retriever in tight and small spaces, useful in separating sutures before tying during a labral repair.	
Knot pusher	Knot pushers help to deliver knots (Duncan sliding or half-hitches) when tying. The type shown requires sutures to be threaded through the aperture.	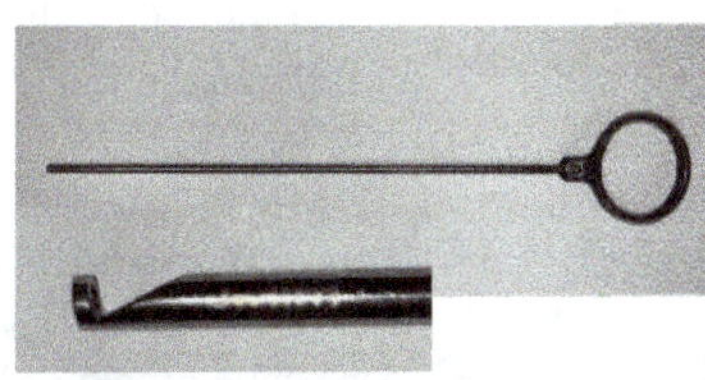
Suture cutter	Sutures are slipped in obliquely in this cutter which is half-closed to prevent the suture from slipping out. The cutter is then used to cut the sutures about 1 cm above the knot.	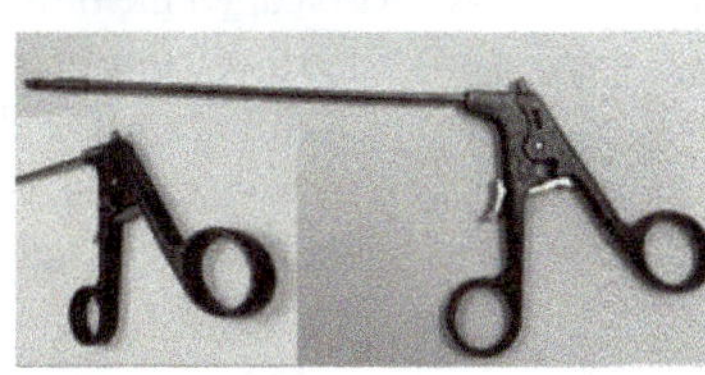

Table 2: Table showing the common instruments used in a cuff repair.

Standard Instruments for Cuff Repairs		
Cortical awl and tap	The 4.5 and 5.5 mm awl/tap are used to prepare for the insertion of the Healix medial row of anchors.	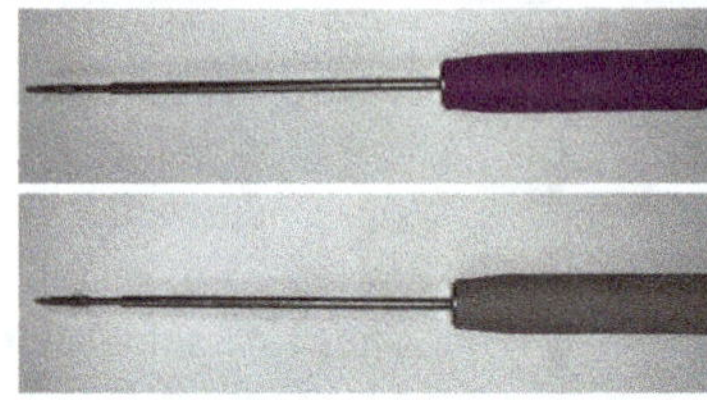
Express Sew III	This is an antegrade suture passer that captures sutures. The larger handle closes the jaw, the smaller handle deploys the flexible needle that threads the suture across the tendon. The suture is trapped in the diving board of the upper jaw.	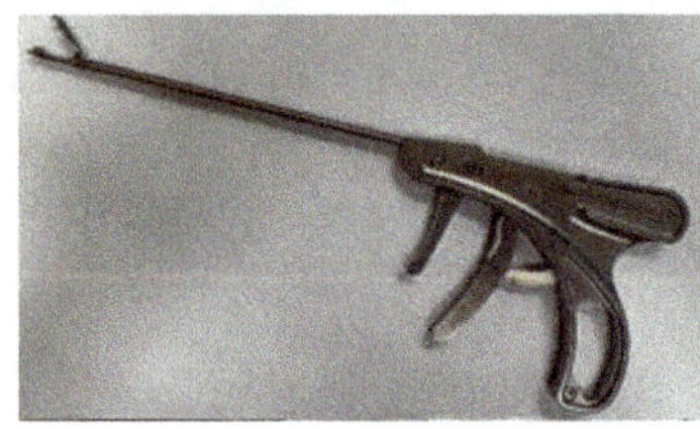
Cleaver hooks	Also called SixTers, these are antegrade suture passers and can be used both in cuff and labral repairs. They come in right and left-sided curves.	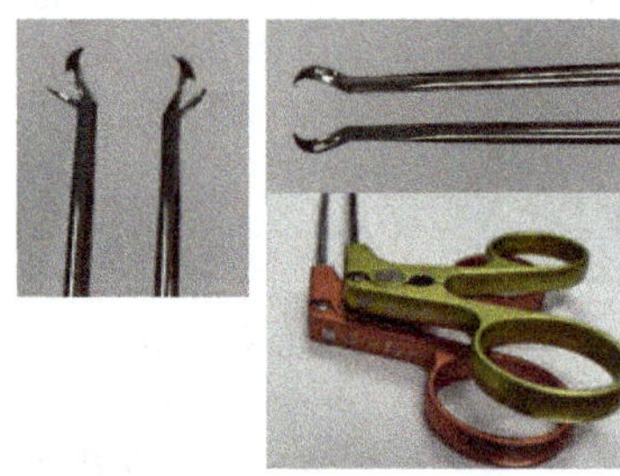
Penetrating grasper	Also called the bird beak retriever, this grasper is useful to retrogradely retrieve sutures. Hence it is useful in both labral and cuff repairs.	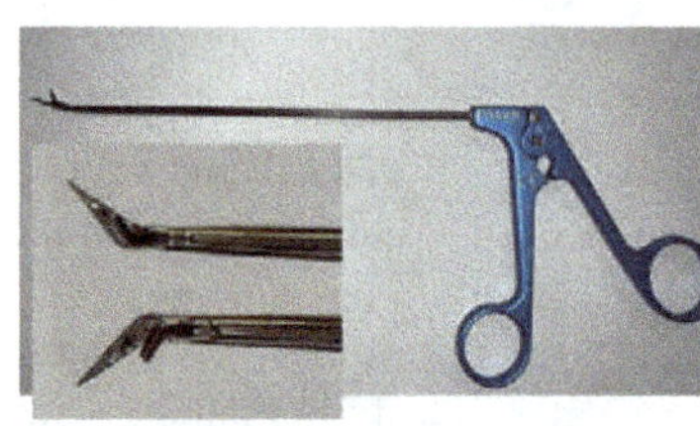
Tissue grasper	Tissue graspers are used to mobilize cuff tendons after debridement. They aid in assessing reparability and useful to hold tendons before securing them.	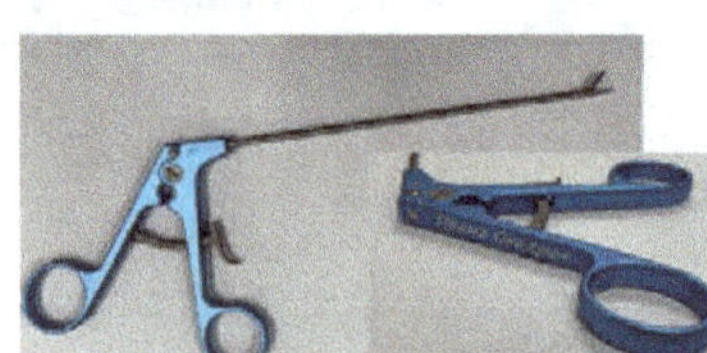

Table 2: (*Continued*)

Standard Instruments for Cuff Repairs		
Suture retrievers	Suture retrievers are important to separate sutures into different portals, to ensure sutures exit within the same soft tissue portal (opening) prior to tying sutures and for general suture management.	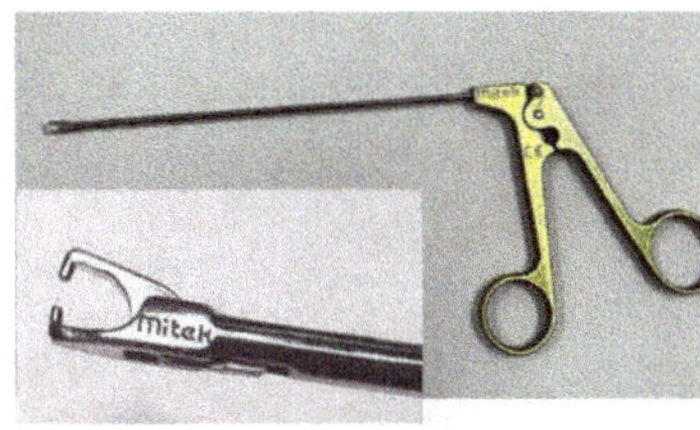
Knot pusher	Knot pushers help to deliver knots (Duncan sliding or half-hitches) when tying. The type shown requires sutures to be threaded through the aperture.	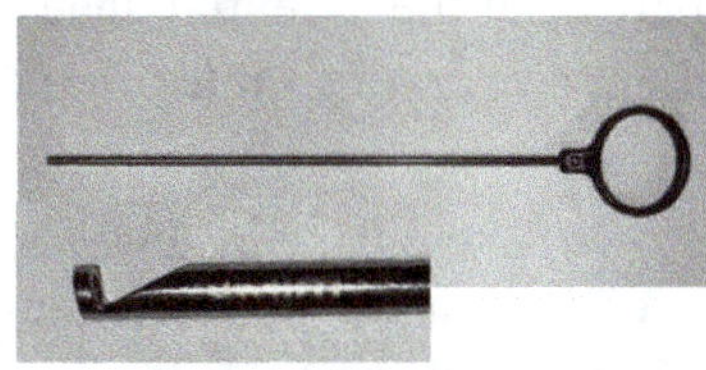
Versalok deployment gun	This deployment gun was specially designed for the Versalok anchor in the lateral row. The gun is inserted into the anchor inserter in the unlocked position (lever down). After locking (lever up) the sutures are tightened in the spool, then the anchor is deployed by depressing the gun.	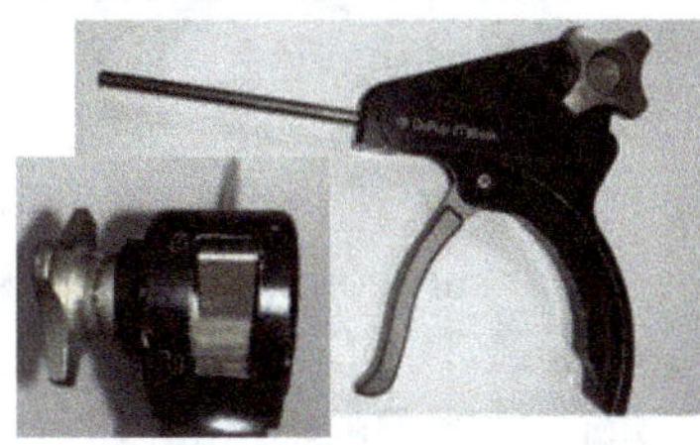
Suture cutter	Sutures are slipped in obliquely in this cutter which is half-closed to prevent the suture from slipping out. The cutter is then used to cut the sutures about 1 cm above the knot.	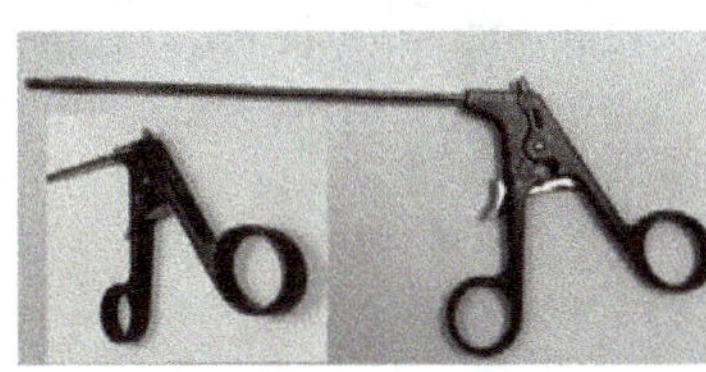

5. Other OT Preparations

5.1 *OT Requirements for Shoulder Arthroscopic Surgery*

A standard Operating Theatre is sufficient, no laminar flow is required for arthroscopic surgery.

5.2 *Functional Lay-out of the OT*

Apart from the essential anaesthesia trolleys and set-up, surrounding the patient's operating table are the following:

(a) The camera stack, monitor and video recording; this should be positioned on the opposite side of the surgeon, about 30° in the caudal direction, or at the level of the pelvis of the patient, on the opposite side. The shaving system and RF console should be integrated as one stack with the camera.
(b) Fluid system and extra bags: this trolley is positioned on the opposite of the surgeon and should be constantly monitored by the circulating nurses. The first two 3L bag of saline should be infused with 1 g epinephrine. Bags should be replaced **BEFORE** the fluid runs out, lest air bubbles be introduced into the sterile fluid system.
(c) The assisting nurse is positioned at the foot of the patient's bed on the same side as the surgeon, surrounded by 2–3 trolleys of surgical instruments.
(d) The anaesthesia team remains at the head of the patient. IV access is maintained from the contralateral hand.

References

1. Salazar DH, Davies W, Zirolgu N, *et al*. Cerebral desaturation events during shoulder arthroscopy in the beach chair position. *JAAOS Glob Res Rev* 2019;3(8):e007.
2. Riazi S, Carmichael N, Awad I, *et al*. Effect of local anaesthetic volume (20 vs 5 ml) on the efficacy and respiratory consequences of ultrasound-guided interscalene brachial plexus block. *Br J Anaesth* 2008;101(4):549–556.

3. Kang R, Jeong JS, Chin KJ, *et al.* Superior trunk block provides noninferior analgesia compared with interscalene brachial plexus block in arthroscopic shoulder surgery. *Anesthesiology* 2019;131(6):1316–1326.
4. Guo CW, Ma JX, Ma XL, *et al.* Supraclavicular block versus interscalene brachial plexus block for shoulder surgery: A meta-analysis of clinical control trials. *Int J Surg* 2017;45:85–91.
5. Benjamin FH Ang, Henry Soeharno, Kong Hwee Lee, Shirlena TK Wong, Denny TT Lie, Paul CC Chang. Camera cover perforation after arthroscopic surgery. *Ann Acad Med Singap* 2018;47(7):263–265.

https://doi.org/10.1142/9789811249846_0004

Chapter 4

The Normal Shoulder: The Arthroscopic Routine in the Gleno-humeral Joint and the Subacromial Space

Denny T.T. Lie and Bryan Wang

Summary of Chapter

1. History of shoulder arthroscopy
2. Indications for arthroscopy, when to do open surgery
3. Surface markings of the shoulder
4. Portals commonly used
5. The shoulder arthroscopic routine

1. History of Shoulder Arthroscopy

The beginnings of shoulder arthroscopy date back to 1806, when the German urologist Philipp Bozzini built an instrument that could be introduced in the human body to visualise the internal organs using a candle as a source of light. He called this instrument "Lichtleiter" and was credited to be the inventor of the first endoscope [1]. The first recorded application of an endoscope to examine a joint was in 1912, when the Danish surgeon

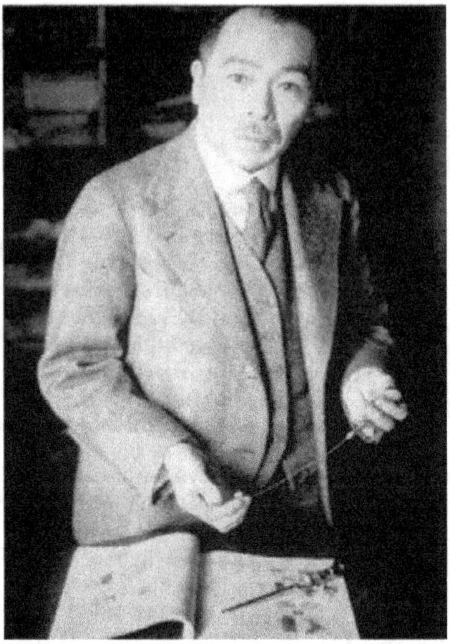

Fig. 1: Professor Kenji Takagi (1888–1963) [27].

Severin Nordentoft used a laparoscope to examine the interior of a knee joint [2]. In 1919, Professor Kenji Takagi, a Japanese orthopaedic surgeon, used a 7.3-mm cystoscope to examine knees of patients affected by tuberculosis in 1918 [3] (see Fig. 1). Other pioneers in the development of arthroscopy include the Swiss surgeon Eugen Bircher, who was the first to perform diagnostic knee arthroscopies on live patients, publishing his series of 21 patients in 1922 [4], and Masaki Watanabe, a former student of Takagi, who was the first to carry out intervention arthroscopy of the knee. He is best remembered for making fundamental improvements to the design of the arthroscope, including pioneering the use of fibre optics in arthroscopy [5].

As a result of their work in the development of arthroscopic technology, Samuel Burman was able to perform the first diagnostic shoulder arthroscopy on a cadaver in USA in 1931. He performed 90 arthroscopies on different cadaver joints, amongst which were 25 shoulders, and compared the arthroscopic findings with those seen when the joint was opened [6]. However, it was not until some 35 years later that the first clinical use of this procedure was described [7]. The use of arthroscopy in shoulder surgery only really started taking off in the 1980s when James Andrews performed arthroscopic debridement of partial supraspinatus tears in 36 patients [8], and Harvard Ellman performed subacromial decompression in 50 consecutive patients in 1985 [9]. These surgeries are considered routine arthroscopic procedures today.

Johnson and Detrisac performed the first arthroscopic shoulder stabilisation procedure in 1980, using a capsular stapling technique [10]. Patients were placed in the lateral decubitus position, and a staple was used to engage the Bankart lesion and portions of the subscapularis and anterior capsule. Arthroscopic stapling, however, offered only a single-point fixation and suffered from a 16% to 33% recurrence rate in addition to a 26% rate of staple loosening [11].

In 1987, Morgan and Bodenstab [12] introduced the arthroscopic trans-osseous suture technique, later modified by McIntyre and Caspari [13]. A Beath pin was placed from anterior to posterior through the IGHL and trans-glenoid drill holes made. Polydioxanone suture was then pulled through the scapula and tied posteriorly through a separate incision. The original authors reported excellent results with no recurrences through 2 years [13]. However, subsequent studies reported recurrence rates as high as 44% [14]. Other disadvantages included the risk of scapulothoracic joint penetration [15] and injury to the suprascapular nerve, and as such, this technique has since fallen out of favour.

Arthroscopic suture anchor placement was first described by Eugene Wolf in 1993 [16] and later modified by Snyder and Strafford [17] who used permanent sutures. Multiple anchors allowed multiple points of fixation, and their pull-out strength was similar to that of trans-osseous sutures [18]. Anchors also facilitated fixation along the glenoid articular edge, as opposed to the medial neck, which had previously re-created anterior labral periosteal sleeve avulsion (ALPSA) lesions. In 2002, Abrams *et al.* [19] reported just a 5% recurrence rate in 662 patients after 2 years, and additional literature has continued to show recurrence rates below 10% for classic Bankart lesions [20]. For this reason, suture anchors remain the most popular mode of arthroscopic repair today.

In 1990, Howard J. Levy suggested combining shoulder arthroscopy with arthrotomy to better diagnose and repair rotator cuff lesions and reported results of 25 patients treated with this "arthroscopically assisted" or "mini-open" technique at a minimum of 1 year of follow-up [21]. This "arthroscopically-assisted" technique served as a transition phase in rotator cuff surgery, which soon evolved to an all-arthroscopic technique in the later part of the 1990s. In the 1990s, shoulder arthroscopy involved predominantly removing loose bodies, treating instability, calcific tendonitis, and septic arthritis. After a preliminary report by Steve Snyder [22], Raymond Thal published a technical note on how to place mattress sutures arthroscopically [23], paving the way for modern arthroscopic rotator cuff repairs.

The understanding of shoulder disorders and their treatment has advanced significantly in the last few decades as a result of arthroscopy, which has fast progressed from diagnosis to ablative procedures and now to reconstructive surgery. It can be used for the diagnosis and management of shoulder instability, rotator cuff disease, fractures and other soft tissue trauma. With increasing expertise in the field of shoulder arthroscopy, this has also allowed us to perform an increasing number of challenging procedures using these minimally-invasive techniques.

2. Indications for Arthroscopy, When to Do Open Surgery

The evolution of shoulder arthroscopy has advanced our understanding of shoulder anatomy and pathology. It has given us the ability to evaluate and address pathology of the shoulder joint using minimally-invasive techniques, with concomitant decrease in post-operative pain, less stiffness, and potential cost-savings as they can be performed in the outpatient setting. Shoulder arthroscopy also minimises the risk of deltoid muscle damage that can sometimes be seen with open surgeries. With the increasing expertise in shoulder arthroscopy, this has also allowed us to develop a new array of techniques in managing complex shoulder problems, which may have once been only amenable to open surgery.

The indications for shoulder arthroscopy include but not limited to:

- Diagnostic surgery;
- Removal of loose bodies;

- Subacromial decompression;
- Rotator cuff debridement or repair;
- Instability repair (including superior labrum);
- Acromioclavicular joint pathology;
- Distal clavicle excision;
- Release of scar tissue in adhesive capsulitis;
- Biceps tenotomy/tenodesis;
- Release of suprascapular nerve entrapment.

Although arthroscopic surgery has become more routine, open shoulder surgery still has its place and remains an important skillset for surgeons. Depending on the training of a surgeon, arthroscopic surgery can potentially have a steeper learning curve, which may translate to longer operating time, weaker repairs and potentially poorer clinical outcomes.

In a systematic review published by Hohmann in 2017, it was found that despite advances in surgical techniques and devices over the past 20 years, either open or arthroscopic surgical treatment of anterior shoulder dislocation results in similar clinical outcomes [24]. The recurrence rate for arthroscopic surgical stabilisation has only marginally decreased, from 16.8% to 14.2%. However, during the earlier decade from 1995 through 2004, patients treated with arthroscopic surgery had twice the risk of recurrence compared with an open procedure. With regards to the surgical management of the rotator cuff, both open and arthroscopic groups showed similar clinical outcomes. Rotator cuff integrity is comparable for small tears, but large tears have twice the re-tear rate after an arthroscopic repair [25]. In a study comparing mini-open versus arthroscopic rotator cuff repair, it was found that the mini-open rotator cuff repair required significantly less operative time and is significantly less expensive than the all-arthroscopic repair [26], which may have a bearing on cost-utilisation in hospitals.

As such, it is imperative to maintain the skillset of open shoulder surgery as they still retain a role today despite the advancement of shoulder arthroscopy. In addition, there are certain pathologies of the shoulder which may not be amenable to shoulder arthroscopy, including the surgical management of some complex fractures of the shoulder, as well as shoulder arthroplasty.

3. Surface Markings on the Shoulder

- Begin from the posterior: using a skin marker, mark the **outer border of the spine** of the scapula, continuing laterally as the **lateral border of the acromion** and anteriorly, mark the **outer border of the clavicle**.
- The **inner border of the spine** of the scapula is then marked, this makes a sharp inflexion at the lateral edge to continue as the **inner border of the clavicle**.
- At the lateral inflexion point of the inner borders, mark the **prominence of the ACJ**.
- The protruding **tip of the coracoid** is also marked.
- From the postero-lateral corner of the acromion, make a marking about 2 cm medial and inferior to it, this is the position of the **posterior portal**.
- The **anterior portal** is positioned and marked just lateral to the tip of the coracoid. A variation of it is slightly higher, described as high **antero-superior portal**.
- Extend a line from the inner border of the spine of the scapula to the lateral acromion, about 2 cm below it marks the **antero-lateral portal.** Another variant is just anterior to this portal, where it enters the joint just anterior to the biceps, called the **biceps portal** (see Fig. 2).

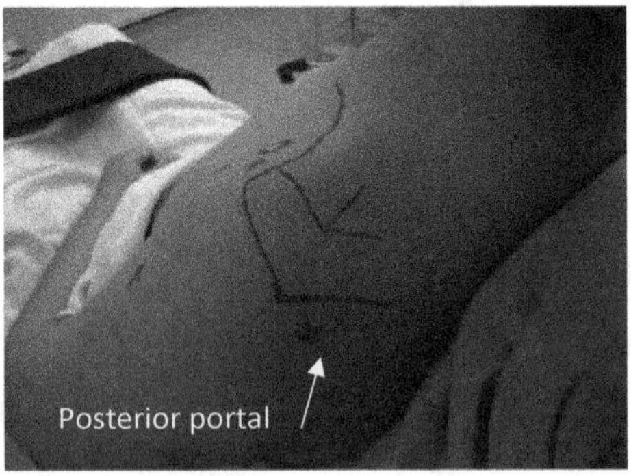

Fig. 2: Surface marking of the shoulder: the outer borders of the spine of the scapula, acromion and clavicle; and the inner borders of the spine and clavicle are seen. The posterior portal (arrow) is 2 cm medial and inferior to the postero-lateral corner of the acromion.

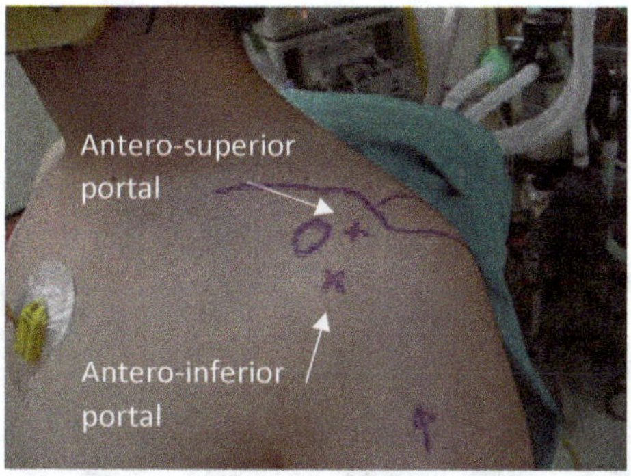

Fig. 3: The tip of the coracoid is marked. The antero-superior portal is just lateral to it and the antero-inferior portal is about 2–3 cm distal to it.

- Similarly, extend a line from the inner border of the clavicle to the acromion, about 1–2 cm below it is the **postero-lateral portal**.
- Midway between these two portals above is the **lateral portal**.
- About 2–3 cm below the antero-superior portal, and about 1 cm lateral is the **antero-inferior portal** (see Fig. 3).

4. Portals Commonly Used

(1) **Routine arthroscopy, debridement and SAD:** Posterior portal for viewing, anterior portal as the working portal, lateral portal as accessory for the SAD.

(2) **Labral repair:** Posterior portal for viewing, high antero-superior portal for SLAP repairs and suture management, main working portal is the antero-inferior portal (see Fig. 4).

(3) **Simple cuff repairs:** Posterior portal for viewing, anterior and antero-lateral portals are the main working ones; an optional viewing portal is the high postero-lateral portal (see Fig. 5).

(4) **Large cuff repairs and SCR:** Initially begin with posterior portal for viewing, this is then shifted to the postero-lateral portal. Main working portals are the antero-lateral and lateral portals, accessory ones are the anterior and posterior portals.

(5) **A tear portal:** It is created from the outside-in, right over the tear. Hence its location is not pre-determined but located when the tear is

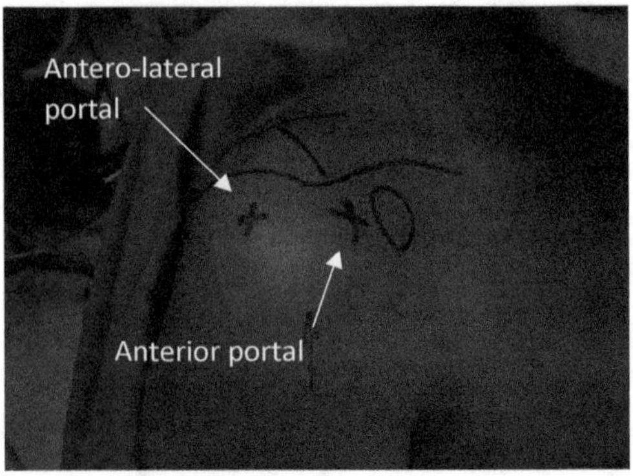

Fig. 4: The anterior and antero-lateral portals used in a typical cuff repair.

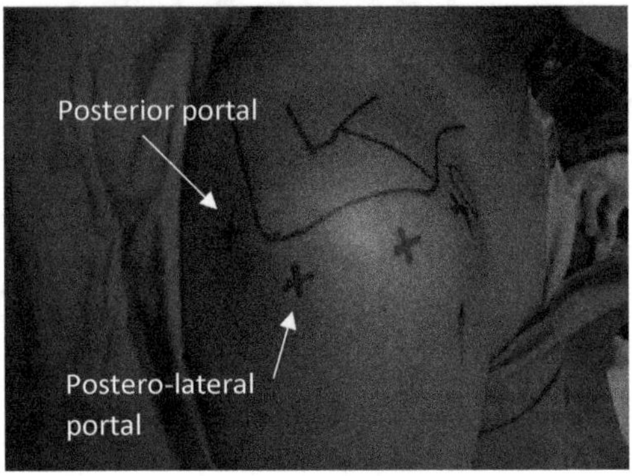

Fig. 5: Side view showing the posterior, postero-lateral and antero-lateral portals.

seen from the gleno-humeral joint. It is usually near the antero-lateral portal.

5. The Arthroscopic Surgery Routine

5.1 *The Glenohumeral Joint*

5.1.1 *From the posterior portal*

With the camera from the posterior portal, create an antero-superior portal and insert a probe or an obturator to assess the following structures (see Fig. 6):

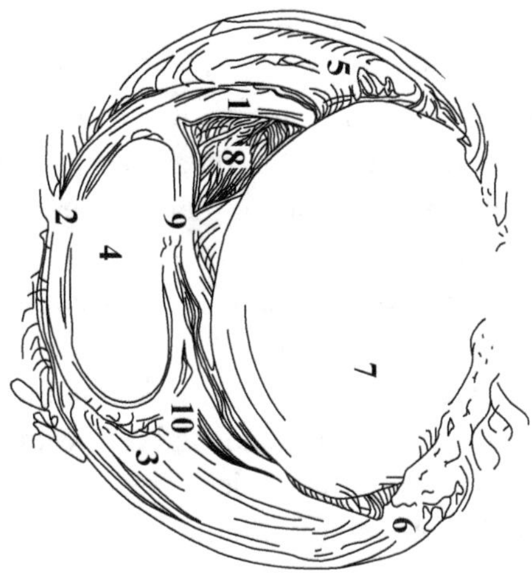

Fig. 6: Schematic drawing showing the routine of shoulder arthroscopy and what to look for, from the posterior portal.

FEATURES IN NORMAL SHOULDER SCOPE
From posterior view: 1. Biceps tendon 2. Posterior labrum 3. Inferior labrum and pouch 4. Glenoid 5. Undersurface of Supraspinatus tendon 6. Infraspinatus tendon 7. Humeral head 8. Rotator interval 9. Anterior labrum and MGHL 10. IGHL From antero-superior view: 1. Articulating surface 2. Posterior labrum 3. Posterior capsule 4. Subscapularis tendon

(1) The biceps tendon and its origin:
- The normal biceps tendon is firmly attached to the superior labrum and remains so when the biceps is firmly tugged. Type I injuries cause fraying but the biceps remains attached and does not droop onto the articulating glenoid surface.

(2) The superior labrum.
(3) The anterior labrum, till the antero-inferior labrum.
(4) The inferior labrum and pouch.
(5) The biceps tendon as it enters the groove, the biceps sling:
- Swing the camera to look lateral and follow the biceps as it enters the bicipital groove. Pull the biceps tendon into the joint space, it is normal to observe slight inflammation at the inflexion.

(6) The subscapularis tendon.
(7) The MGHL, anterior IGHL and anterior capsule.
(8) The rotator interval (within which runs the SGHL):
- The rotator interval is bounded medially by the labrum, inferiorly by the subscapularis and supero-laterally by the biceps tendon. The SGHL is a condensation of the fascia and runs along the biceps tendon.

(9) The articular surface of the supraspinatus tendon:
- To look for small tears, abduct and slightly rotate the arm externally.

(10) The humeral head and the bare area:
- The bare area is a small area on the humeral head devoid of cartilage. It is best seen by externally rotating the arm and bringing it to slight abduction. This is different from the Hills Sachs lesion which is often larger, more medial, bare of cartilage and often decorticated as well.

5.1.2 *From the antero-superior portal*

Transfer the camera to the antero-superior portal to have a better view of the posterior structures of the glenohumeral joint (see Fig. 7):

(1) The glenoid articulating surface:
- Examine the overall morphology of the glenoid which is described as pear-shaped. It is important that the lower portion, at

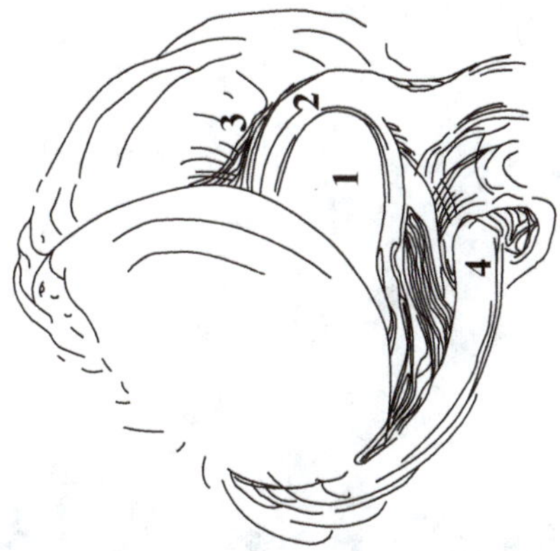

Fig. 7: Posterior structures to inspect from the antero-superior portal.

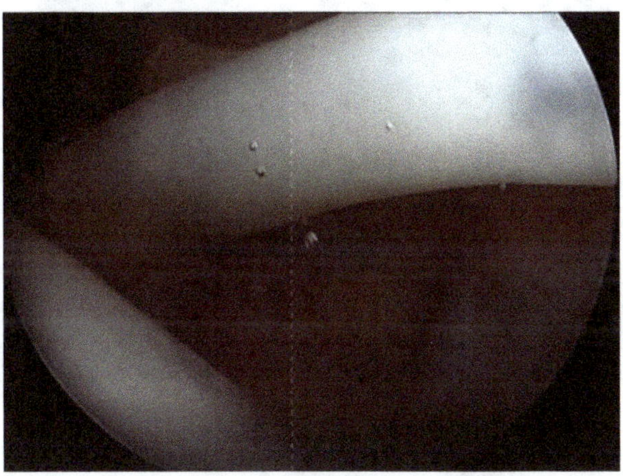

Fig. 8: The intact long head of biceps tendon.

the equator, the glenoid is wider that at the upper part (top hat). Observe the bare spot in the geometric centre of the glenoid. Measure the AP diameter at the bare spot, taking note of the distance from the bare spot to the posterior and anterior edge of the glenoid (see Figs. 8–13).

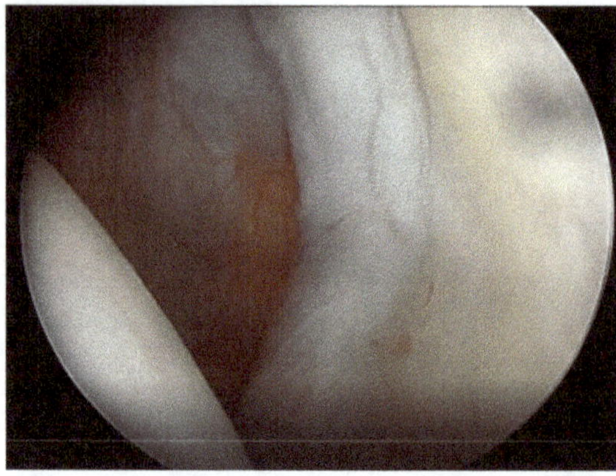

Fig. 9: Normal-looking anterior labrum.

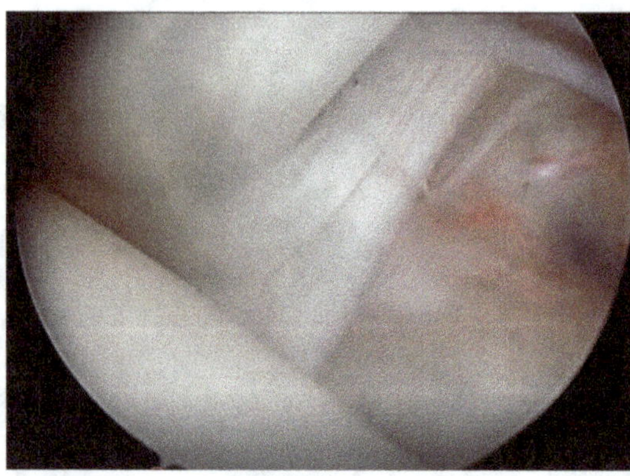

Fig. 10: Intact biceps sling.

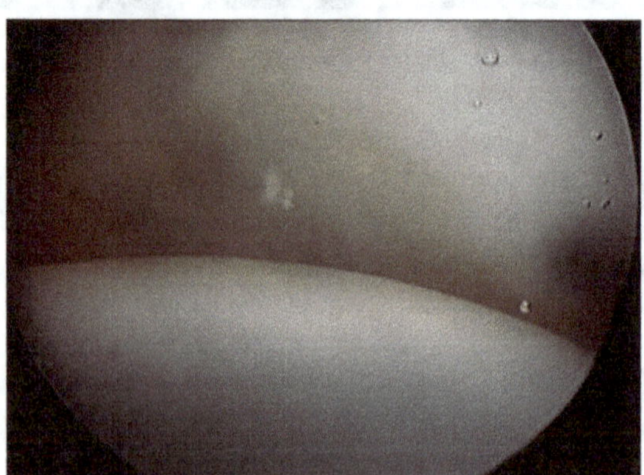

Fig. 11: Undersurface of an intact supraspinatus tendon.

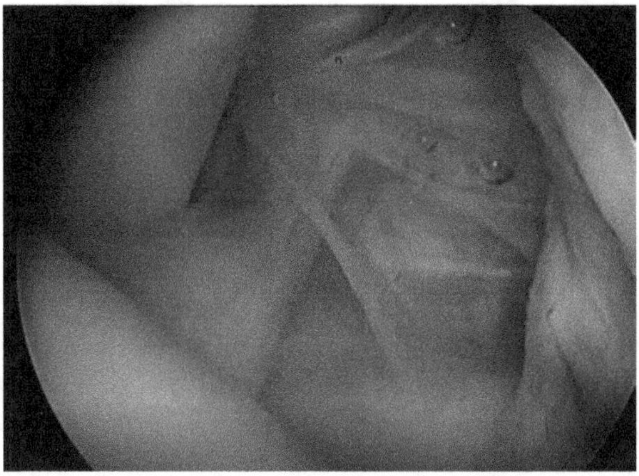

Fig. 12: The rotator interval is bounded by the biceps, subscapularis and anterior labrum.

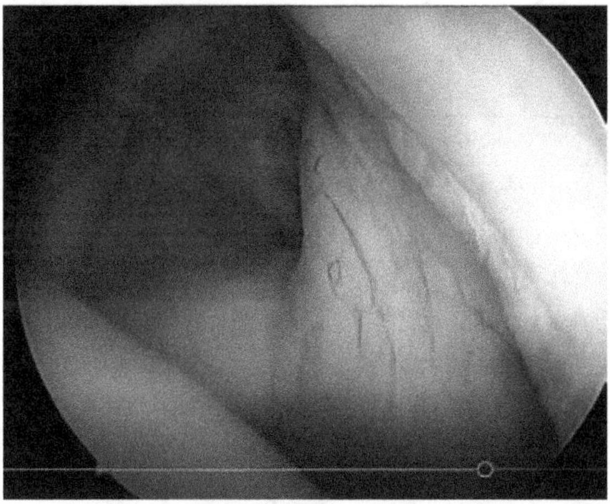

Fig. 13: Intact MGHL.

(2) The posterior labrum.
(3) The posterior capsule.

5.2 *The Subacromial Space*

The camera enters from the posterior portal but angled about 45 degree superiorly and runs just below the acromion, hugging the under-surface

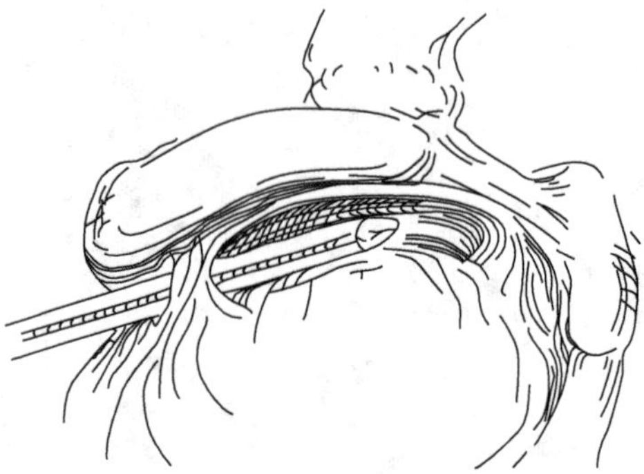

Fig. 14: The subacromial space is entered by running the obturator on the undersurface of the acromion.

of the acromion as it is pushed forwards. The structures to observe are listed below and will be discussed as limits of the subacromial decompression in Chapter 13 (see Fig. 14).

STRUCTURES IN THE SUBACROMIAL SPACE
1. Subacromial bursa
2. Acromion
3. CA ligament
4. AC joint
5. Fat pad medially
6. Supraspinatus tendon
7. Posterior bursa

(1) The subacromial bursa.
(2) Superiorly the roof of the space is the acromion and deltoid muscle.
(3) Anteriorly the coraco-acromial ligament (CAL) is seen.
(4) Medial to it is the acromio-clavicular joint (ACJ) and lateral edge of the clavicle.
(5) Medial to the subacromial space is the fat pad which hides the rich blood supply.
(6) The floor of the space is the thick whitish and tough supraspinatus tendon.

(7) The posterior limit of the space is the bursa which is seen as a curtain.

References

1. Bush RB, Leonhardt H, Bush IV, Landes RR. Dr. Bozzini's Lichtleiter. A translation of his original article (1806). *Urology* 1974;3(1):119–123.
2. Kieser CW, Jackson RW. Severin Nordentoft: the first arthroscopist. *Arthroscopy* 2001;17(5):532–535.
3. Takagi K. The classic arthroscope. Kenji Takagi. J Jap Orthop Assoc, 1939. *Clin Orthop Relat Res* 1982;167:6–8.
4. Kieser C. Eugen Bircher — Schweizer Pionier der Arthroskopie (1883–1956). *Arthroskopie* 2004;17:272–276.
5. DeMaio M. Giants of orthopaedic surgery: Masaki Watanabe MD. *Clin Orthop Relat Res* 2013;471:2443–2448.
6. Burman MS. Arthroscopy or the direct visualization of joints: an experimental cadaver study. 1931. *Clin Orthop Relat Res* 2001;390:5–9.
7. Andren L, Lundberg BJ. Treatment of rigid shoulders by joint distention during arthroscopy. *Acta Orthop Scand* 1965; 36: 45–53.
8. Andrews JR, Broussard TS, Carson WG. Arthroscopy of the shoulder in the management of partial tears of the rotator cuff: a preliminary report. *Arthroscopy* 1965;1:117–122.
9. Ellman H. Arthroscopic subacromial decompression: analysis of one- to three-year results. *Arthroscopy* 1987;3:173–181.
10. Johnson LL. Arthroscopy of the shoulder. *Orthop Clin North Am* 1980;11:197–204.
11. Hawkins RB. Arthroscopic stapling repair for shoulder instability: a retrospective study of 50 cases. *Arthroscopy* 1989;5:122–128.
12. Morgan CD, Bodenstab AB. Arthroscopic Bankart suture repair: technique and early results. *Arthroscopy* 1987;3:111–122.
13. McIntyre LF, Caspari RB. The rationale and technique for arthroscopic reconstruction of anterior shoulder instability using multiple sutures. *Orthop Clin North Am* 1993;24:55–58.
14. Green MR, Christensen KP. Arthroscopic versus open Bankart procedures: a comparison of early morbidity and complications. *Arthroscopy* 1993;9: 371–374.
15. Shea KP, Lovallo JL. Scapulothoracic penetration of a Beath pin: an unusual complication of arthroscopic Bankart suture repair. *Arthroscopy* 1991;7:115–117.

16. Wolf EM. Arthroscopic capsulolabral repair using suture anchors. *Orthop Clin North Am* 1993;24:59–69.
17. Snyder SJ, Strafford BB. Arthroscopic management of instability of the shoulder. *Orthopedics* 1993;16:993–1002.
18. Pope EJ, Ward JP, Rokito AS. Anterior shoulder instability — a history of arthroscopic treatment. *Bull NYU Hosp Jt Dis* 2011;69:44–49.
19. Abrams JS, Savoie FH, Tauro JC, Bradley JP. Recent advances in the evaluation and treatment of shoulder instability: anterior, posterior, and multidirectional. *Arthroscopy* 2002;18(Suppl 2):1–13. http://dx.doi.org/10.1016/S0749-8063(02)80110-4.
20. Cole BJ, Romeo AA. Arthroscopic shoulder stabilization with suture anchors: technique, technology, and pitfalls. *Clin Orthop Relat Res* 2001;(390):17–30.
21. Levy HJ, Uribe JW, Delaney LG. Arthroscopic assisted rotator cuff repair: preliminary results. *Arthroscopy* 1990;6(1):55–60.
22. Snyder SJ, Bachner EJ. Arthroscopic fixation of rotator cuff tears: a preliminary report. Paper presented at the *12th Annual Meeting of the Arthroscopy Association of North America Palm Desert*, CA, 1993.
23. Thal R. A technique for arthroscopic mattress suture placement. *Arthroscopy* 1993;9(5):605–607.
24. Hohmann E, Tetsworth K, Glatt V. Open versus arthroscopic surgical treatment for anterior shoulder dislocation: a comparative systematic review and meta-analysis over the past 20 years. *J Shoulder Elbow Surg* 2017;26(10):1873–1880.
25. Bishop J, Klepps S, Lo I, Bird J, Gladstone J, Flatow E. Cuff integrity after arthroscopic versus open rotator cuff repair: a prospective study. *J Shoulder Elbow Surg* 2006;15:290–299.
26. Churchill S, Ghorai J. Total cost and operating room time comparison of rotator cuff repair techniques at low, intermediate, and high volume centre: mini-open versus all-arthroscopic. *J Shoulder Elbow Surg* 2010;19(5): 716–712.
27. Robert W Jackson. A history of arthroscopy. *Arthroscopy* 2010;26(1): 91–103.

https://doi.org/10.1142/9789811249846_0005

Chapter 5

Arthroscopic Capsular Release for Adhesive Capsulitis

Denny T.T. Lie and Mak Wai Keong

Summary of Chapter

1. Introduction and epidemiology of adhesive capsulitis
2. Clinical presentation of the frozen shoulder
3. Pathophysiology of adhesive capsulitis, phases
4. Diagnosis & Imaging, is there any?
5. Surgical technique of the arthroscopic capsular release
6. Rehabilitation
7. Clinical outcomes

1. Introduction and Epidemiology

- Adhesive capsulitis affects 2–5% of the general population [1].
- Affecting women more than men, often occurring between the ages of 40 to 60 years old.
- Incidence is also higher amongst diabetics as compared to the general population.
- About 20–30% of those affected will develop the condition in the opposite shoulder.

- Diabetics suffer from greater ROM restrictions and poorer treatment outcomes.
- Other systemic conditions such as obesity, thyroidal dysfunction, cardiac diseases, Dupuytren's contracture, breast cancer therapy have been described to be association with increased risk of developing adhesive capsulitis [2,3].

2. Clinical Presentation

- Patients usually first present with shoulder pain before developing loss of both active and passive range of motion joint.
- Shoulder pain is usually worse at extremes of motion due to tensioning of capsule.
- Adhesive capsulitis of the shoulder is characterised by a progressive painful loss of passive and active shoulder range of motion.
- Painful stiffness of the shoulder can adversely affect activities of daily living and consequently impair quality of life. 40% of patients experience persistent symptoms of more than 2 years and about 7–15% experience some degree of permanent functional loss [2].
- Most cases of adhesive capsulitis are primary (idiopathic cause), some may be secondary to extrinsic causes (disuse due to trauma, CVA) and others to intrinsic causes (cuff tendinosis and tears, biceps tendinosis) [3]. It is thus imperative to exclude these secondary causes before treating a patient as idiopathic primary adhesive capsulitis.

3. Pathophysiology of Problem

- Once described as "difficult to define, difficult to treat and difficult to explain from the point of view of pathology [4]."
- The principle pathology is excessive fibrosis and therefore contracture of the shoulder capsule resulting in stiffness, pain and dysfunction.
- About 20–30% of patients report history of trauma to shoulder but evidence of adhesive capsulitis as a post-traumatic (secondary) condition is not well proven.

It is postulated that development of adhesive capsulitis starts with an inflammatory process that eventually leads to fibrotic changes involving inflammatory and growth factors such as TGF-beta [5].
- The three phases of adhesive capsulitis are well known: freezing phase (up to 9 months) characterised by pain rather than stiffness, frozen phase (up to 12 months) in which the pain diminishes but stiffness is profound and the thawing phase (up to 36 months) when the stiffness seems to spontaneously resolve [6].

4. Diagnosis and Imaging

- Diagnosis of shoulder capsulitis is often clinical and by exclusion of secondary causes.
- Other causes such as rotator cuff pathologies, arthritis, infections or radicular pain should be investigated and considered prior.
- Imaging studies are often used for exclusion of other pathologies as opposed to confirmation of adhesive capsulitis.

5. Arthroscopic Surgery

5.1 *Indications for Surgery*

- Persistent pain and stiffness of 6 months duration or more
- Failed physiotherapy
- Stiffness affecting ADL despite physiotherapy and injections

5.2 *Positioning & Portals*

- Posterior portal
- Antero-superior portal

5.3 *Arthroscopic Capsular Release for Adhesive Capsulitis*

Conceptually the procedure consists of 6 steps:

(1) Clearing the rotator interval

Using a 90° RF wand or shaver inserted through the anterior portal, the **rotator interval** is first cleared. (The interval is bound superior-laterally by the biceps tendon, medially by the labrum and inferiorly by the subscapularis tendon.)

- Clear the fascia in the rotator interval. In normal shoulders this fascia is thin and is easily shaved off. In adhesive capsulitis however, this layer is thickened and more difficult. Use RF to ablate (Fig. 1).
- **Avoid** the biceps sling which is found at the lateral corner of the interval, hugging the biceps tendon as it plunges into the groove.
- **Avoid** the SGHL which runs along the biceps tendon. Clear the interval till the whitish conjoint tendon and muscle of the anterior deltoids are visible.

(2) Debriding and clearing the middle glenohumeral ligament (MGHL)

- Switch to hook RF wand, insert through the anterior portal. With the hook pointing towards the camera (remember to keep the tip of the hook in your sight!) use the shoulder of the hook as a knife to

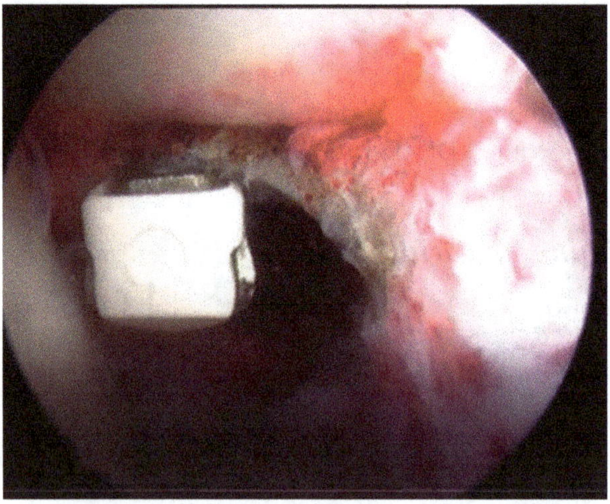

Fig. 1: Rotator Interval. In step 1, an RF wand is used to clear the thickened fascia in the rotator interval.

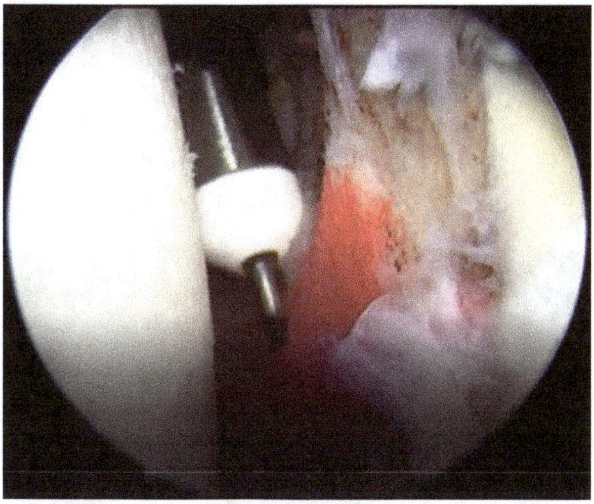

Fig. 2: MGHL. In step 2, a hook wand is used to incise the MGHL.

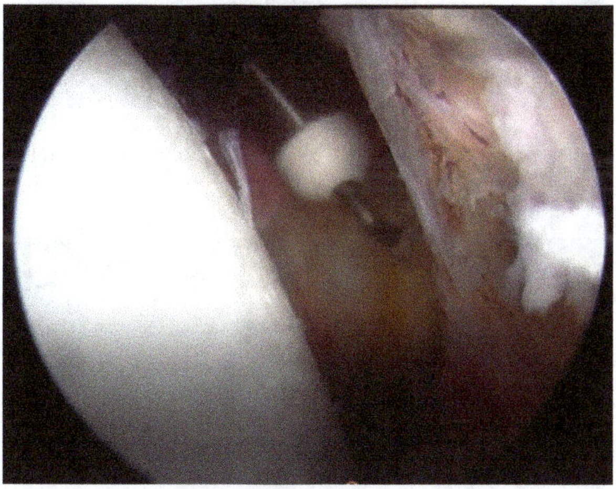

Fig. 3: Subscapularis. In step 3, the tendinous part of the upper subscapularis is released.

incise the MGHL, which is found running diagonally across the subscapularis.

- Completely divide the MGHL (Fig. 2). Use a shaver to debride the MGHL on both sides of the incision, to create a gap between 2–5 mm wide (Fig. 3). This will help to reduce chances of recurrence.

(3) Partial release of the Subscapularis

Use the hook to incise deeper, to ablate the capsule and tendinous portion of the subscapularis (Fig. 4), till the muscle layers are visible (Figs. 5 and 6).

The superior tendinous portion of the subscapularis is the more important portion, hence incise only the articular aspect of the tendon

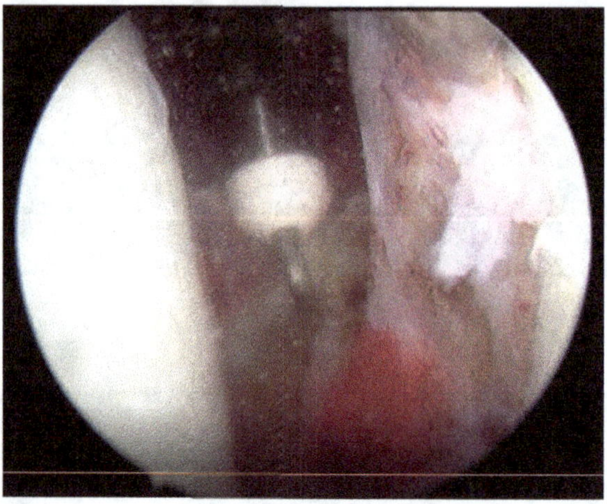

Fig. 4: Anterior Capsule. In step 4, this release is continued inferiorly to release the anterior capsule.

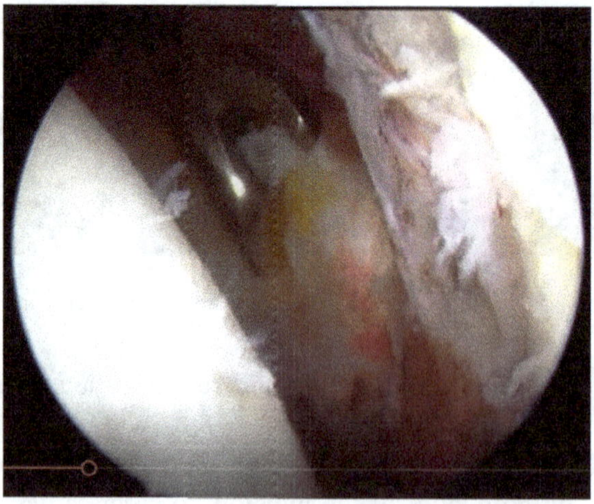

Fig. 5: Widening the release. An arthroscopic punch is used to debride the edges of the release, to widen the gap.

(about one-third of its thickness). This will not reduce the strength of the subscapularis.

Bring the arm to external rotation progressively, to assess the effectiveness of the release so far. This manoeuvre will also allow the surgeon to debride the plane between the glenoid and the subscapularis, just lateral to the labral edge.

This will improve the release and this plane is safe, the radial and musculocutaneous nerves being in the plane external to the subscapularis.

(4) Releasing the antero-inferior capsule

Use the hook RF wand to continue incising the anterior capsule just inferior to the MGHL, of which the border between the structures blend imperceptibly.

- Using the hook wand and keeping the tip visible, move the wand inferiorly millimetre by millimetre, progressively going deeper till there is a give, or if the muscle layers are visible. *Bring the arm to slight external rotation and to forward flexion, this will bring the antero-inferior capsule up towards the camera (in a beach chair*

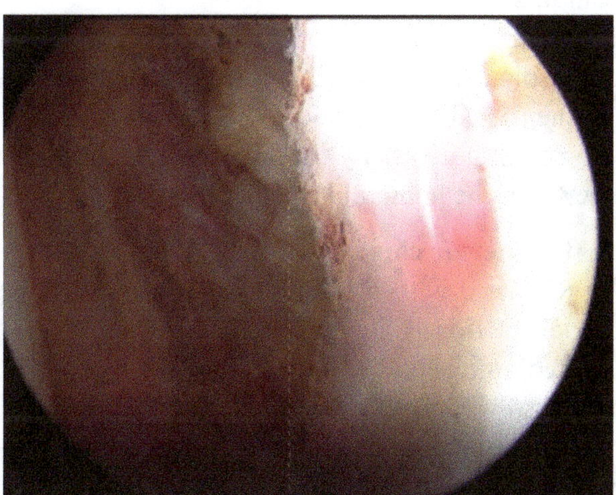

Fig. 6: Subscapularis. The fascia over the subscapularis is debrided till the muscle belly is seen.

position) and so enable easier access of the shaver or RF wand to the capsule.

- Work the wand inferiorly till about the 5–6 o'clock position (right shoulder), incising the peri-labral capsule about 1–2 mm just lateral to the labrum.
- *The camera is removed and a switching stick is then inserted in the trocar to maintain patency of the posterior portal. The trocar is then removed and inserted into the anterior portal. ROM can then be assessed: forward flexion, abduction, external rotation and internal rotation in abduction. Be mindful not to perform excessive MUA at this stage, as it can cause bleeding and the inferior capsule is not released yet.*

(5) Releasing the posterior capsule

- With the camera viewing from the anterior portal, the switching stick in the posterior portal is visible. Widen the skin incision of the posterior portal, then use the switching stick to bluntly widen the posterior portal and insert a large (8 mm) cannula.
- Use a shaver to debride the posterior capsule. Withdrawing the cannula so that it sits just at the aperture or opening of the portal would increase the manoeuvrability of the working instrument, the shaver in this case.
- Debride the posterior capsule till muscle is seen, from superiorly (the supraspinatus tendon) to the inferior capsule. A switching stick is then used to assess the drive-through sign (Fig. 7), the switching stick must easily traverse the glenohumeral joint in the plane between the humeral head and glenoid.

(6) Releasing the inferior capsule

- A hook RF wand is then inserted from the posterior portal and a slight axial traction is applied to the arm. The inferior capsule is then incised along the peri-labral line, just lateral to the inferior labrum (Fig. 8).
- In normal or lax shoulders, the inferior capsule falls away to create an inferior pouch. This pouch is obliterated in adhesive capsulitis, bringing the inferior capsule more accessible to the RF wand. *Bringing the arm to forward flexion also helps to pull the inferior capsule upwards.*

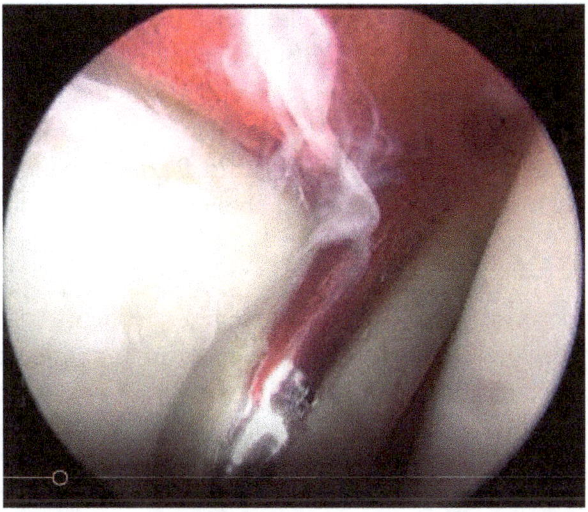

Fig. 7: Posterior capsule. A switching stick is inserted in the posterior portal, the posterior capsule is released as above.

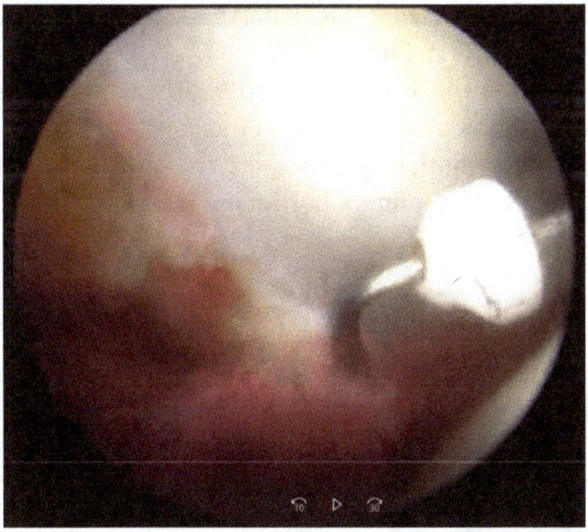

Fig. 8: Inferior capsule. A hook wand continues the release from posterior capsule to the inferior capsule.

- With the tip of the hook visible, incise the inferior capsule slowly, from posterior to anterior till the capsule is completely released. The camera can then be removed, and a switching stick inserted in the posterior portal.
- Assess the range of motion: forward flexion, abduction, external rotation and internal rotation in abduction. Any residual bands are released by a directed and limited MUA doing this ROM manoeuvre.
- A single dose of 20 mL of Marcaine & Shincort is then injected into the glenohumeral joint to reduce inflammation and prevent recurrence of adhesions.

6. Post-operative Management and Rehabilitation

- Fine balance is required between immobilisation to allow for healing of surgical wound versus early rehabilitation to prevent arthrofibrosis.
- Post-operative pain management is crucial to allow for comfortable engagement in physical therapy.
- As with the described technique, intra-articular marcaine provides significant and much required pain relief.
- Passive range of motion exercises are initiated once pain control is achieved so as to minimise post-operative capsular adhesions and improve range of motion.

7. Outcomes

In our cohort, all patients (diabetics and non-diabetics) undergoing arthroscopic capsular demonstrate significant improvements in range of motion, pain and shoulder function scores [7]. Our patients demonstrated about 40° improvement in forward flexion and abduction planes.

Patients also demonstrate and approximately four levels of improvements in the active function composite scores for measure of internal and external rotation. Although achieving significant improvement as compared to preoperatively, diabetic patients achieved poorer internal rotation and forward flexion as compared to their non diabetic counterparts [7].

References

1. Tighe CB, Oakley WS. Jr. The prevalence of a diabetic condition and adhesive capsulitis of the shoulder. *South Med J* 2008;101(6):591–595. doi:10.1097/smj.0b013e3181705d39. PMID: 18475240.
2. Robinson CM, Seah KT, Chee YH, *et al*. Frozen shoulder. *J Bone Joint Surg* 2012;94:1–9. https://doi.org/10.1302/0301-620X.94B1.27093.
3. Gregory P. Nicholson. Arthroscopic capsular release for stiff shoulders, Arthroscopy. *J Arthroscop Related Surg* 2003;19(1):40–49. https://doi.org/10.1053/jars.2003.50010.
4. Codman EA. *The Shoulder: Rupture of the Supraspinatus Tendon and Other Lesions in or About the Subacromial Bursa*. T Todd Company, Boston MA, 1934.
5. Le HV, Lee SJ, Nazarian A, Rodriguez EK. Adhesive capsulitis of the shoulder: Review of pathophysiology and current clinical treatments. *Shoulder Elbow* 2017 Apr;9(2):75–84. doi: 10.1177/1758573216676786.
6. Grey RG. The natural history of "idiopathic" frozen shoulder. *J Bone Joint Surg Am* 1978;60:564.
7. Geraldine Lei Yanlei, Mak Wai Keong, Denny Lie Tijauw Tjoen. Do diabetic patients have different outcomes after arthroscopic capsular release for frozen shoulder? *J Orthop* 2019;16(3). https://doi.org/10.1016/j.jor.2019.02.003.

https://doi.org/10.1142/9789811249846_0006

Chapter 6

Arthroscopic Labral Repair and Capsular Shift — The Hybrid Technique Using Modified Mason-Allen Suture Configuration

Denny T.T. Lie and Lai Mun Chun

Summary of Chapter

1. Introduction and epidemiology of shoulder instability
2. Clinical presentation of the unstable shoulder
3. Pathophysiology of shoulder instability
4. Diagnosis & Imaging
5. Surgical technique of the arthroscopic labral repair using the hybrid suture technique
6. Rehabilitation
7. Clinical outcomes

1. Introduction and Epidemiology of Shoulder Instability

Shoulder dislocations are one of the common shoulder injuries encountered by the orthopaedic surgeon. The reported incidence for first time-time shoulder dislocation is approximately 8.0–8.2 per 100,000 people per year and the prevalence is around 2%. Anterior shoulder dislocations make up 96–98% of all shoulder dislocations [1]. The recurrence episode depends on the patient's age during the first episode and the reported risk of re-dislocation is approximately 80%, especially in male patient younger than 20 years. Therefore, surgical treatment is usually recommended compared to conservative management, in view of the high recurrence rate [2,3].

2. Clinical Presentation and Examination of the Unstable Shoulder

Clinical history and physical examination are crucial in the diagnosis of shoulder dislocation. Patients with shoulder dislocation may describe a popping sensation, sudden onset of pain with limited range of motion or the sensation of joint rolling out of the socket, after a single traumatic event. Meanwhile, patients with recurrent shoulder dislocations may describe multiple previous dislocations or apprehension when performing overhead activities. Additional information with regards to the mechanism of injury, number of recurrences, and whether patient required reduction in the emergency room should be documented as well. It is also important to find out the level of activity that caused the instability episode. For instance, did the dislocation happen in extreme positions of abduction and external rotation or did it occur during activities of daily living? This may provide information with regards to the severity of the soft tissue or bony injury of the shoulder. Lastly, clinicians should assess for any numbness or weakness of the dislocated shoulder, which may indicate nerve injury [4].

The shoulder should be inspected from the front, side and back. We should look for any asymmetry, muscle wasting of the shoulders, winging of the scapula and scars from previous injuries or surgeries. A patient with anterior dislocation usually presents with a "squared off" shoulder due to loss of deltoid muscle contour compared with contralateral site. The arm is classically held in slight abduction and external rotation. After inspection, clinicians should palpate the bony prominence and look for any tenderness at area such as acromioclavicular (AC) joint, sternoclavicular (SC) joint, acromion, spine of the scapula, biceps tendon and greater tuberosity.

The active and passive range of motion of the shoulder should then be assessed. The planes of motions include forward flexion, extension, abduction, internal and external rotation at the side, and internal and external rotation in abduction. The patient with dislocated shoulder usually has limited range of motion or may resist any attempt to move the shoulder.

There are several provocative exam manoeuvres described to detect instability in shoulder dislocation (see Chapter 1). The **sulcus sign** is one of the common manoeuvres performed. The patient is positioned upright with arms at their side. The examiner will stabilize the shoulder and apply downward traction on the elbow. If a dimple is seen at the lateral edge of the acromion, then the test is considered positive.

For **load and shift test**, the patient is seated or lies supine with shoulder abducted at 40–60° and elbow flexed at 90°. The examiner will load the humerus axially into the glenoid fossa and apply anterior and posterior translation forces. The test is considered positive when there is increase translation compared to the contralateral side.

The **apprehension test** performed by abducting the arm to 90° and full external rotation. A positive finding is when patient experiences the sensation of instability. The examiner can perform a **relocation test** after the apprehension test. This test is performed by applying posterior directed force on the humeral head. Resolution of guarding and apprehension is considered a positive relocation test.

3. Pathophysiology of Shoulder Instability

The **static stabilisers** consist of the congruency of the humeral head and glenoid, the glenoid labrum, negative intraarticular pressure and the glenohumeral ligaments. The glenohumeral ligaments comprise the superior glenohumeral ligament (SGHL), the middle glenohumeral ligament (MGHL) and the inferior glenohumeral ligament (IGHL). The **dynamic stabilisers** include the rotator cuff muscles which produce a stabilising effect by compressing the humeral head against the glenoid. The tendon of the long head of the biceps, and periscapular muscles are also part of the dynamic stabilisers. Any disruption in the static and dynamic structures can lead to dislocation, or recurrent instability [5].

The mechanism of injury is usually a fall on the outstretched arm, with the shoulder abducted and externally rotated. In this position, the IGHL is the primary restraint to anterior translation of the humeral head. Injury to the anterior band of IGHL and anteroinferior labrum results in a Bankart lesion. The bony Bankart lesion is seen if there is an avulsion fracture of the anteroinferior glenoid, which is the insertion for IGHL. A Hill-Sachs lesion can be seen due to impaction of the posterior humerus head against the glenoid rim. A study by Owen *et al.* on patients with a first-time anterior shoulder dislocation showed that 96% of the patients had a Bankart lesion and 92.5% had a Hill-Sachs lesion [6].

4. Diagnosis and Imaging

Plain radiographs with anteroposterior (AP), scapula Y and axillary views are first line radiologic studies for patients with anterior shoulder dislocation. A Valpeau view can be obtained if the patient is unable to do an axillary view due to acute pain. In acute anterior shoulder dislocation, the humeral head is dislocated anteriorly and rests under the coracoid process on AP view (Fig. 1). On scapula view, the humeral head is displaced anterior to the scapula (Fig. 2). On axillary view, the humeral head is displaced anteriorly in front of the coracoid process. A Hill-Sachs lesions are best

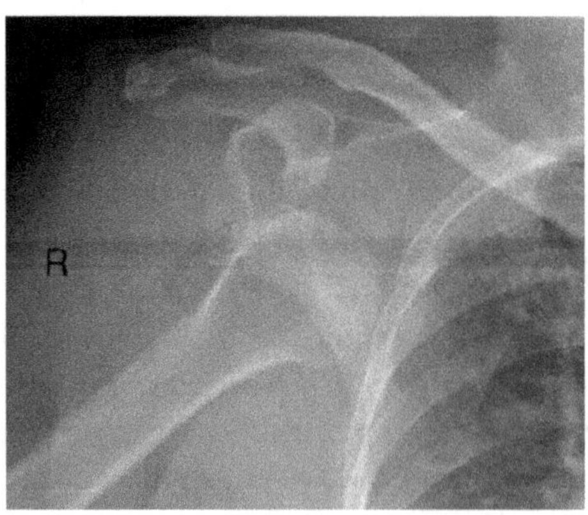

Fig. 1: AP Xray of the shoulder showing antero-inferior dislocation of the humeral head.

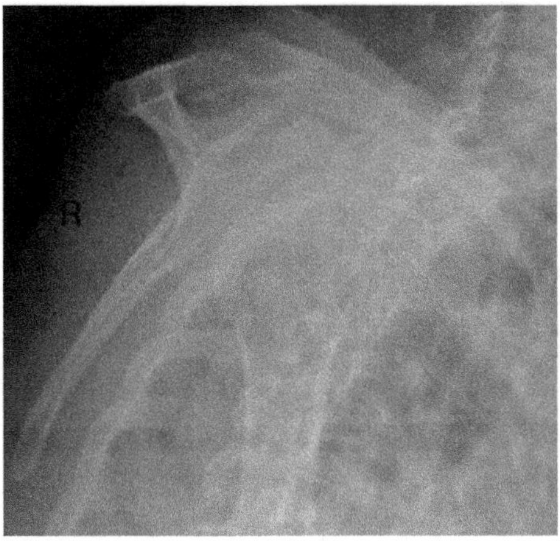

Fig. 2: Y-scapula view of the shoulder showing the dislocated humeral head.

view on the AP radiographs in internal rotation and Stryker notch views. The Stryker view is taken with the patient in supine position and arm forward flexed to 100° with the X-ray beam centered over the coracoid and tilted 10° cephalad [7].

Recurrent dislocations can lead to erosion of the glenoid rim. Loss of 20% of the glenoid rim is biomechanically highly unstable and usually require bony procedures, together with soft tissue stabilisation [8]. This defect may be seen on the axillary view and may be suggested by a break in the sclerotic line encircling the glenoid rim on the AP view of the shoulder (Fig. 3). Additional views such as the West Point view can be considered if further investigation is required. The West Pont view is done with patient lying prone, and shoulder abducted at 90° and the elbow flexed 90° and forearm off the table. The X-ray beam is directed at 25° medial and 25° caudal [9].

Advanced imaging modalities such as computed tomography (CT) and magnetic resonance imaging (MRI) are useful when the diagnosis is uncertain. Computed tomography is useful to evaluate glenoid bone loss or fractures, glenoid version and humeral head abnormalities [4]. MRI is used to evaluate soft tissue injuries or bony contusion. MR arthrograms have shown to have greater sensitivity in detecting soft tissue pathology such as labral tears and capsular damage in chronic cases (Figs. 4–6). Soft

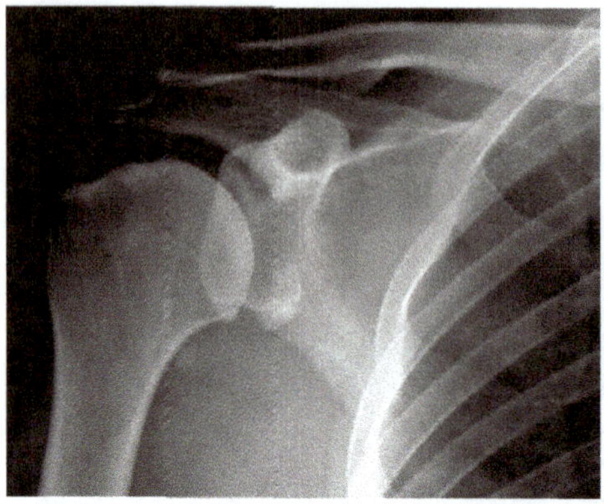

Fig. 3: Xray showing bony Bankart of the anterior glenoid.

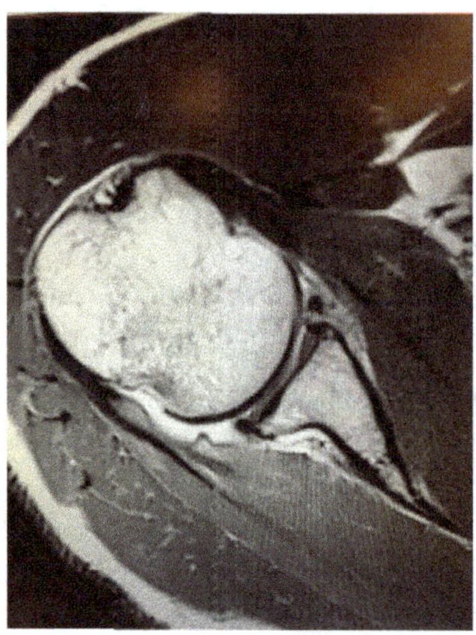

Fig. 4: T1-weighted MRI of the shoulder showing torn anteror labrum and Hill-Sachs lesion on the posterior humeral head.

tissue injuries such as anterior periostial sleeve avulsion (ALPSA) or a humeral avulsion of glenohumeral ligament (HAGL) can also be detected by MRI and MR arthrogram. These lesions are associated with higher recurrence rates if undetected and can lead to higher post-surgical failure [10,11].

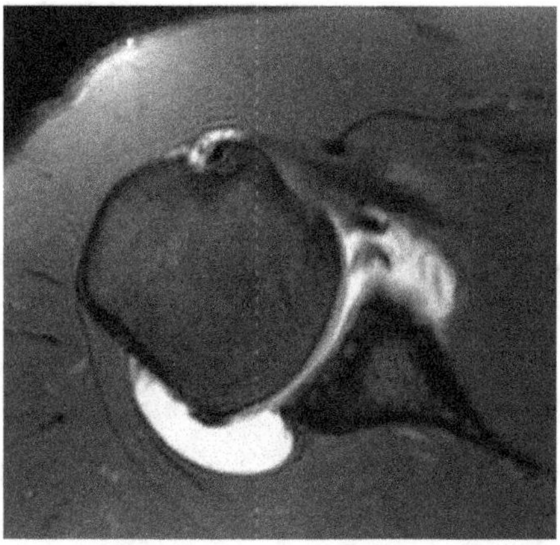

Fig. 5: T2 weighted MRI showing torn anterior labrum.

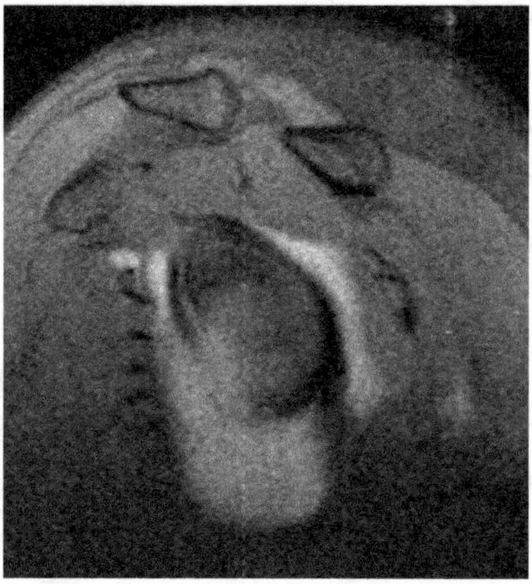

Fig. 6: MRI of the shoulder sagittal view showing torn anterior labrum with large patolous anterior capsule.

5. Arthroscopic Surgery

5.1 *Indications for Surgery*

- Patient with first time dislocation with confirmed Bankart lesion on MRI and younger than 25 years of age (higher recurrence rate 90% in this age group if treated conservatively).

- Recurrent dislocation.
- High demand athletes.

5.2 *Positioning and Portals*

Position: Beach chair.

Portals:

Posterior portal: Standard portal for viewing.

Antero-superior portal: This portal is surface marked just lateral to the tip of the coracoid and will enter the joint high, between the biceps and superior labrum. Useful for suture management. A 5.5 mm cannula is inserted.

Antero-inferior portal: This portal lies inferior and lateral to the antero-superior portal, it enters the joint space at the lateral corner of the rotator interval. The trajectory of this portal is about 45°oblique in 2 planes; superior to inferior, lateral to medial, and must be able to access the lower most anchor position, at about 5:30 o'clock position. An 8.5 mm cannula is used here.

5.3 *Arthroscopic Labral Repair and Capsular Shift (the Hybrid Technique Using Modified Mason-Allen Suture Configuration)*

(a) **Mobilising the labrum**

- Transfer the camera to the antero-superior portal which provides a good view of the anterior labrum. Inspect the entire labrum from the superior, anterior and down to the inferior pouch. Check for HAGL (humeral avulsions of gleno-humeral ligaments) lesions.
- A liberator from the antero-inferior portal can be used to free the labrum. The torn labrum is partially healed in a recessed position behind the glenoid surface, and is thus an ineffective stabiliser. Completely liberate the labrum till the normal attachments;

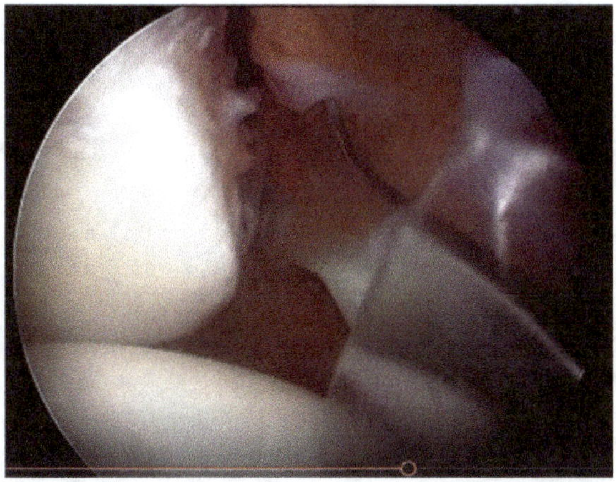

Fig. 7: A liberator is used to free the labrum and capsule, viewed from the anterosuperior portal.

superiorly till about the 1 o'clock position (unless there is a SLAP tear) and inferiorly, to about 5 o'clock position (Fig. 7). Ensure that the labrum can be freely mobilised to the edge or onto the glenoid surface.

(b) **The lower most anchor (5:30 o'clock position)**

- The camera is then transferred back to the posterior portal. A dual-loaded anchor (5 mm Gryphon BR anchor) is inserted from the antero-inferior portal (Fig. 8). Remember the direction of the anchor as it is inserted; 45° oblique superior to inferior, lateral to medial, pointing slightly posteriorly.
- Retrieve three of the four suture limbs to the antero-superior portal, both limbs from suture (A) and one limb from suture (B).

(c) **Hybrid suture configuration**

- A grasper from the antero-superior portal is used to tent up the antero-inferior labrum and anterior IGHL. A suture passer (70° straight Acupass) from the antero-inferior portal is used to take a deep bite of the labrum and IGHL, as low as possible (Fig. 9). This is the **first bite** and it will shift the inferior capsule superiorly. Often the bite may need to be taken in parts, IGHL first then the labrum. Keep the arm in the neutral rotation position, to

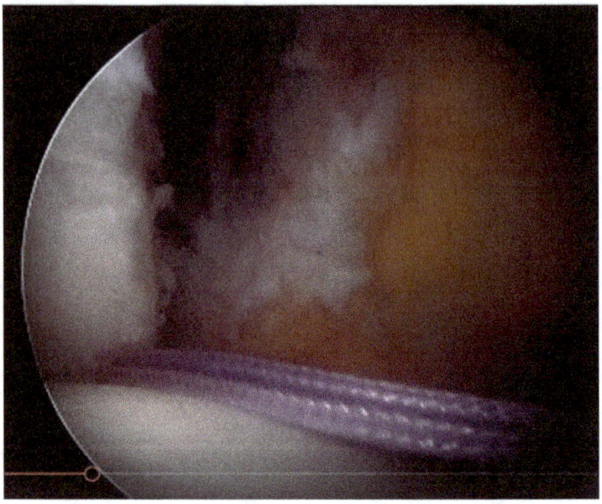

Fig. 8: The lowest 5–6 o'clock anchor is inserted.

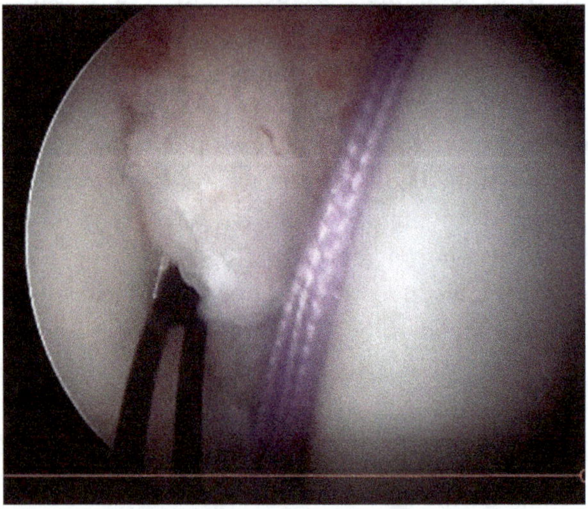

Fig. 9: A large first bite of the labrum and capsule is taken to pass a filament, to shuttle the suture.

achieve adequate tension without over-tensioning the shift. A suture limb from suture (A) is then shuttled (Fig. 10).

- Still tenting the labrum superiorly, the **second bite** is taken, incorporating the labrum, anterior IGHL and capsule (Figs. 11 and 12).

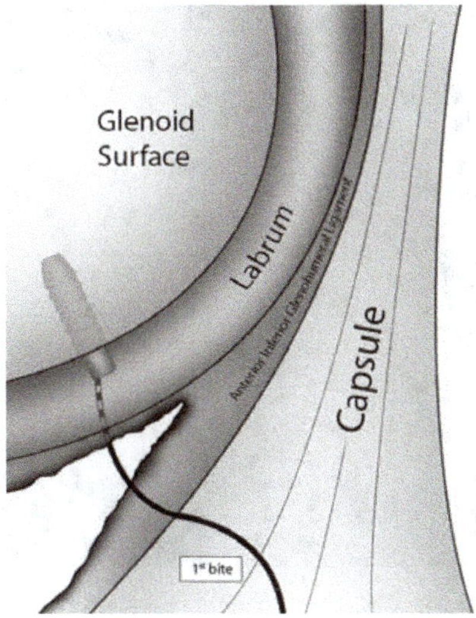

Fig. 10: Diagram of the 1st bite.

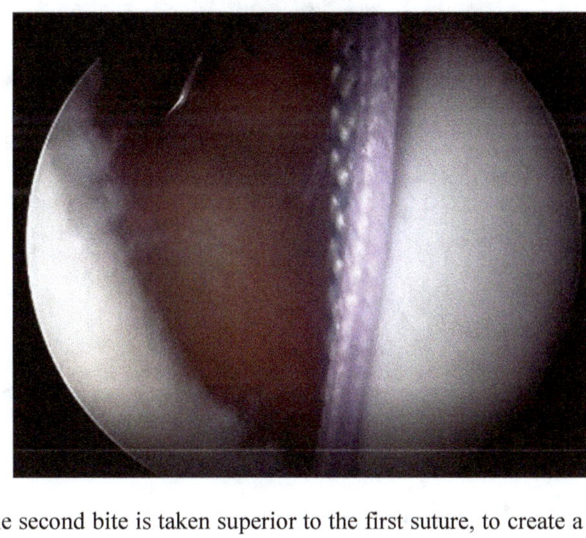

Fig. 11: The second bite is taken superior to the first suture, to create a mattress stitch.

This bite is taken about 10–15 mm above (superior to) the first bite, but because it incorporates capsule, it lies in a different tissue plane. This reduces the risk of the sutures cutting out. The second limb from suture (A) is then retrieved (Fig. 13).

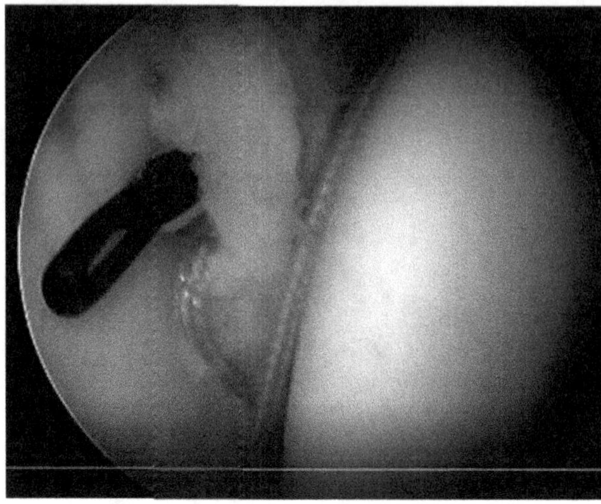

Fig. 12: The second pass similarly takes a large bite of the labrum and capsule.

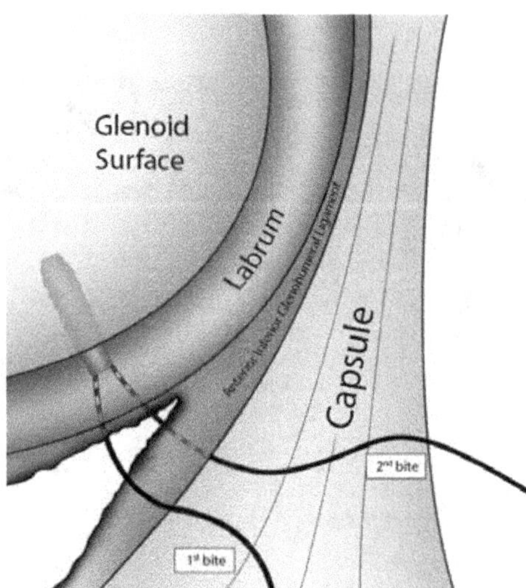

Fig. 13: Diagram showing the 2nd bite.

- The **third bite** is taken roughly perpendicular to a line drawn between the first two suture bites, and like the second bite, incorporates labrum, IGHL and some capsule (Fig. 14). A suture limb from suture (B) is retrieved (Fig. 15). *(The remaining suture limb from suture (B) is from the anchor).*

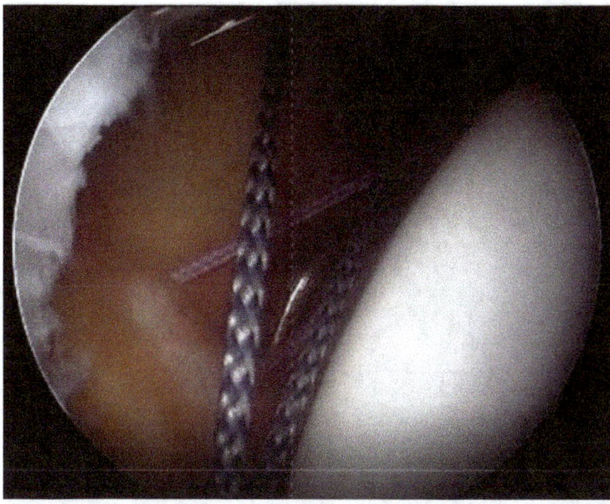

Fig. 14: The third bite begins between the first 2 sutures.

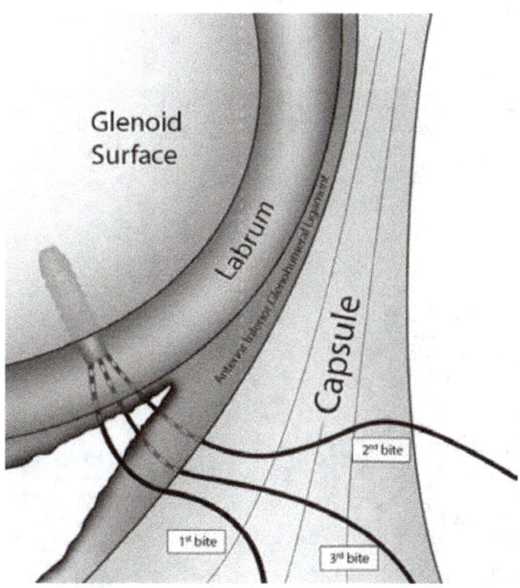

Fig. 15: Diagram showing the 3rd bite.

- Both limbs of suture (A), parked in the antero-superior portal (Figs. 16 and 17), are then tied first, to create the **horizontal mattress stitch** (Fig. 18). It will create a large bumper.
- Suture limbs from suture (B), (one from the third bite and the other from the anchor) are then tied to create a **simple stitch**, perpendicular to and over the mattress stitch.

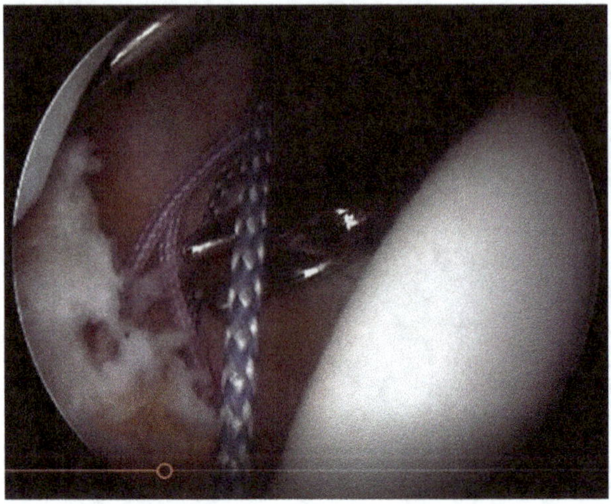

Fig. 16: The shuttled suture from the third bite is retrieved behind the mattress stitch formed by the first 2 sutures.

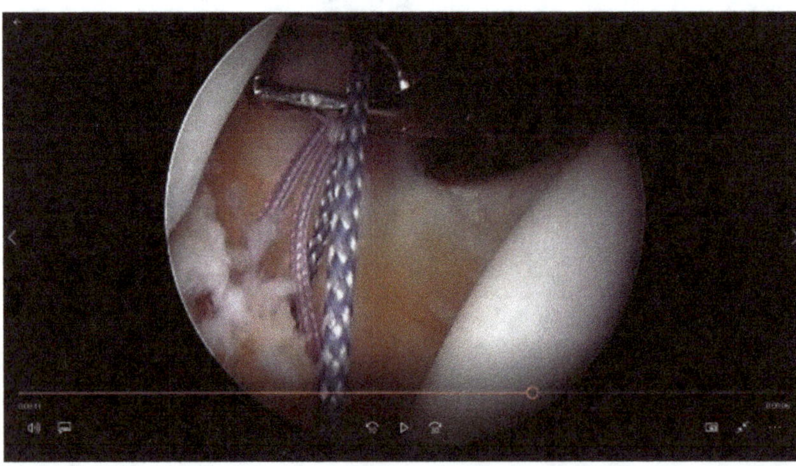

Fig. 17: The combination of the simple stitch formed by the blue suture and the mattress stitch (purple sutures) creates a hybrid pattern, forming a Mason Allen-like pattern.

This combined configuration of horizontal mattress and simple stitches (hence called hybrid) effectively creates a modified Mason-Allen suture configuration (Figs. 20 and 21).

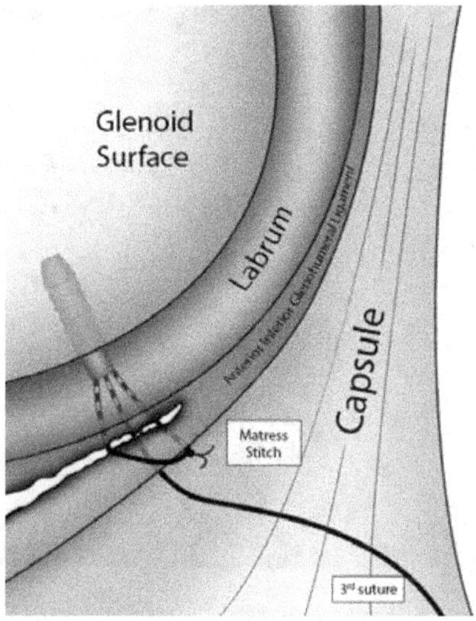

Fig. 18: Diagram showing the mattress stitch created by tying the first 2 sutures.

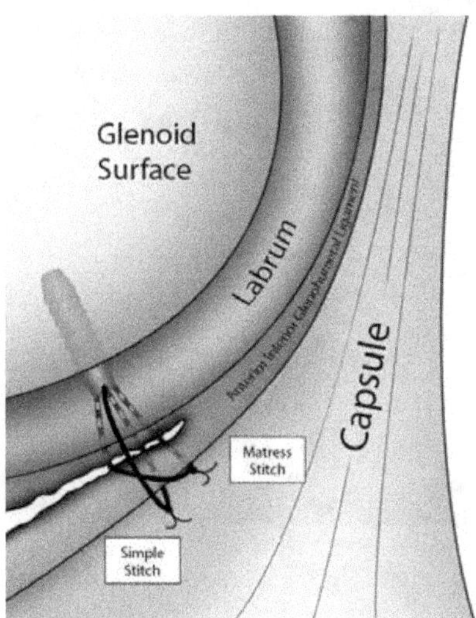

Fig. 19: Diagram showing the third suture tied as a simple stitch over the mattress stitch

(d) The middle anchor (4 o'clock position)

- A second anchor (5 mm dual-loaded Gryphon BR anchor) is inserted at roughly the 4 o'clock position, about 7–10 mm

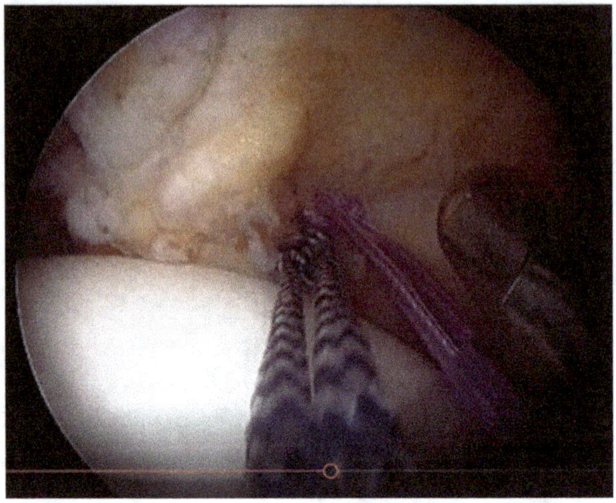

Fig. 20: View of the hybrid suturing from the anterosuperior portal.

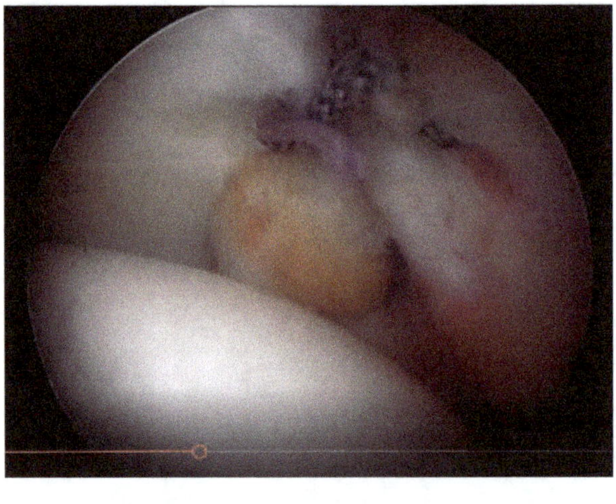

Fig. 21: View of the anteroinferior labrum, seen from posterior portal.

superior to the lowest anchor. One limb from both sutures (A) and (B) are then retrieved (Fig. 22).

- A suture passer from the antero-inferior portal is used to bite the labrum and a sliver of capsule (avoid biting the MGHL), one bite below the anchor and another, above the anchor. Pass one suture limb from each of the sutures, tie simple stitches above and below the anchor, to stabilise the labrum (Figs. 23 and 24).

(e) **The upper anchor (3 o'clock position)**

- A third anchor, if needed, can be deployed at the 2–3 o'clock position. A single-loaded anchor (Gryphon BR anchor or Gryphon Pro-knot) is adequate.

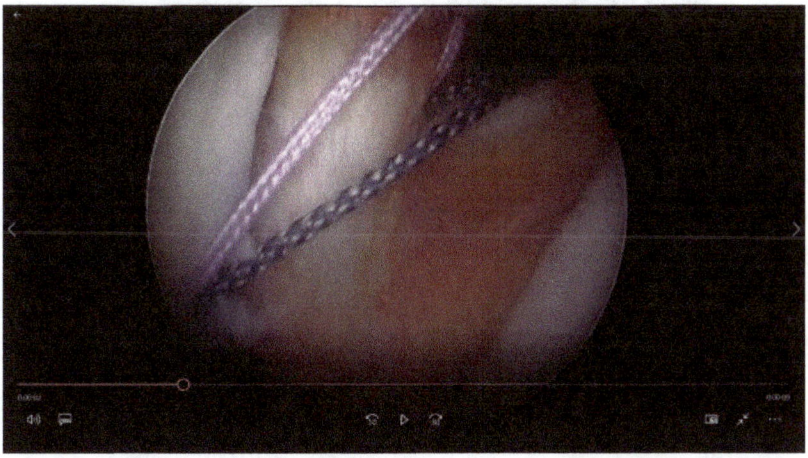

Fig. 22: The middle 4 o'clock anchor is placed and sutures shuttled to create 2 simple stitch patterns.

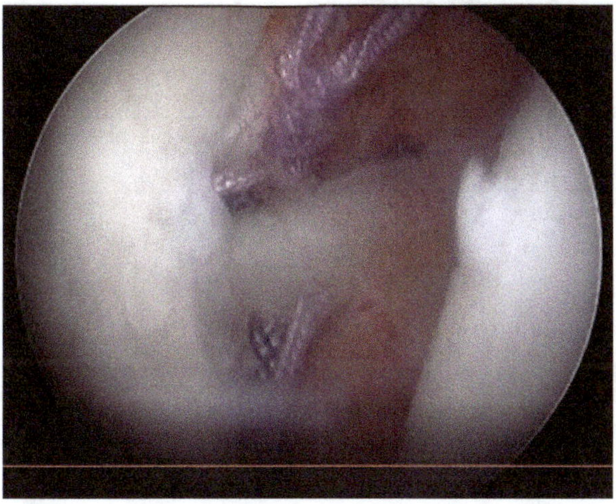

Fig. 23: View of the labrum after tying the sutures from the middle anchor.

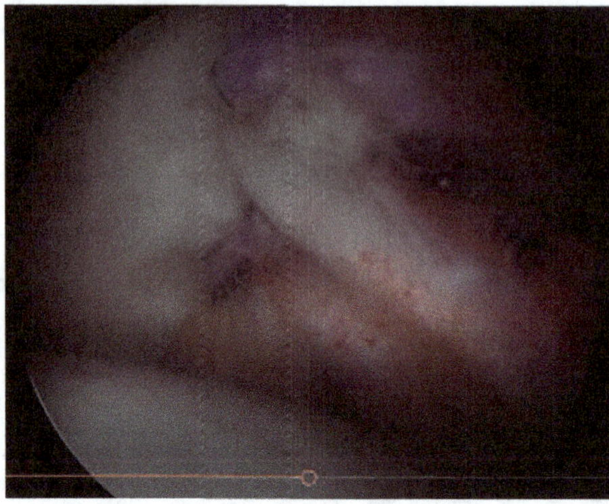

Fig. 24: View from the anterosuperior portal showing the labrum re-attached along with a significant capsular shift to re-create the anterior wall.

	Labrum	IGHL	Capsule	
1st				Simple conventional repair
2nd				Mattress stitch
3rd				Simple suture perpendicular to mattress suture, Mason Allen like
4th				Capsule envelopes repair

Fig. 25: Concept of the hybrid suture pattern.

- It is adequate to take a bite of the labrum only, without any capsule, and securing it with a simple stitch.

This hybrid suturing technique creates a modified Mason-Allen configuration and respects the anatomy of the glenohumeral joint, taking bites of the labrum, IGHL and capsule sequentially. This is summarised in Fig. 25.

6. Post-op Management and Rehabilitation

After the arthroscopic Bankart repair, patients routinely will be on arm sling for 6 weeks. The early rehabilitation exercise encourages neck exercises with freedom of motion of the elbow and wrists, while the shoulder continues to be immobilised for the first three weeks. Limited pendular exercises are then permitted in the second three weeks. Full shoulder mobilisation can be started after six weeks. In general, the focus of the first 3 months is restoration of motion. Strength training is started only after that and may continue up to 6 months. Resumption of overhead sports is usually encouraged after 6 months post-surgery.

7. Clinical Outcomes

There are two studies that have reported the functional outcomes of the hybrid technique. In 2013, Lee *et al.* published a case series consist of 76 arthroscopic Bankart repairs using the hybrid suture technique. At two years follow up, most of the patients reported the strength of the supraspinatus and the range of motion were either maintained or restored. There were 6 reported recurrence of dislocation after surgery, of which five shoulders required revision surgeries, representing a recurrence rate of about 7.8% [12].

The second study is a comparative study which assessed the clinical outcomes of hybrid suture technique versus simple suture technique. This study demonstrated the hybrid sutures technique showed superior improvement in Constant Shoulder Score, UCLA shoulder score and Oxford Instability score compared to simple suture group at 3 months follow up. The postoperative recurrence rate was comparable between both groups (hybrid suture group 7.81% vs simple suture group 7.84%) [13].

References

1. Kirkley A, Werstine R, Ratjek A, Griffin S. Prospective randomized clinical trial comparing the effectiveness of immediate arthroscopic stabilization versus immobilization and rehabilitation in first traumatic anterior dislocations of the shoulder: Long-term evaluation. *Arthroscopy* [Internet]. 2005;21(1):55–63. Available from: https://doi.org/10.1016/j.arthro.2004.09.018.

2. Jakobsen BW, Johannsen HV, Suder P, Søjbjerg JO. Primary repair versus conservative treatment of first-time traumatic anterior dislocation of the shoulder: A randomized study with 10-year follow-up. *Arthroscopy* 2007;23(2):118–123.
3. Rowe CR, Patel D, Southmayd WW. The Bankart procedure: A long-term end-result study. *JBJS* [Internet]. 1978;60(1). Available from: https://journals.lww.com/jbjsjournal/Fulltext/1978/60010/The_Bankart_procedure__a_long_term_end_result.1.aspx.
4. Gil JA, DeFroda S, Owens BD. Current concepts in the diagnosis and management of traumatic, anterior glenohumeral subluxations. *Orthop J Sport Med.* 2017;5(3):1–6.
5. Lippitt S, Matsen F. Mechanisms of glenohumeral joint stability. *Clin Orthop Relat Res* 1993;20–28.
6. Owens BD, Nelson BJ, Duffey ML, Mountcastle SB, Taylor DC, Cameron KL, *et al.* Pathoanatomy of first-time, traumatic, anterior glenohumeral subluxation events. *J Bone Jt Surg Am* 2010;92(7):1605–1611.
7. Pavlov H, Warren RF, Weiss CB, Dines DM. The roentgenographic evaluation of anterior shoulder instability. *Clin Orthop Relat Res* 1985; 194(2):153–158.
8. Itoi E, Lee SB, Berglund LJ, Berge LL, An KN. The effect of a glenoid defect on anteroinferior stability of the shoulder after Bankart repair: A cadaveric study. *J Bone Jt Surg Am* 2000;82(1):35–46.
9. Rokous JR, Feagin JA, Abbott HG. Modified axillary roentgenogram. A useful adjunct in the diagnosis of recurrent instability of the shoulder. *Clin Orthop Relat Res* 1972;82:84–86.
10. Ozbaydar M, Elhassan B, Diller D, Massimini D, Higgins LD, Warner JJP. Results of arthroscopic capsulolabral repair: Bankart lesion versus anterior labroligamentous periosteal sleeve avulsion lesion. *Arthroscopy* 2008;24(11):1277–1283.
11. Kim DS, Yoon YS, Chang Ho Yi. Prevalence comparison of accompanying lesions between primary and recurrent anterior dislocation in the shoulder. *Am J Sports Med* 2010;38(10):2071–2076.
12. Lee KH, Soeharno H, Chew CP, Lie D. Arthroscopic bankart repair augmented by placation of the inferior glenohumeral ligament via horizontal mattress suturing for traumatic shoulder instability. *Singapore Med J* 2013;54(10):555–559.
13. Lai MC, Ang FHB, Lee KH, Chang CCP, Lie TTD. Hybrid suture technique vs simple suture technique for antero-inferior labral tears: Two years' clinical outcomes. *Asia-Pacific J Sport Med Arthrosc Rehabil Technol* 2019;18:6–10. Available from: https://doi.org/10.1016/j.asmart.2019.08.002.

https://doi.org/10.1142/9789811249846_0007

Chapter 7

Approach to Glenoid Bone Loss Arthroscopic Remplissage Procedure Using TransTend Anchor System

Andrew Chou and Denny T.T. Lie

Summary of Chapter

1. Introduction and epidemiology of glenoid bone loss
2. Clinical presentation of the unstable shoulder
3. Pathophysiology of glenoid bone loss, glenoid tracking
4. Diagnosis and Imaging
5. Surgical technique of the arthroscopic Remplissage procedure
6. Rehabilitation
7. Clinical outcomes

1. Introduction and Epidemiology

Although the soft tissue (e.g. glenoid labrum, glenohumeral ligaments) is most frequently injured in shoulder dislocations, glenohumeral bone loss is also commonly found in patients with recurrent shoulder instability [1]. In fact, Hill-Sachs lesions (HSLs), a posterolateral bony defect of the humerus, are found in up to 51% of patients on plain radiographs and up to 90% of patients on diagnostic arthroscopy [2,3]. Similarly, glenoid bone loss (GBL) is found in up to 78.8% of patients after a dislocation event [4]. However, as both glenoid and humeral bone loss contribute to glenohumeral articulation and GBL increases the risk of an HSL dislocating, both articular surfaces need to be considered when predicting risk of dislocation [1]. Bipolar bone loss of the shoulder, defined by concurrent glenoid and humeral bone loss, is found in up to 84% of patients with chronic shoulder instability [5]. However, despite anatomical studies indicating significant differences in shoulder morphology for Asian populations, which has had clinical impact on shoulder arthroplasty design, no studies to date have studied the incidence of bipolar bone loss in Asian populations [6,7].

As the arthroscopic Bankart repair, a soft tissue reconstructive procedure, is typically first line treatment for anterior shoulder instability, glenohumeral bone loss is usually overlooked in initial surgical management [1]. However, growing evidence suggest that bipolar bone loss is strongly correlated to post-Bankart repair recurrent instability and should be addressed early [1,3]. Failure to address an engaging HSL not only increases risk of post-operative instability, but may also further aggravate bone loss and likely will worsen symptoms [1,8].

2. Pathophysiology of Glenoid Bone Loss

Bipolar bone loss is thought to contribute to post-Bankart repair instability due to a deficit in the articular arc of the glenohumeral joint [3]. HSLs increase the risk of an indented humeral surface of dislocation, while GBL results in reductions in the glenoid surface with greater propensity for engaging the HSL. Previous biomechanical studies indicate that HSLs with monopolar humeral bone loss of 20–37.5% result in risk of dislocation [9–11]. While initial cadaveric studies suggested a GBL threshold of 20–25%, recent literature have shown that as little as 13.5% of GBL can result in poor outcomes after Bankart repair [11–14].

To better predict which HSLs are at risk of dislocation, Itoi *et al.* introduced the concept of the glenoid track (GT), which is the area of the posterior humeral articular surface in contact with the glenoid when the arm moves along the posterior end-range of motion [8,15]. Using measurements from a diagnostic arthroscopy or 3D CT scan, Itoi defined the width of glenoid track by multiplying the diameter of the inferior glenoid by 0.83 and subtracting the width of the anterior glenoid bone loss, as shown in Fig. 1. The Hill-Sachs interval (HSI) was calculated as the sum of the width of the Hill-Sach lesion and the width of the bone bridge between the rotator cuff attachments and the lateral aspects of the Hill-Sachs lesion, as shown in Fig. 1 [8]. If HSI < GT, then an HSL remains contained within the margins of the GT and it is considered an "on track" lesion and not a risk of dislocation, as shown in Fig. 2 [8]. Conversely, if HSI > GT, then it is considered an "off track" lesion and at risk of dislocation, as shown in Fig. 3 [8].

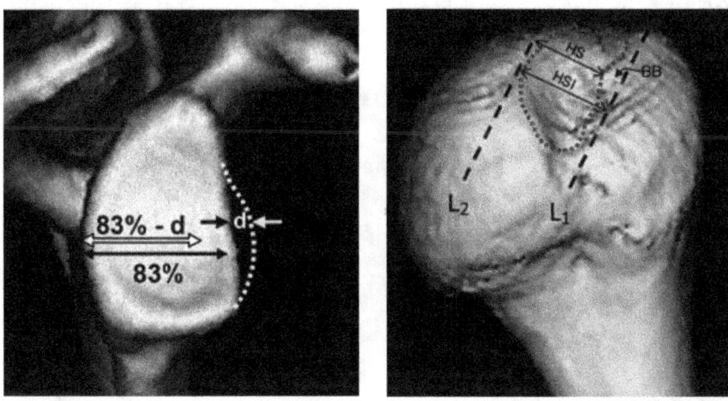

Fig. 1: Quantifying the GT and HSL. Using measurements from either a 3D CT scan or diagnostic arthroscopy, the GT and HSI can be calculated. If HSI < GT, then the lesion is "on track" and not at risk of dislocation. If HSI > GT, then the lesion is "off track" and at risk of dislocation.

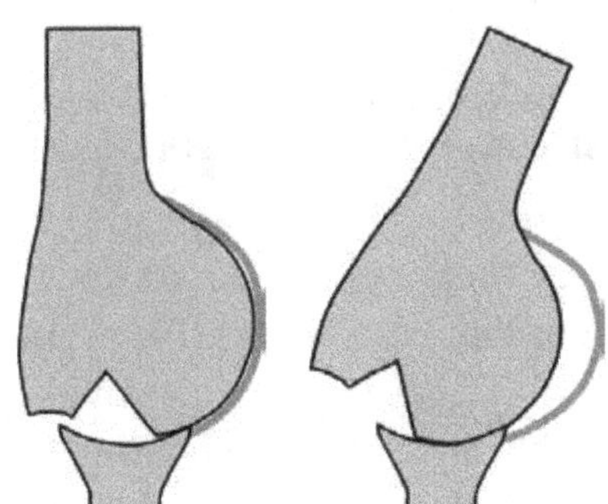

Fig. 2: "On track" lesion. If HSI < GT, then an HSL remains within the margins of the glenoid track, it is considered at low risk of dislocation.

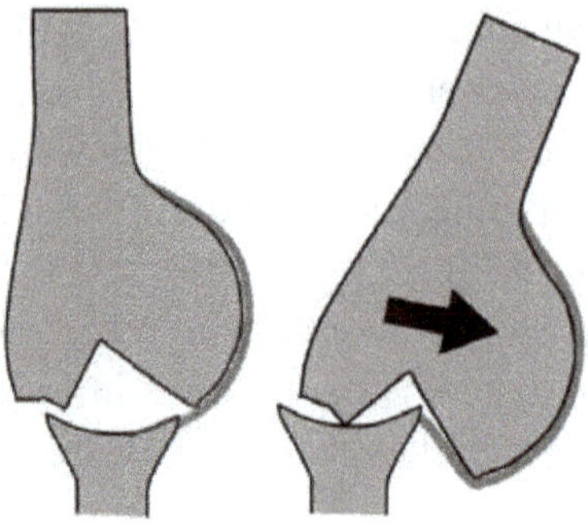

Fig. 3: 'Off-track' lesion. If HSI > GT, then the size of an HSL is sufficiently large or the glenoid bone loss has reduced the glenoid track sufficiently, it is considered at risk of dislocation.

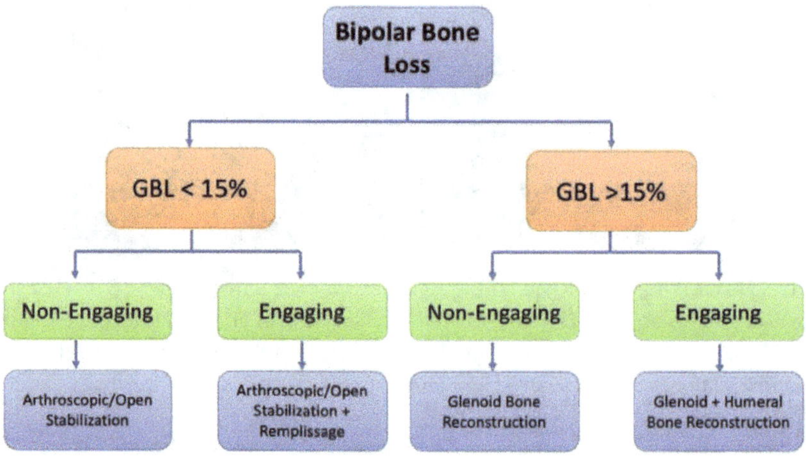

Fig. 4: Bipolar bone loss treatment algorithm. Gowd *et al.* recommended basing treatment on the quantity of GBL and whether or not the HSL is at risk of engagement.

Using the results of their systematic review, Gowd *et al.* recommended a treatment algorithm based on a GBL threshold of 15% and risk of engagement as per the GT equation, as shown in Fig. 4 [1] . However, although multiple treatment algorithms accounting for GBL, HSL, and the GT have been proposed, none have been validated with clinical studies thus far [1,27].

3. Clinical Presentation

Patients with bony shoulder instability typically present after a high energy trauma to the shoulder with frequent, easy dislocations of the shoulder that occur with activities of daily living or even with sleep [16]. Compared to patients with purely soft tissue injuries of the shoulder, they may experience numerous dislocation events occurring at comparatively lower degrees of abduction and external rotation than the "position of athletic function", which is described as 90° of abduction and 90° of external rotation [17,18]. It's also important to take a thorough past medical and surgical history, as patients with bony instability often require reduction for the initial trauma and may have had previous failed surgical interventions with persistent instability [3].

The physical examination should include a general inspection to look for scars suggestive of previous surgical intervention, as well as muscular atrophy, bony deformity, and a neurovascular assessment. The rotator cuff is frequently injured in dislocation events and should be assessed accordingly [16]. While numerous clinical tests — anterior apprehension, relocation, release, and load-and-shift — can be performed to assess for instability, the bony apprehension test, performed at 45° of abduction and 45° of external rotation, as compared to the usual 90/90, has been noted in the literature to be more specific [16]. In particular, it's important to recognise that a sense of apprehension — not pain — should be used as a positive result in these tests [19,20]. For patients undergoing surgery, examination under anaesthesia can be useful to perform a comprehensive physical assessment without causing the patient undue distress and pain.

4. Imaging of the Shoulder

Each patient with shoulder instability should be assessed initially with a series of radiographs, including a shoulder anteroposterior, internal and external rotation views, a Y-scapular view, an axillary lateral view, and an apical oblique view [21,22]. A West-Point and Stryker view can be useful for better visualising bony deformities if needed [23]. However, up to 60% of bony lesions are missed on plain radiographs, thus X-rays alone are

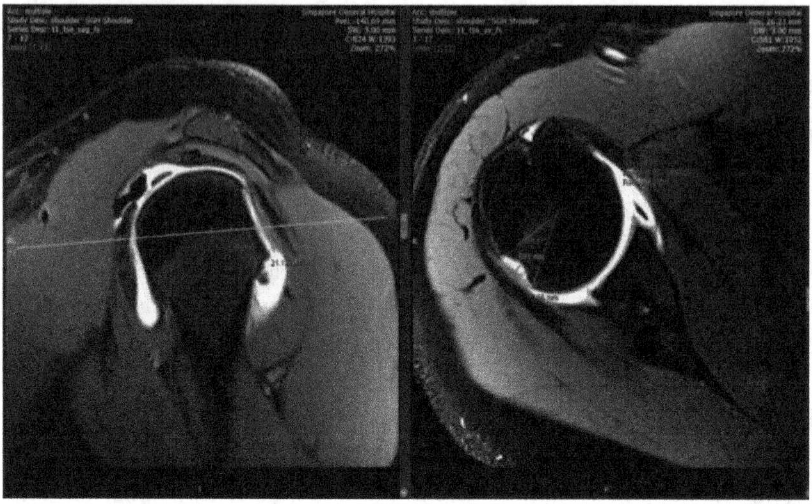

Fig. 5: Hill Sachs lesion: MRI shows it is wide as seen in the sagittal view and deep on the transverse view.

rarely sufficient for planning of treatment and advanced imaging with either an MRI or CT is required [24]. MRI scans better visualise soft tissue structures and can be useful in delineating other associated shoulder pathology (e.g. rotator cuff tears, biceps pathology, labral tears), while CT scans better define the bony anatomy in terms of size, location, an extent. While Itoi *et al.* described calculating the GT using CT scans, the same concept has been successfully applied to MRI scans with moderate to high accuracy [25] (Fig. 5).

5. Arthroscopic Surgery

(1) **Indications for surgery:** A large and engaging (off-track) lesion would warrant a Remplissage procedure at the time of soft tissue stabilisation
(2) **Special instruments:** TransTend anchors (Figs. 6 and 7)
(3) **Positioning and portals**
  - **Position:** Beach chair
  - **Portals:** Standard posterior for viewing, antero-superior and antero-inferior portals for labral repair. The HSL is accessed from

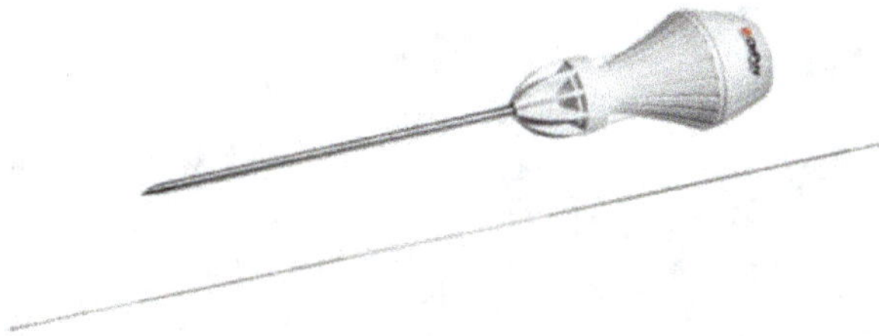

Fig. 6: The TransTend system: the wire is first inserted over which the cannula is inserted. The cannula enables the anchor to be inserted without direct visualization.

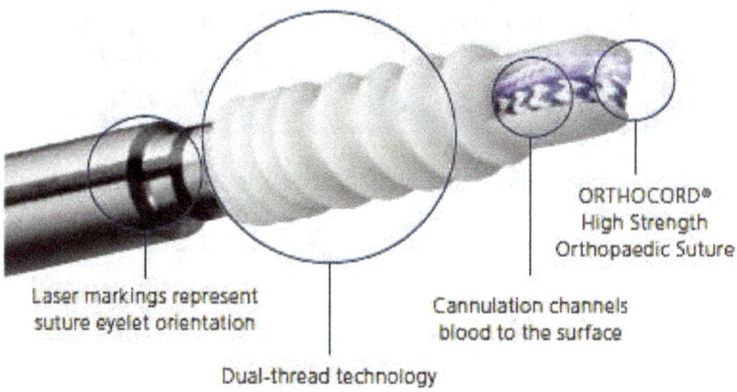

Fig. 7: The TransTend anchor. Enlarged view of the anchor, similar to the Healix anchor in construction.

a position about 2 cm below the postero-lateral corner of the acromion. Finally, a lateral portal in the subacromial space may be needed to retrieve and tie the sutures.

(4) **Arthroscopic Remplissage procedure:**

This procedure is usually performed together with anterior labral stabilisation and/or glenoid reconstruction. The anchors are first placed but not tied. After all anterior stabilisation is completed, only then are the sutures tied. A good Remplissage procedure will collapse the posterior space and will obscure visualisation.

(a) **Preparing the Hill Sachs lesion**

- The HSL is best visualised from the posterior portal, with the arm in varying angles of external rotation and slight abduction (Figs. 8 and 9).

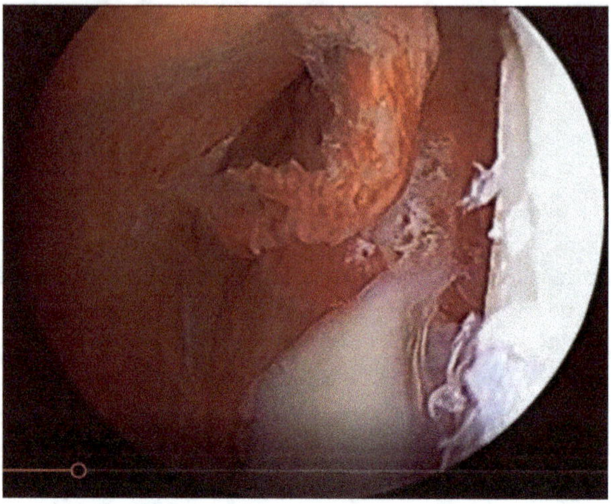

Fig. 8: Hill Sachs lesion. The large cavitatory lesion is seen from the posterior portal, with the viewer facing left.

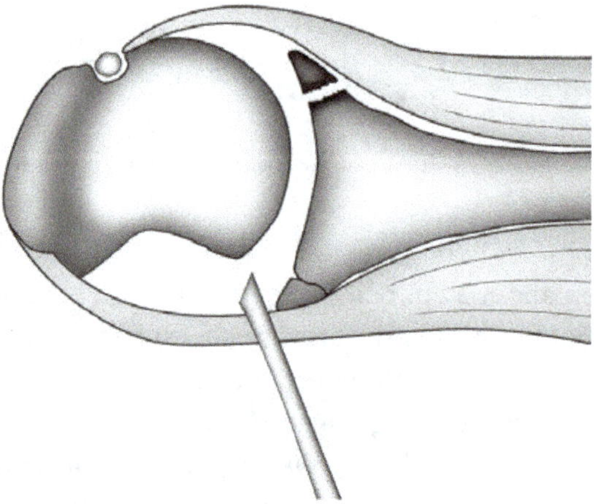

Fig. 9: Viewing the Hill Sachs. Schematic diagram showing the camera from the posterior portal viewing the HSL.

- Assess whether the lesion is on or off-track, does the lesion engage and cause the humeral head to sublux or dislocate as the arm is brought to abduction and external rotation? The lesion stays on-track if the head does NOT dislocate. An off-track lesion needs the Remplissage, some large on-track lesions may also require this procedure.

- If possible, debride the Hill Sachs lesion using a shaver from the antero-superior portal. Access may be difficult in smaller lesions.

(b) **Deploying the TransTend anchors**

- A wire is first inserted from the postero-lateral corner of the acromion, directed to the Hill Sachs lesion. Every lesion has its unique orientation depending on the injury mechanism. The lesion is usually vertical, though some are more oblique with the superior end pointing lateral (Fig. 10). The wire is first directed to the superior end of the lesion (or the end of the lesion further away from the camera) (Figs. 11 and 12).
- A 2 cm skin incision is made over the wire and the custom cannulated guide inserted over the wire. When the bulbous end of the guide is seen, withdraw the inner guide. Ensure the end of the outer guide remains in view, keep the arm in external rotation and slight abduction for best visualisation (Fig. 13).

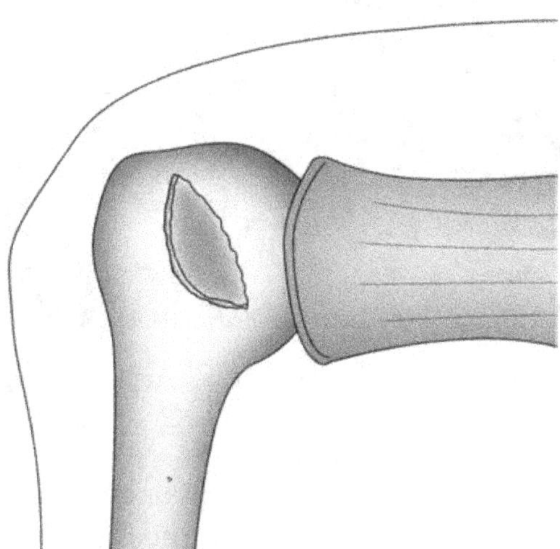

Fig. 10: HSL. Schematic diagram of a large Hill Sachs lesion, each of which usually is oriented obliquely.

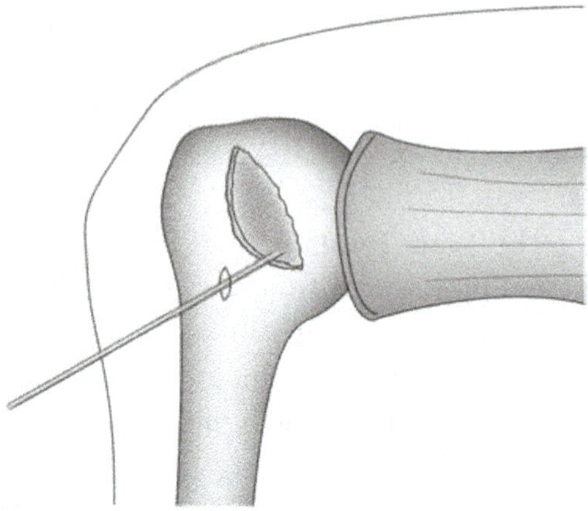

Fig. 11: TransTend wire. A TransTend wire is inserted cutaneously, directed to either end of the HSL.

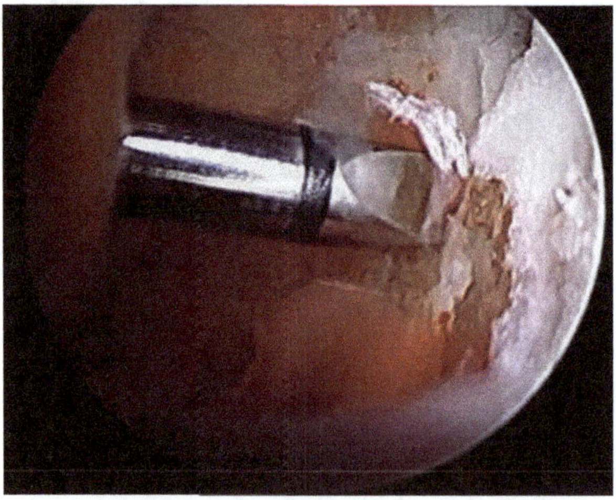

Fig. 12: TransTend wire. Arthroscopic view of the TransTend wire at one end of the lesion.

- The outer guide is kept in position at the upper more lateral end of the Hill Sachs, an awl is used to start a hole (Fig. 14), into which a single-loaded 4 mm TransTend anchor is inserted.
- Estimate the size and orientation of the Hill Sachs. On the skin, walk the same distance and orientation from the skin incision where the anchor was placed; then insert the wire

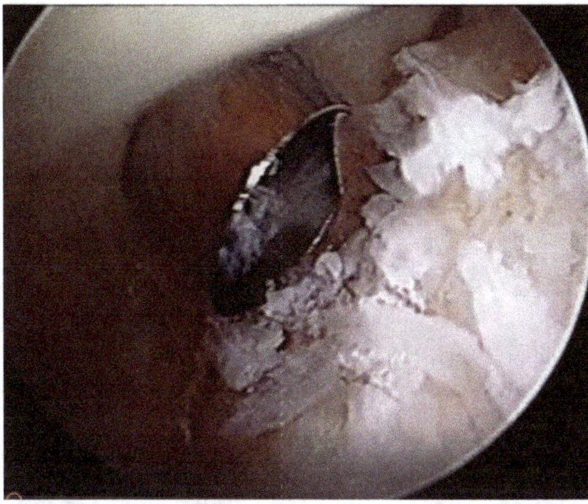

Fig. 13: TransTend cannula. A cannula is inserted over the wire.

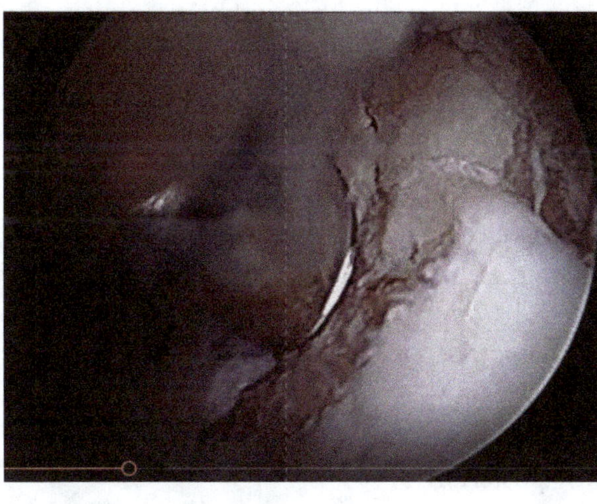

Fig. 14: TransTend anchor. After awling, the anchor is inserted whilst keeping the cannula in the same position.

directed to the inferior (more medial) end of the lesion. Similarly, a skin incision is made to allow access of the guide, to awl and insert the single-loaded suture anchor (Fig. 15).

- If the distance between the skin incisions is less than the Hill Sachs lesion, a divergent suture trajectory is created, thus the

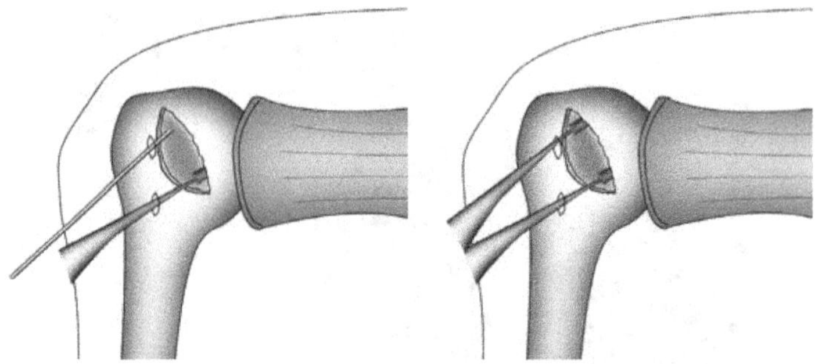

Fig. 15: Placement of TransTend anchors. After one anchor is inserted, the wire is inserted cutaneously at the other end of the lesion. The cannula is inserted over the wire and the anchor is inserted.

posterior capsule is made to "fill" and stretch over a larger bony lesion. If instead, a convergent trajectory is created, a wider area of posterior capsule is made to "fill" and secure the instability. This, in the author's opinion, is a stronger stabilisation.

(With the anchors placed and sutures parked in the postero-lateral corner of the shoulder, anterior stabilisation can now proceed.)

(c) **Retrieving the sutures in the subacromial space**

- The subacromial space is then entered with the camera at the posterior portal. A lateral portal is created, and a shaver is used to debride and clear the bursa *under direct visualisation.* Be careful to avoid cutting the sutures which are in the postero-lateral corner of the space. The sutures can be protected by inserting them in knot pushers and tucking them away posteriorly.
- Once a clearing of the bursa is made, deliver the sutures using the knot pushers into this clearing. Then retrieve all sutures from the lateral portal. *Remember to mark the suture limbs from each anchor and separate the sutures from the 2 anchors.*

(d) **Tying the sutures and compressing the Remplissage**

- Take one suture limb from each anchor, and tie them together as a transverse suture. The other suture limbs are then pulled. By this double-pulley system, a suture bridge between the

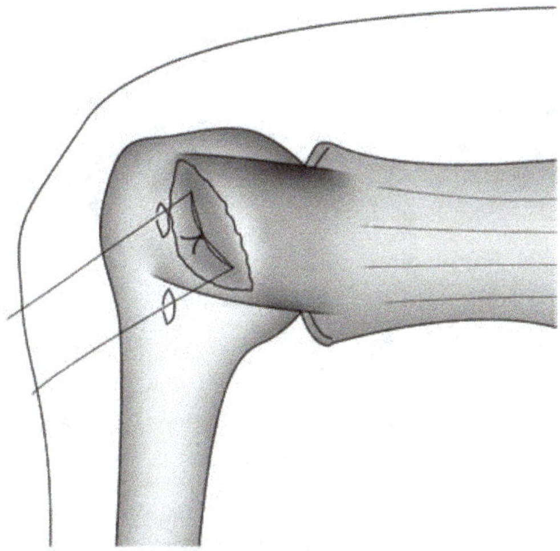

Fig. 16: The horizontal tie. One suture limb from each anchor is retrieved and tied together to form the horizontal tie, which fills up the HSL in this double-pulley system.

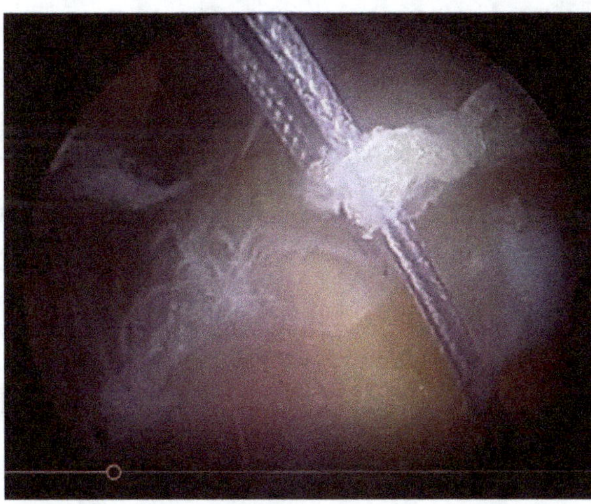

Fig. 17: The horizontal tie. The tighter the loose suture limbs are pulled, the more compressed will the infraspinatus be in the HSL.

anchors is created to fill and thus compress the posterior capsule into the Hill Sachs lesion (Figs. 16 and 17).

- The pulling suture limbs can now be tied together over the transverse suture bridge (Fig. 18). Alternatively, both the

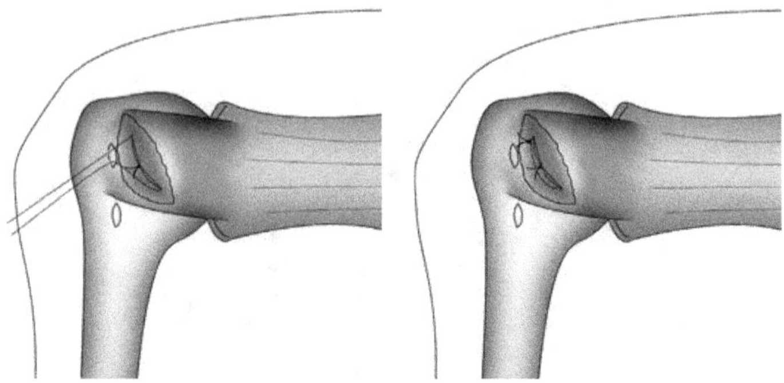

Fig. 18: The Remplissage procedure. The loose suture limbs are then retrieved via the same soft tissue portal and tied as firmly as possible.

pulling sutures can be tied to a Versalok knotless anchor, positioned roughly perpendicular to the transverse suture bridge. The higher the sutures are tensioned in the Versalok anchor, the more compression will be exerted on the transverse suture which would fill the Hill Sachs lesion, thus ensuring a secure Remplissage procedure.

6. Post-operative Management and Rehabilitation

The main goals of post-operative rehabilitation for patients who have undergone anterior shoulder stabilisation procedures are to restore glenohumeral compression stability, scapulohumeral motion synchrony, and proprioceptive mechanisms [26]. Accordingly, physiotherapy should be tailored based on the individual patient's pathology, procedure performed, and activity level of the patient. Generally, a minimum of six weeks of activity limitation are advised to minimise stress to the repaired structures and allow for adequate healing, usually with a sling for at least three to four weeks [26]. In particular, combined external rotation and abduction should be avoided during this period. However, active range of motion and use of uninvolved joints (e.g. elbow, wrist, fingers) is advised to reduce incidence of stiffness.

After the third post-operative week, assisted range of motion and isometric exercises can be started to prevent adhesion formation and muscle inhibition respectively [26]. External rotation should be progressively increased to prevent overstressing the repair. After the six weeks of immobilisation is over, rehabilitation via muscle retraining, range of motion exercises, and proprioceptive training aims to restore full active range of motion by 12 weeks post-operatively. Resistance exercises using bands may be useful after 8–10 weeks post-operatively under supervision by a physical therapist [26]. Generally, patients can return to throwing exercises after 18 weeks and back to sports after 32 weeks if cleared by a physiotherapist.

7. Outcomes

In a study of 103 patients from a multi-ethnic Asian population who underwent surgery for shoulder instability, patients were stratified into soft tissue injury only, monopolar bone loss (either glenoid or humeral bone loss), and bipolar bone loss. Patients were assessed pre-operatively and post-operatively based on the Constant-Murley score, UCLA Shoulder Score, the Visual Analogue scale for pain, and two questions adapted from the North American Spine Society low back instrument on expectations regarding and satisfaction about surgery. Additionally, patients were assessed post-operatively only for the presence of complications, which were defined as wound infection, numbness, pain, or recurrent dislocations.

Of these patients, 31% were found to have bipolar bone loss, but fewer than 3% of them were found to have “off-track” HSLs. Mean GBL was 10.9%, while mean HSL was 548.66 mm^2. Although patients with soft tissue injury only were found to be significantly younger than the other patients, there were no statistically significant difference in clinical outcomes, patient expectation, patient satisfaction and post-operative complications 2-years post-operatively. While limited by a modest patient size, small number of patients with bipolar bone loss, and the use of MRI instead of CT imaging, these findings suggest that minor bone loss, or GBL less than 15% and a non-engaging HSL, soft tissue reconstruction alone may be adequate for the treatment of bipolar bone loss in Asian populations.

References

1. Gowd AK, Liu JN, Cabarcas BC, Garcia GH, Cvetanovich GL, Provencher MT, *et al.* Management of recurrent anterior shoulder instability with bipolar bone loss: A systematic review to assess critical bone loss amounts. *Am J Sports Med* 2018:0363546518791555.
2. Yiannakopoulos CK, Mataragas E, Antonogiannakis E. A comparison of the spectrum of intra-articular lesions in acute and chronic anterior shoulder instability. *Arthroscopy* 2007;23(9):985–990.
3. Burkhart SS, De Beer JF. Traumatic glenohumeral bone defects and their relationship to failure of arthroscopic Bankart repairs: significance of the inverted-pear glenoid and the humeral engaging Hill-Sachs lesion. *Arthroscopy* 2000;16(7):677–694.
4. Edwards TB, Boulahia A, Walch G. Radiographic analysis of bone defects in chronic anterior shoulder instability. *Arthroscopy* 2003;19(7):732–739.
5. Patel RM, Walia P, Gottschalk L, Kuklis M, Jones MH, Fening SD, *et al.* The effects of Latarjet reconstruction on glenohumeral kinematics in the presence of combined bony defects: A cadaveric model. *Am J sports Med* 2016;44(7):1818–1824.
6. Zhang Q, Shi LL, Ravella KC, Koh JL, Wang S, Liu C, *et al.* Distinct proximal humeral geometry in Chinese population and clinical relevance. *JBJS.* 2016;98(24):2071–2081.
7. Yanke AB, Shin JJ, Pearson I, Bach Jr BR, Romeo AA, Cole BJ, *et al.* Three-dimensional magnetic resonance imaging quantification of glenoid bone loss is equivalent to 3-dimensional computed tomography quantification: cadaveric study. *Arthroscopy* 2017;33(4):709–715.
8. Di Giacomo G, Itoi E, Burkhart SS. Evolving concept of bipolar bone loss and the Hill-Sachs lesion: from "engaging/non-engaging" lesion to "on-track/off-track" lesion. *Arthroscopy* 2014;30(1):90–98.
9. Kurokawa D, Yamamoto N, Nagamoto H, Omori Y, Tanaka M, Sano H, *et al.* The prevalence of a large Hill-Sachs lesion that needs to be treated. *J Shoulder Elbow Surg* 2013;22(9):1285–1289.
10. Sekiya JK, Wickwire AC, Stehle JH, Debski RE. Hill-Sachs defects and repair using osteoarticular allograft transplantation: biomechanical analysis using a joint compression model. *Am J Sports Med* 2009;37(12): 2459–2466.
11. Yamamoto N, Muraki T, Sperling JW, Steinmann SP, Cofield RH, Itoi E, *et al.* Stabilizing mechanism in bone-grafting of a large glenoid defect. *JBJS* 2010;92(11):2059–2066.

12. Dickens JF, Owens BD, Cameron KL, DeBerardino TM, Masini BD, Peck KY, *et al.* The effect of subcritical bone loss and exposure on recurrent instability after arthroscopic Bankart repair in intercollegiate American football. *Am J Sports Med* 2017;45(8):1769–1775.
13. Shaha JS, Cook JB, Song DJ, Rowles DJ, Bottoni CR, Shaha SH, *et al.* Redefining "critical" bone loss in shoulder instability: functional outcomes worsen with "subcritical" bone loss. *Am J Sports Med* 2015;43(7): 1719–1725.
14. Itoi E, Lee S-B, Berglund LJ, Berge LL, An K-N. The effect of a glenoid defect on anteroinferior stability of the shoulder after Bankart repair: a cadaveric study. *JBJS* 2000;82(1):35–46.
15. Itoi E. 'On-track'and 'off-track'shoulder lesions. *EFORT Open Reviews* 2017;2(8):343–351.
16. Bushnell BD, Creighton RA, Herring MM. Bony instability of the shoulder. *Arthroscopy* 2008;24(9):1061–1073.
17. Miniaci A, Gish MW. Management of anterior glenohumeral instability associated with large Hill–Sachs defects. *Tech Shoulder Elb Surg* 2004; 5(3):170–175.
18. Burkhart SS, Lo IK, Brady PC. *Burkhart's view of the shoulder: A cowboy's guide to advanced shoulder arthroscopy*, 1st edn. Lippincott Williams & Wilkins, 2006.
19. Lo IK, Nonweiler B, Woolfrey M, Litchfield R, Kirkley A. An evaluation of the apprehension, relocation, and surprise tests for anterior shoulder instability. *Am J Sports Med* 2004;32(2):301–307.
20. Farber AJ, Castillo R, Clough M, Bahk M, McFarland EG. Clinical assessment of three common tests for traumatic anterior shoulder instability. *JBJS* 2006;88(7):1467–1474.
21. Garth Jr WP, Slappey C, Ochs C. Roentgenographic demonstration of instability of the shoulder: the apical oblique projection. A technical note. *JBJS* 1984;66(9):1450–1453.
22. Bushnell BD, Creighton RA, Herring MM. Hybrid treatment of engaging Hill-Sachs lesions: arthroscopic capsulolabral repair and limited posterior approach for bone grafting. *Tech Shoulder Elb Surg* 2007;8(4):194–203.
23. Pavlov H, Warren RF, Weiss JC, Dines DM. The roentgenographic evaluation of anterior shoulder instability. *Clin Orthop Relat Res* 1985(194): 153–158.
24. Bushnell BD, Creighton RA, Herring MM. The bony apprehension test for instability of the shoulder: a prospective pilot analysis. *Arthroscopy* 2008;24(9):974–982.

25. Gyftopoulos S, Hasan S, Bencardino J, Mayo J, Nayyar S, Babb J, *et al.* Diagnostic accuracy of MRI in the measurement of glenoid bone loss. *Am J Roentgenol* 2012;199(4):873–878.
26. Hayes K, Callanan M, Walton J, Paxinos A, Murrell GA. Shoulder instability: management and rehabilitation. *J Orthop Sports Phys Ther* 2002;32(10):497–509.
27. Di Giacomo G, Pugliese M, Lie DTT, Chou ACC, Chen J, Rosenberg N *et al.* How to handle minor and major bone loss in the shoulder? Current concepts. *JISAKOS*, 2020;5(3):117–122.

https://doi.org/10.1142/9789811249846_0008

Chapter 8

Approach to Major Bone Loss of the Glenoid: Arthroscopic Repair of the Bony Bankart Arthroscopic Glenoid Reconstruction Using Iliac Crest Bone Graft — Eden-Hybinette Procedure

Denny T.T. Lie and Abby Choke

Summary of Chapter

1. Introduction and epidemiology of major glenoid bone loss
2. Clinical presentation of the unstable shoulder with bony defects
3. Diagnosis and imaging
4. Surgical technique of the arthroscopic bony Bankart repair
5. Surgical technique of glenoid reconstruction using iliac crest bone graft (ICBG) — the Eden-Hybinette procedure
6. Rehabilitation
7. Clinical outcomes

1. Introduction and Epidemiology of Problem

Recurrent anterior shoulder instability can result from soft tissue labral injuries or from glenoid bone loss. The most common lesion following an initial traumatic dislocation is an inferior capsule-labral tear of the glenoid rim, known as a Bankart lesion. A fracture of the glenoid rim, or referred to as bony Bankart lesion, contributes to further instability by altering the glenohumeral contact area. Bony Bankart lesions are seen in approximately 22–41% of initial anterior dislocation and in up to 73–86% of recurrent instability [1,2]. Up to 22% of those who suffered from initial traumatic shoulder dislocation had some degrees of bone loss due to fracture of the glenoid rim [3]. Glenoid bone loss has also been noted in up to 89% of failed prior stabilisation procedures, and the failure rate for such surgery has been shown to significantly increase from 4% to 67% in those with significant glenoid bone loss [3,4]. The degree of bone loss can increase over time as a consequence of repeated dislocations and attritional changes.

2. Clinical Presentation

The most common traumatic glenohumeral dislocations is anterior in direction (85–95%) and the remainder are usually posterior and inferior [5]. The mechanism of an anterior dislocation involves a fall with an anteriorly directed force on the arm when the shoulder is abducted and externally rotated. The individual typically presents with a clinical history of recurrent dislocation, feeling of instability, and occasional shoulder pain. Examination of the unstable shoulder is described in Chapter 7, and was elaborated in Chapter 1.

3. Diagnosis and Imaging, Algorithm

Plain radiograph of the shoulder may not accurately demonstrate glenoid bone loss (Fig. 1). A bony Bankart fragment can sometimes be visualised on a standard AP view or in axillary view, but the highest yield projection would be the apical oblique view. A Hill-Sachs lesion can be visualised on the Stryker notch view or AP view with the shoulder in internal rotation.

The best modality for quantifying glenoid bone loss is a CT (computed tomography) scan. A digital subtracted 3D CT scan can accurately quantify the percentage of glenoid bone loss by using the "circle of best fit" method, where a circle is drawn on the inferior two-third of the

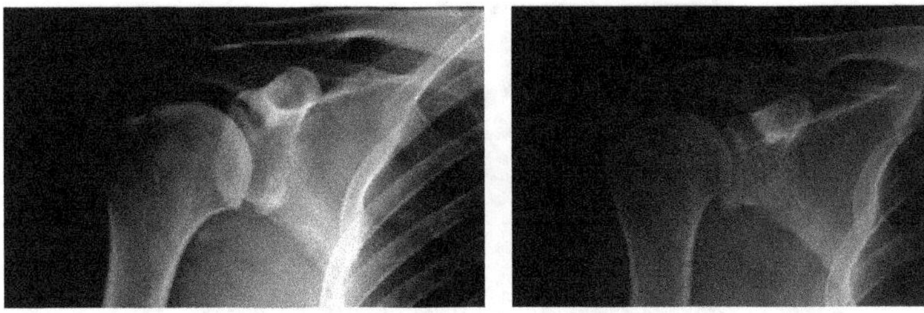

(a) (b)

Fig. 1: X-rays of glenoid bone loss. (a) The broken contour of the anterior glenoid and the fragment. (b) However looks surprisingly normal. MRI of the same shoulder is shown in Fig. 2.

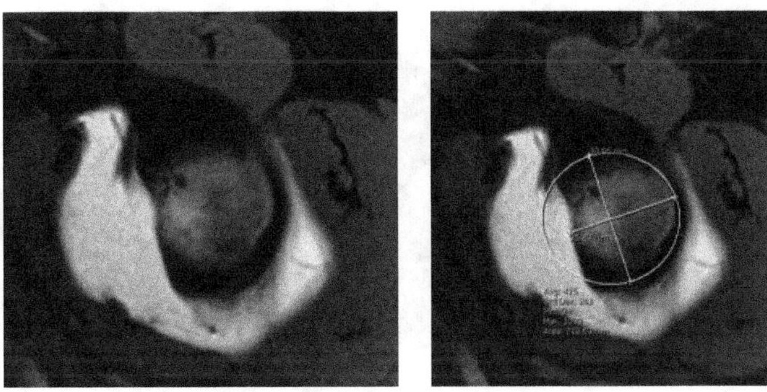

(a) (b)

Fig. 2: MRI of glenoid bone loss. (a) Sagittal view of MRI of shoulder from Fig. 1(b), shows a significant bone loss. The circle of best fit estimates the loss to be 20%, shown in (b).

glenoid and the total surface area of the missing bone is digitally measured [6]. Magnetic resonance imaging (MRI) or arthrography can also be utilised in the same way (see Figs. 2, 3 and 4). Biomechanical studies have suggested that 20% is the critical percentage bone loss of the glenoid surface area that can result in significant instability [7]. In such cases, anatomic reconstruction of the glenoid rim is necessary (see algorithm shown in Fig. 5).

The concept of glenoid bone augmentation was first described by Eden-Hybinette in 1918 where a tibial bone autograft was used as mechanical barrier to extend the anterior glenoid rim [8]. The iliac crest bone graft subsequently replaced the tibial graft due to its easier access and lesser

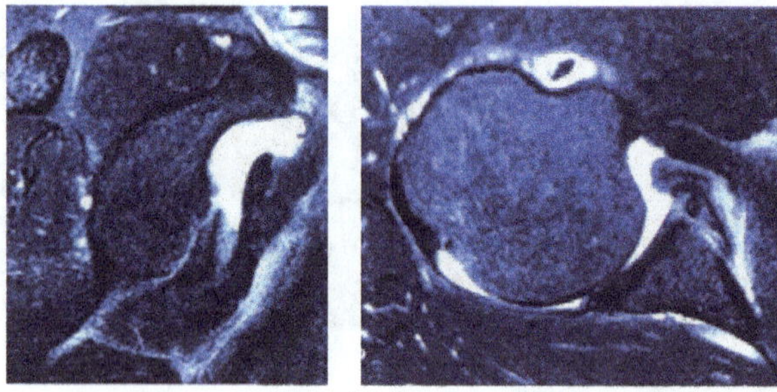

(a) (b)

Fig. 3: MRI of glenoid with bony Bankart. (a) is the sagittal view of MRI of a shoulder with bony Bankart, estimated to be about 17%. (b) is the transverse view, showing the anterior bony Bankart.

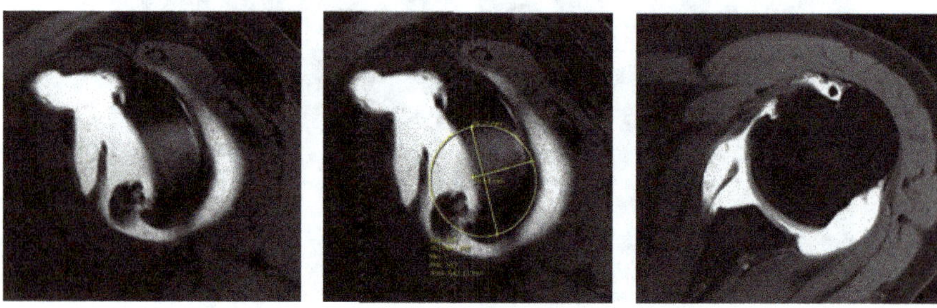

(a) (b) (c)

Fig. 4: MRI of large glenoid bone loss. (a) The sagittal view of a glenoid with a large bone loss, estimated to be about 45% as shown in (b). (c) The transverse view shows the significant glenoid bone loss and a large Hill Sachs lesion.

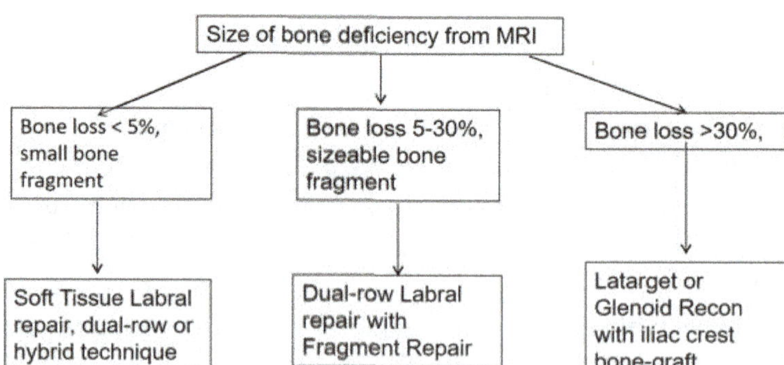

Fig. 5: Algorithm showing approach to glenoid bone loss and bony Bankart.

donor site morbidity. With the advancement of arthroscopic techniques and instruments, an all-arthroscopic bone block technique is now routinely being performed [9]. In 2008, Taverna *et al.* described his arthroscopic approach for an extracapsular iliac crest bone grafting on a cadaveric model [8]. In 2014, Kraus *et al.* published the first case series of 15 patients who undergone an all-arthroscopic approach: ICBG fixation using compression screws showing good to excellent early clinical results [10].

4. Arthroscopic Repair of the Bony Bankart — The Dual-Row Labral Repair

(1) **Special instruments:** Knotless Bio-Raptor anchors by Smith & Nephew.

(2) **Positioning and portal**
- **Position:** Beach chair.
- **Posterior portal:** The standard landmarks are used to keep the trajectory in the plane of the glenoid.
- **Anterosuperior portal:** This is made just lateral to the tip of the coracoid and directed vertically downwards. This portal is for suture shuttling and management.
- **Anteroinferior portal:** This is made above the subscapularis tendon, inferior to the portal above, in the plane of the glenoid surface. It is more medial than the usual anteroinferior portal, and can be done inside-out. As long as the portal is kept lateral to the conjoint tendon, the nerves are safe.
- **Anterolateral portal:** This is the additional portal for this procedure and is surface-marked just below the anterolateral corner of the acromion. The trajectory is anterior to the biceps tendon and this provides an excellent viewing portal for the procedure.

(3) **Step 1: Preparation of the glenoid rim and bony Bankart**
- Debride the synovitis and liberate the labrum from the anterior glenoid to mobilise it well. Liberate the bony Bankart fragment from the anterior glenoid but be careful not to allow it to float freely, this will make it harder to repair it later. Osteotomise any partial bony union if needed, to mobilise the bone fragment (Fig. 6(a)).

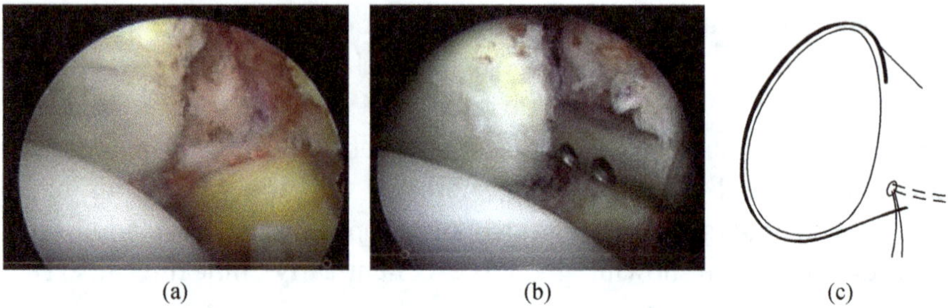

Fig. 6: The bony Bankart fragment and the AIM anchor. (a) The bony fragment still adherent to the labrum and anterior capsule. This has to be well debrided to allow a antero-inferior medial (AIM) anchor to be inserted about 7–10 mm from the glenoid edge, as in (b). This schematic is shown in (c).

- Shift the camera to the antero-lateral portal for better viewing.
- The anterior rim of the glenoid is then decorticated using a shaver to create a bleeding bony surface.

(4) **Step 2: The anteroinferior medial (AIM) anchor**

- The drill guide is positioned as low as possible (5:30 o'clock position for the right shoulder) about **7–10 mm medial** to the rim of the glenoid (Figs. 6(b) and 6(c)).
- A dual-loaded suture anchor (Gryphon BR anchor or equivalent) is then inserted. Often the vault of the glenoid slopes away sharply, causing the anchor or equivalent to skive off. Hence it is imperative to keep the trajectory of the anchor placement in the plane or medial to the glenoid. Widen the antero-inferior portal to allow a more medialised anchor placement.
- An alternative is the curved suture anchor system (Conmed Y-knot dual-loaded anchor).

(5) **Step 3: Repair of the bony Bankart and soft tissue envelope**

- For large bony fragments (about 1 cm long and at least 4 mm thick) an Acupass suture passer (30° straight) from the antero-inferior portal is used to pierce the fragment from the anterior face (Figs. 7(a)–7(c)). A grasper from the antero-superior portal can be used to stabilise the fragment, but be careful NOT to break the fragment. All four suture limbs from the anchor are then shuttled through the fragment (Figs. 8(a) and 8(b)). Then park all four suture limbs in the antero-superior portal.

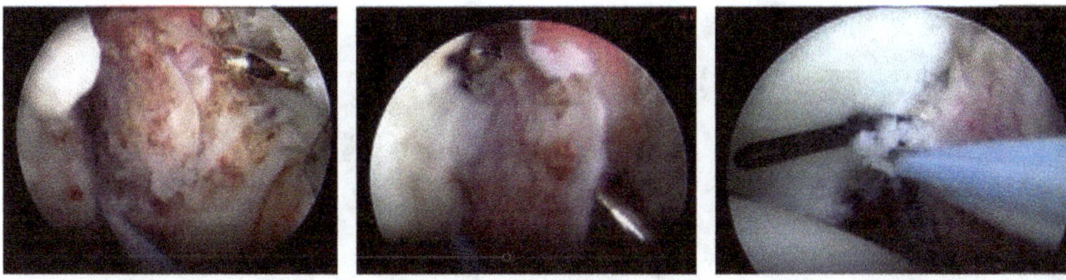

(a) (b) (c)

Fig. 7: Piercing the bony fragment. (a) A Acupass suture passer piercing the middle of the bony fragment, as in (b). A filament is passed (c) to shuttle all 4 sutures through the bony fragment.

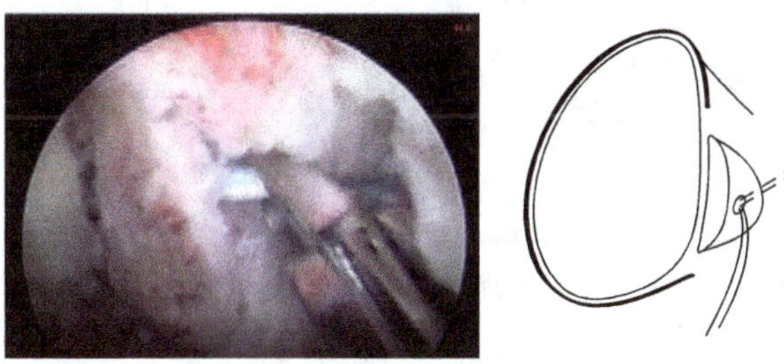

(a) (b)

Fig. 8: Fixing the bony fragment. The sutures are retrieved after piercing the bony fragment, as shown in (a) and schematically in (b). This ensures the fragment is not permitted to shift in the soft tissue envelope and will aid healing.

(Note that in thick bony fragments, thicker than 10 mm, it may be necessary to drill the fragment with a 16 mm drill bit first before the suture passer is negotiated through the fragment.)

- A deep bite of the labral-capsule complex above the bony fragment is taken and both limbs of the blue sutures are shuttled through (Fig. 9(a)).
- Tent the antero-inferior labrum-complex up with a grasper from the antero-superior portal, then using 70° straight suture passer from the antero-inferior portal, take a deep bite of the labrum-capsule, including the anterior IGHL, below the bony fragment. Then shuttle both limbs of the white suture (Figs. 9(b)–9(d)).
- For thin fragments (less than 4 mm thick) piercing the fragment as described above can break the fragment and is thus NOT

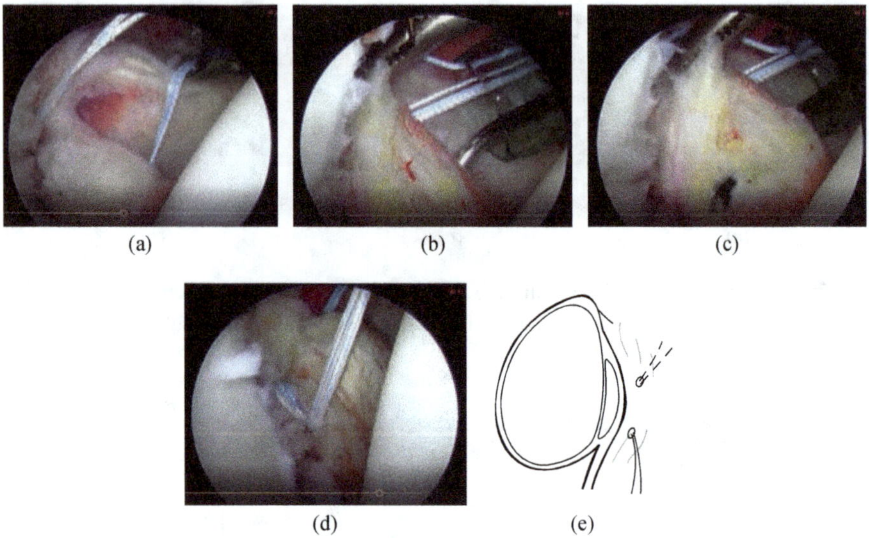

(a) (b) (c) (d) (e)

Fig. 9: The soft tissue envelope. A deep bite of the labrum and capsule is taken to shuttle the blue sutures above the fragment, as shown in (a). (b) and (c) show an Acupass suture passer piercing the labrum and capsule below the fragment and the blue sutures, to retrieve the white sutures (d). This is shown in the schematic diagram (e).

recommended. Instead, keep the thin fragment adherent to the labrum–capsule complex, then pierce the Acupass medial to the fragment, below the fragment to retrieve both limbs of blue sutures, and another bite above the fragment to retrieve white sutures.

- An option here would be to take one limb of the blue suture and one limb of the white suture, then tie them together. Keep the suture ends of this transverse tie long, to incorporate them to the suture bridge later. Pulling the other limbs of blue and white sutures as a double-pulley would compress the bony fragment onto the glenoid, with the labrum-complex soft tissue envelope entombing the bony fragment.

(6) **Step 4: The Rim anchor**

- One limb of the blue suture and another from the white suture are then retrieved and tied to a knotless anchor (BioRaptor 20 mm). This anchor is positioned at the rim or edge of the glenoid face, about 5 mm below the position of the AIM anchor (Fig. 10(a)).

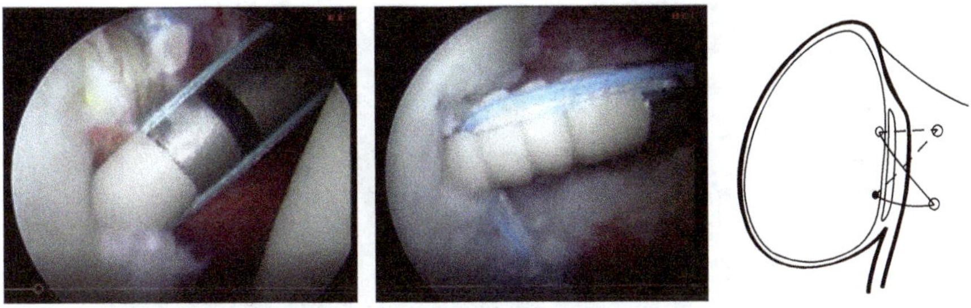

(a) (b) (c)

Fig. 10: The dual-row labral repair. (a) One suture from the blue pair and another from the white are retrieved and anchored to the rim with knotless Bio-Raptor anchor, above the fragment. (b) The other pairs are then secured to another rim anchor, above the bony fragment. This dual-row suture bridge repair is shown in the schematic diagram in (c).

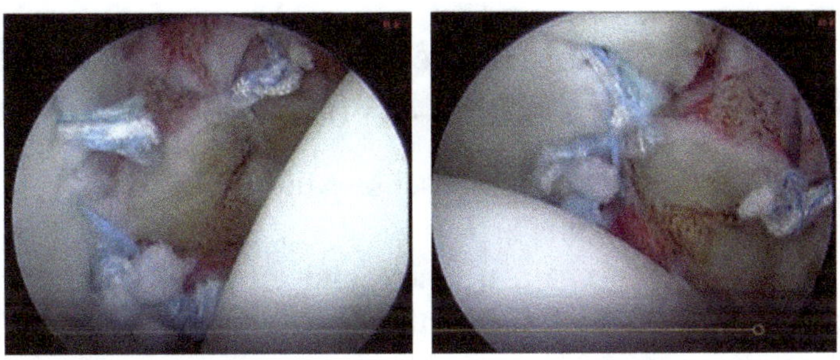

(a) (b)

Fig. 11: The final check, (a) is seen from the posterior portal and (b) is from the anterolateral portal; showing the bony fragment fully enveloped or entombed in the soft tissue envelope, which restored the anterior wall and capsule.

- Similarly, the remaining limbs of the blue and white sutures are retrieved and tied to another knotless anchor at the glenoid rim, about 7–10 mm above the AIM anchor (Fig. 10(b)). This creates a dual-row suture-bridge repair of the labrum-capsule which incorporates and envelopes the bony fragment (Fig. 10(c)).
- The rest of the labrum is repaired in a standard way described in an earlier chapter.
- A final check is shown in Fig. 11 and MRI 6 months after the surgery showed healed bony fragment (Fig. 12).

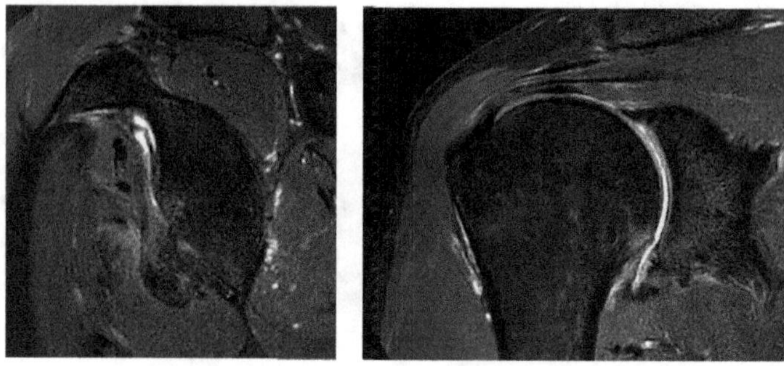

(a) (b)

Fig. 12: Post-op MRI. Six months after surgery, (a) shows the bony fragment in position and healed, with the divergent anchor tracks. (b) shows the reconstructed inferior labrum and capsule.

5. Arthroscopic Glenoid Reconstruction Using Iliac Crest Bone-Block (Eden-Hybinette Procedure)

(1) **Special instruments:** Latarget set by Mitek (Fig. 13)

(2) **Positioning and portals**

- **Position:** Beach chair, **prepare and clean the ipsilateral iliac crest for bone block harvesting.**
- **Posterior portal:** The standard landmarks are used to keep the trajectory in the plane of the glenoid.
- **Anterosuperior portal:** This is made just lateral to the tip of the coracoid and directed vertically downwards. This portal is for suture shuttling and management.
- **Anteroinferior portal:** This is made above the subscapularis tendon, inferior to the portal above, *in the plane of the glenoid surface.* It is more medial than the usual anteroinferior portal, and can be done inside-out. As long as the portal is kept lateral to the conjoint tendon, the nerves are safe. **The incision is widened to at least 2–3 cm. This is the main working portal.**
- **Anterolateral portal:** This is the additional portal for this procedure and is surface-marked just below the anterolateral corner of the acromion. The trajectory is anterior to the biceps tendon and this provides an excellent viewing portal for the procedure.

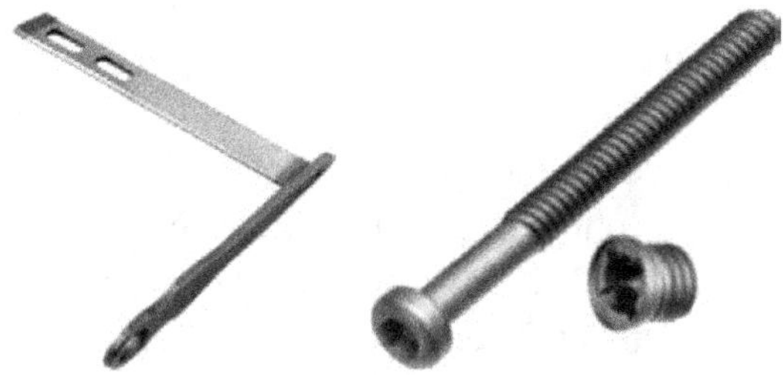

(a) (b)

Fig. 13: The Latarget system. (a) The drill guide, to fix 2 wires into the bone graft. (b) shows the cortical screw and locking head of the system.

(3) **Step 1: Preparation of the Glenoid Rim**
- The labrum is carefully detached using a liberator and any frayed tissue is debrided with a shaver. It is important to completely detach any remnant labrum to create a large enough cavity for the bone block (Fig. 15(a)).
- The camera is then shifted to the antero-superior portal, and a calibrated probe is inserted via the antero-superior portal to measure the length of the bone graft required to fill the bony defect (Fig. 15(b)).
- The anterior glenoid rim is decorticated and flattened with the shaver to create a flat bleeding bone surface for accommodation of the graft. Then, the antero-inferior portal is widened to 2 cm to prepare for delivery of the bone block. *Remember to keep the trajectory of the portal in the plane of the glenoid or medial to the glenoid.*
- The rotator interval is then debrided and cleared, till the conjoint tendon is clearly seen. Bluntly dilate the portal using a pair of forceps. Visualisation can be difficult in muscular patients, and a large cannula may be needed.

(4) **Step 2: Iliac Bone Graft Harvest**
- The tricortical bone graft is harvested from the ipsilateral hip. This can be performed concurrently with the arthroscopic procedure. *We recommend adducting and flexing the shoulder to 30°s to provide sufficient space for both surgical sites.* A 3-cm skin incision is made over the anterior superior iliac crest (ASIS) and dissected down to the outer cortex of the bone.

- The iliac crest bone is marked and sawed into a 2 × 1 × 1 cm bone block. The bone block is cut to fit the sloping vault of the anterior glenoid, such that inner table of the iliac crest conforms to the articulating face of the glenoid. This is usually fashioned as a J-shaped block to match the glenoid slope.
- Using a 2.7 mm hand drill, two drill holes are made 5 mm from each bone edge. The inferior and outer surface of the bone block is marked with a surgical marker (Figs. 14(a) and 14(b)).

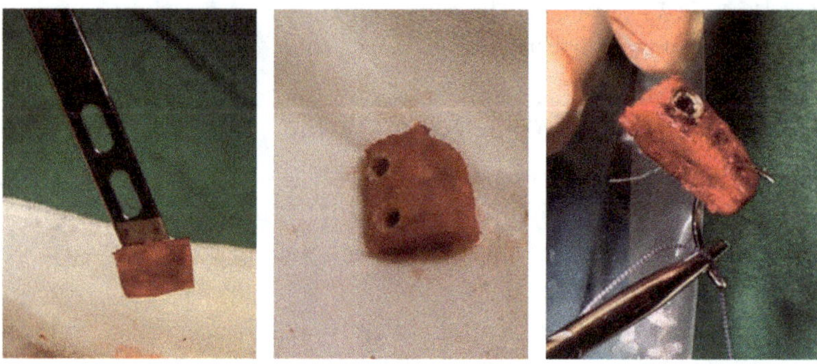

(a) (b) (c)

Fig. 14: Preparing the bone graft. (a) The bone graft, usually 2 × 1 × 1 cm in size, harvested from the anterior iliac crest, prepared using the drill guide. (b) The two screw holes prepared in the graft. (c) The current modification, using 1 screw hole and two small perforations for sutures.

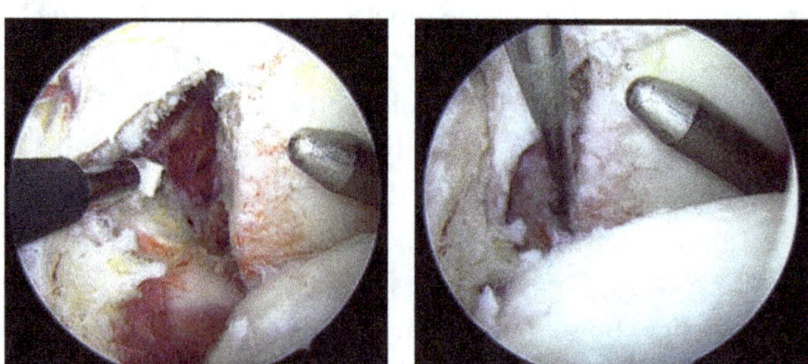

(a) (b)

Fig. 15: Preparing the glenoid defect. (a) The large space due to the bone defect. The anterior glenoid was decorticated and prepared, then the size of the defect measured using a graduated probe (b).

- An alternative is to drill one 2.7 mm hole for the screw prepared with a locking hat, and two small holes for the passage of sutures (Fig. 14(c)).

(5) **Step 3: Securing the Bone Graft**

- A double-loaded suture anchor (Gryphon Healix BR System, Mitek Depuy Synthes, MA, USA) is placed at the 5 o'clock anteroinferior position of the deficient glenoid rim (Fig. 16(a)), and the one pair of sutures is parked in the antero-superior portal (Fig. 16(b)).
- An inferior capsular pouch is first created, by tenting up the inferior capsule and anterior IGHL using a tissue grasper from the antero-superior portal. A deep bite of this tissue is taken using a suture retriever (70° straight Acupass) from the antero-inferior portal. The suture is then shuttled.
- The suture is then returned to the antero-superior portal, from where the sutures are tied to create an inferior capsular pouch, on which the bone block is cradled. The bone block will thus sit no lower than the 6 o'clock position, or even higher. The sutures are preferably parked in the antero-lateral portal, which continues to be the viewing portal.
- The orientation of the bone block is determined, where the convex outer table is matched to the glenoid slope, and the inner concave

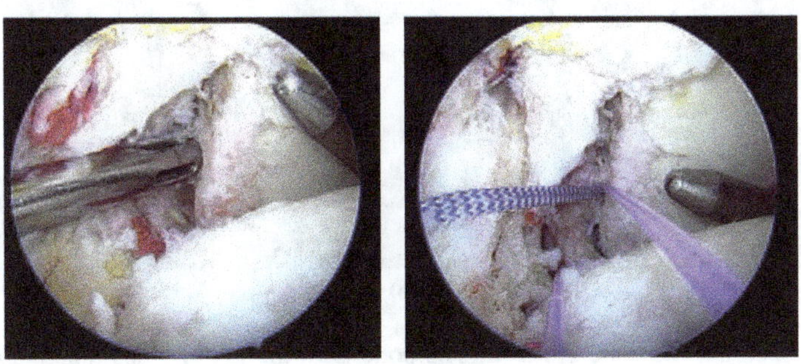

(a) (b)

Fig. 16: The AIM anchor and the inferior pouch. (a) An antero-inferior medial anchor being placed. It is located about 7–10 mm medial to the glenoid edge. (b) shows one purple suture tenting up the inferior labrum and capsule. The striped blue sutures will be used to relay and guide the bone graft into position.

cancellous portion is matched to the decorticated glenoid surface. Using a "chia wire", both limps of the remaining suture are delivered through the drill hole of the bone block.

- Using the suture as a tracking guide, the bone graft is carefully delivered through the antero-inferior portal horizontally first. After it clears over the subscapularis tendon, the sutures are tugged gently and the block is guided into position using a probe from the antero-superior portal (Fig. 17(a)).
- An obturator from the antero-inferior portal can be used to push the bone block to position. The guide sutures are then tied to provide initial stability and sutures cut. Next, a Latarget cortical screw or a 3.5 mm cannulated headless compression screw (Depuy Synthes, PA, USA) is introduced and carefully threaded in to anchor the bone block onto the glenoid rim (Fig. 17(b)). The screw will thus rest at the 9 o'clock position of the glenoid (left shoulder) (Fig. 17(c)).
- Once the graft is fixed, the initial sutures that created the inferior pouch, parked at the antero-lateral portal, are then retrieved. If necessary, they can be used to plicate any patulous anterior capsule, to provide a soft-tissue augment to the bony glenoid reconstruction (Figs. 18(a) and 18(b)).

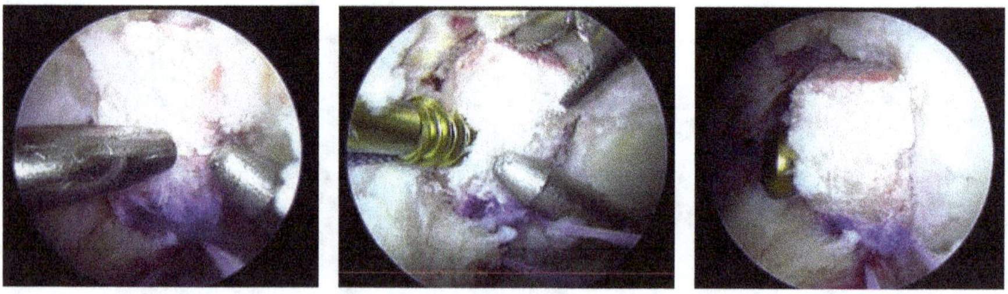

(a) (b) (c)

Fig. 17: Securing the bone graft. (a) The bone graft guided into position. An obturator from the posterior portal keeps the graft flushed with the glenoid surface. (b) A grasper from the antero-superior portal holding the graft in place as it is secured with a partially-threaded cancellous screw, directed from the antero-inferior portal. (c) The well-fixed bone graft in position.

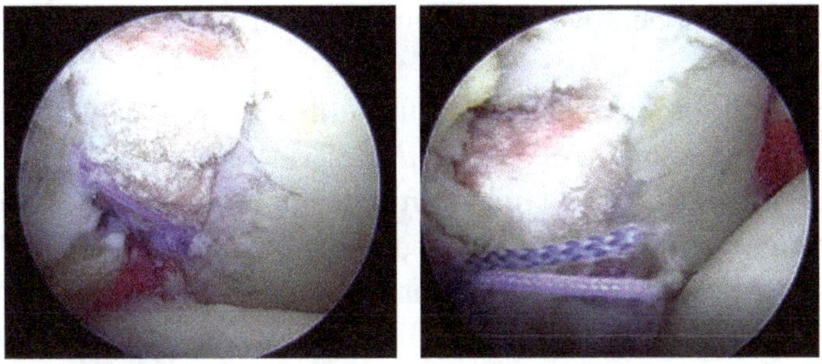

(a) (b)

Fig. 18: The final check. (a) The view from the lateral portal, sutures from the AIM anchor are used to tie the anterior capsule and hence re-create the anterior wall. (b) The view from the antero-superior portal which shows the graft flushed with the glenoid surface.

6. Post-Op Management and Rehabilitation

Post-operatively, all the patients were placed in an arm sling for support. Gentle pendulum exercises were initiated immediately after surgery, followed by passive range of motion at week 2–3 and active assisted range of motion from week 3–4. From week 6 onwards, they were allowed active range of motion and gradual strengthening exercises.

7. Outcomes of Glenoid Reconstruction

The goal in the treatment of glenoid deficiency is to re-establish the bony buttress of the glenoid rim which is pivotal in providing resistance to the axial and shear force in the glenohumeral joint to prevent recurrent instability. The Edin-Hybinette bone block procedure is a reliable technique that is used to restore glenoid rim deficiency. An iliac crest bone graft has the biomechanical merit in providing an anatomic restoration of the glenohumeral arc. The benefits of an all-arthroscopic procedure compared to an open technique are well established. These include lesser soft tissue dissection, reduced risk of infection, better joint visualisation, and earlier return to function [11]. An arthroscopic approach also does not violate the subscapularis function and structural integrity, which is important for postoperative rehabilitation and in maintaining the stability of the shoulder [12].

Several arthroscopic techniques using iliac crest bone graft has been described in literature. Scheibel *et al.* described one of the first arthroscopic techniques for iliac bone grafting using a bio-compression screw for interfragmentary compression combined with capsulolabral repair using suture anchors [11]. Kalogrianitis introduced a knotless fixation technique using an adjustable-length loop cortical suspensory fixation device, or also known as the TightRope-RT (Arthrex) which eliminates the use of screws and their potential problems [13].

Kraus *et al.* reported a case series of 15 patients who underwent arthroscopic glenoid reconstruction using iliac crest bone graft, showing a significant improvement of the mean Constant score, Western Ontario Shoulder Instability Index (WOSI), shoulder function score with no recurrent instability after a mean follow up of 20 months [10]. Most recently in 2018, Bockmann *et al.* presented his clinical results for 32 patients who underwent the same procedure using two double-helix screws (metallic or bioresorbable screws). His cohort demonstrated good functional results with a recurrence rate of 9% at 42 months follow up [14]. In our very own institutional experience using a double screw technique for bone graft fixation for seven patients, all had a significantly improved functional score (Oxford Shoulder Score, UCLA, Constant-Murley Score) with evidence of graft incorporation and no reports of recurrence after 2 years. However, one patient required screw removal due to screw cut out and partial graft resorption [15].

In conclusion, an arthroscopic glenoid reconstruction procedure using iliac crest bone graft is a reliable technique that obviates the risks of open surgery and does not cause permanent change to the anterior shoulder anatomy. However, this technique has a steep learning curve and technical modification as described above can improve the feasibility for an all-arthroscopic approach.

References

1. Chen AL, Hunt SA, Hawkins RJ, Zuckerman JD. Management of bone loss associated with recurrent anterior glenohumeral instability. *Am J Sports Med* 2005;33:912–992.

2. Griffith JF, Antonio GE, Yung PS, *et al.* Prevalence, pattern, and spectrum of glenoid bone loss in anterior shoulder dislocation: CT analysis of 218 patients. *AJR* 2008;190:1247–1254.
3. Burkhart SS, De Beer JF. Traumatic glenohumeral bone defects and their relationship to failure of arthroscopic Bankart repairs: significance of the inverted-pear glenoid and the humeral engaging Hill-Sachs lesion. *Arthroscopy* 2000;16:677–694.
4. Taylor DC, Arciero RA. Pathologic changes associated with shoulder dislocations: arthroscopic and physical examination findings in first-time, traumatic anterior dislocations. *Am J Sports Med* 1997;25:306–311.
5. Kwon YW, Zuckerman JD. Subluxations and dislocations about the glenohumeral joint. In: Rockwood CA, Green DP, Bucholz RW (eds.), *Rockwood and Green's Fractures in Adults*. Lippincott Williams & Wilkins, Philadelphia, PA, 2006.
6. Sugaya H, Moriishi J, Dohi M, Kon Y. Tsuchiya A: Glenoid rim morphology in recurrent anterior glenohumeral instability. *J Bone Joint Surg Am* 2003; 85:878–884.
7. Itoi E, Lee SB, Berglund LJ, Berge LL, An KN. The effect of a glenoid defect on anteroinferior stability of the shoulder after Bankart repair: a cadaveric study. *J Bone Joint Surg* 2000;82(1):35–46.
8. Taverna E, Golano P, Pascale V, Battistella F. An arthroscopic bone graft procedure for treating anterior-inferior glenohumeral instability. *Knee Surg Sports Traumatol Arthrosc* 2008;16:872–875.
9. Anderl W, Kriegleder B, Heuberer PR. All-arthroscopic implant-free iliac crest bone grafting: new technique and case report. *Arthroscopy* 2012; 28(1):131–137.
10. Kraus N, Amphansap T, Gerhardt C, Scheibel M. Arthroscopic anatomic glenoid reconstruction using an autologous iliac crest bone grafting technique. *J Shoulder Elb Surg* 2014;23(11):1700–1708.
11. Scheibel M, Kraus N, Diederichs G, Haas NP. Arthroscopic reconstruction of chronic anteroinferior glenoid defect using an autologous tricortical iliac crest bone grafting technique. *Arch Orthop Trauma Surg* 2008; 128(11):1295–1300.
12. Scheibel M, Nikulka C, Dick A, Schroeder RJ, Popp AG, Haas NP. Structural integrity and clinical function of the subscapularis musculotendinous unit after arthroscopic and open shoulder stabilization. *Am J Sports Med* 2007; 35:1153–1161.
13. Kalogrianitis S, Tsouparopoulos V. arthroscopic iliac crest bone block for reconstruction of the glenoid: a fixation technique using an adjustable-length

loop cortical suspensory fixation device. *Arthrosc Tech* 2016;5(6): e1197–e1202.

14. Bockmann B, Venjakob AJ, Reichwein F, Hagenacker M, Nebelung W. Mid-term clinical results of an arthroscopic glenoid rim reconstruction technique for recurrent anterior shoulder instability. *Arch Orthop Trauma Surg* 2018;138(11):1557–1562.
15. Abby Choke, Erick Wonggokusuma, Mun Chun Lai, Denny Lie. Clinical outcomes of an all-arthroscopic glenoid reconstruction using iliac crest bone graft with a double cannulated screw fixation technique. *Asia-Pac J Sports Med* 2021;24(3):41–48. doi: 10.1016/j.asmart.2021.01.002.

https://doi.org/10.1142/9789811249846_0009

Chapter 9

Arthroscopic Repair of Posterior Labral Tears

Denny T.T. Lie, Bryan Loh and Lim Mui Hong

Summary of Chapter

1. Introduction and epidemiology of posterior labral tears
2. Clinical presentation and examination
3. Pathophysiology and causes of posterior labral injuries
4. Diagnosis and imaging
5. Surgical technique of arthroscopic posterior labral repair in beach chair position
6. Surgical technique of arthroscopic posterior labral repair in lateral decubitus
7. Rehabilitation
8. Clinical outcomes

1. Introduction and Epidemiology of Problem

Posterior shoulder instability is a relatively rare cause of recurrent instability with its incidence at 2–10% [1–3]. It tends to affect athletes in contact sports (Rubgy/Football players) or those engaged in overhead sports [4].

2. Clinical Presentation

Symptoms reported by these individuals tend to be vague, ranging from deep seated posterior shoulder pain, weakness of the arm after overhead activity to generalised instability [1, 5]. In suspected cases of posterior shoulder instability, a thorough physical examination is important. To determine the extent and direction of instability, the following tests have been reported: Jerk test [6], Kim test [7], posterior apprehension test and the load and shift test [8] (see Chapter 1). Unlike its anterior counterpart, the posterior apprehension test is not as sensitive in detecting posterior shoulder instability [9]. Kim *et al.* found that a combination of the Kim test and Jerk test showed a 97% sensitivity in detecting posterior shoulder instability (Figs. 1 and 2) [7].

3. Pathophysiology of Problem

It is a result of either repetitive microtrauma, traumatic dislocations or subluxations and less commonly from seizure or electrocution injuries [8]. The most common cause is due to repetitive microtrauma or a posterior force directed towards the shoulder in the flexed, adducted and internal rotated position [10].

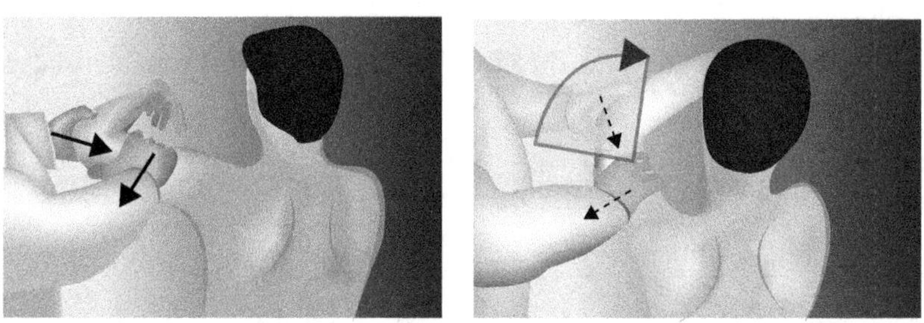

(a) (b)

Fig. 1: Kim test for posteroinferior instability, (a) the patient is first placed in a seated position and the arm abducted to 90° (b) The examiner cups the elbow with his left hand while applying an axial load to the elbow while his right hand applies a downward and posterior force to the upper arm. He then elevates the arm an additional 45° and a positive examination is represented by a clunk, click or pain expressed by the patient.

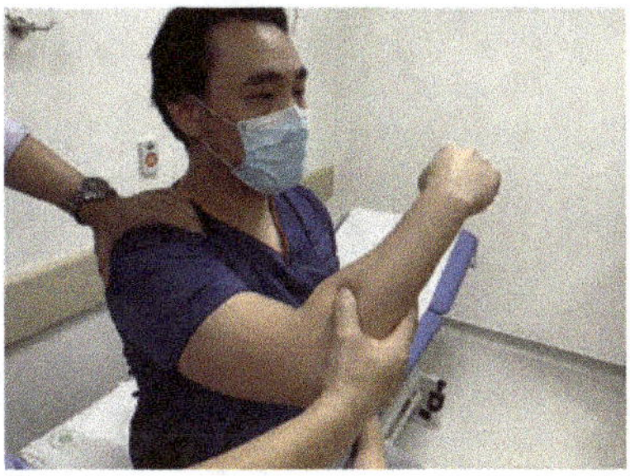

(a)

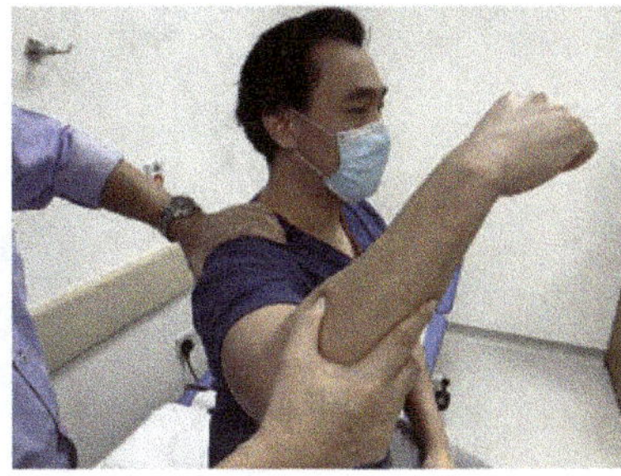

(b)

Fig. 2: Jerk test for posteroinferior instability. (a) The patient is seated upright with the arm in forward flexion, adduction and internal rotation. The examiner's right hand stabilises the shoulder girdle while his left hand applies a posterior-directed force along the humerus. (b) A positive examination is represented by a clunk, click or pain expressed by the patient as the humerus head relocates on the glenoid.

4. Diagnosis and Imaging

In terms of diagnostic imaging, a routine AP Xray of the shoulder may miss a posterior dislocation of the shoulder (Fig. 3(a)). A CT scan of the same patient shows the posteriorly dislocated humeral head (Fig. 3(b)). A Magnetic Resonance Imaging (MRI) is often adequate to detect abnormalities in the posterior capsulolabrum (reverse bankart lesion and Kim lesion) (Fig. 3(c)) as well as the presence of any concomitant reverse Hill-Sachs lesions [11]. Glenoid retroversion (15–17°), which has shown to be a significant risk factor for posterior shoulder instability [12, 13], can also be measured on MRI scan (Fig. 3(d)). In severe cases of instability, a CT scan may be useful in evaluating glenoid bone loss.

5. Arthroscopic Surgery

5.1 *Indications for Surgery*

- Symptomatic isolated posterior instability.
- Post traumatic posterior dislocations.
- Part of multi-directional stabilisations.
- Posterior instability post epilepsy are relative indications.

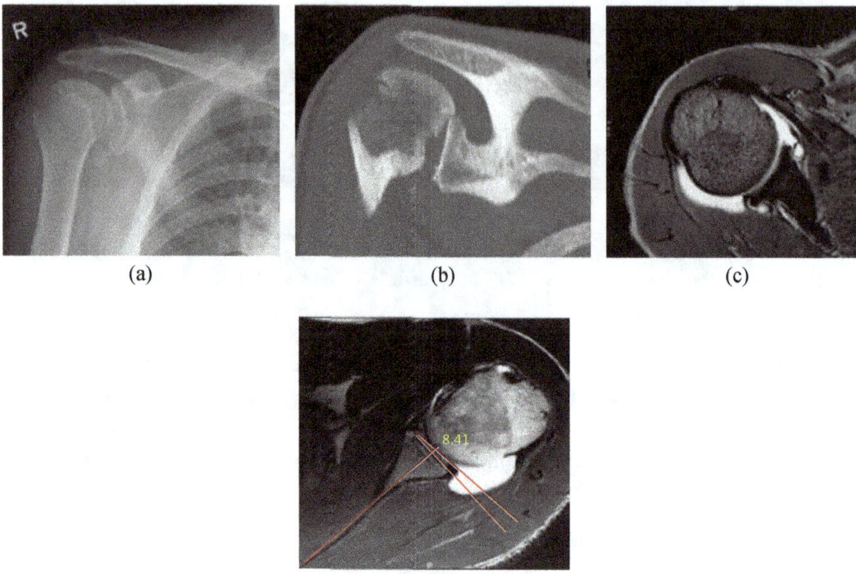

(a) (b) (c)

(d)

Fig. 3: (a) AP Xray of the shoulder of an elderly man who suffered an electric shock, may be passed off as unremarkable, missing the posterior dislocation. (b) CT scan evidently showed the posteriorly dislocated humeral head with a shallow reverse Hill Sachs lesion. (c) MRI showing the Kim lesion in the posterior labrum. (d) shows MRI axial cuts with measurement of the osseous glenoid version based on the criteria used by Kim *et al.* (Angle between the perpendicular drawn from the plane of scapula and the plane of the osseous portion of glenoid –8.41° anterior in this shoulder).

5.2 *Arthroscopic Repair of Posterior Labral Tears in Beach Chair Position*

Conventionally posterior labral repairs are performed with the patient in the lateral decubitus position. This technique is done in the beach chair position and increasingly more common and popular, as it enables anterior labral repair and conversion to open surgery.

- **Position:** Beach chair with the ipsilateral arm free to flex forwards and rotate.

- **Posterior portal:** The standard posterior portal is often described as 1 inch medial to and inferior to the postero-lateral corner of the acromion. For posterior labral repairs in the beach chair, the posterior portal is sited about 1 cm more **lateral**; this will bring its trajectory about 30°–45° oblique to the plane of the glenoid. *Too lateral will result in the trajectory hitting the humeral head and cannot enter the glenohumeral joint. Too medial will mean that the trajectory is parallel to the plane of the glenoid, and insertion of anchors is difficult.* The trajectory from the posterior portal must be oblique to the plane of the glenoid.
- **Antero-superior portal:** This is high in the rotator interval and is the main viewing portal.
- **Antero-inferior portal:** For posterior labral repairs this portal is more **medial** than the standard anterior labral repairs. It is above the subscapularis, in the plane of the glenoid, and is the suture management portal.
- **Optional postero-inferior (7 o'clock) portal:** This is established about 2 cm inferior to the posterior portal and it traverses the infraspinatus muscle. This is not commonly used and has a small risk of nerve injury.

(1) **Glenohumeral debridement, preparation of the posterior labrum.**
   - The glenohumeral joint is first viewed from the posterior portal as the relevant anterosuperior and anteroinferior portals are established. A 5 mm cannula is inserted in the anteroinferior portal.
   - A thorough inspection is first performed and synovitis debrided. It is not necessary to clear the rotator interval, only the synovitis that may block visualisation.
   - The camera is then switched to the anterosuperior portal where the posterior labrum can be clearly seen. *Remember to keep the plane of the glenoid vertical in front of the viewing camera.* The posterior portal is kept patent with a switching stick, over which an 8 mm cannula is inserted (Fig. 4).

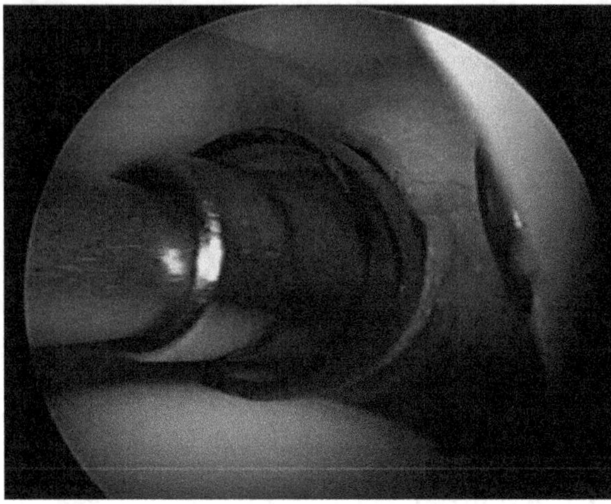

Fig. 4: Viewed from anterolateral portal, a cannula is inserted into the main working posterior portal.

- The posterior labrum is then debrided and its attachment to the glenoid rasped and roughened. The labrum needs to be mobilised so that it sits on top of the glenoid surface, at the posterior edge. *It should not be tethered to the posterior glenoid beneath the surface of the glenoid (ALPSA-like lesion).*

(2) **The low posterior anchor**

- From the posterior portal the drill is directed obliquely, to the posterior edge of the glenoid at about the 5 or 5:30 o'clock position (left shoulder) (Fig. 5).
- The anchor must be directed at about 45° angle oblique to the plane of the glenoid. *Too horizontal (a common mistake) and the anchor will run beneath the cartilage, causing a bump, damage the cartilage, and the anchor can easily be pulled off. Too vertical and the anchor can skive off the posterior glenoid as the posterior vault of the glenoid slopes away sharply.*
- A double loaded suture anchor is recommended (Gryphon BR 4 mm) (Fig. 6). One limb of both blue and purple sutures are then

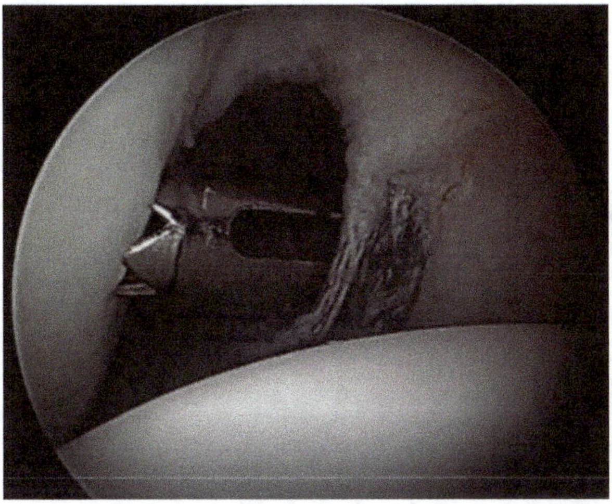

Fig. 5: A drill guide is placed at the posterior glenoid edge, at about 45° to the surface.

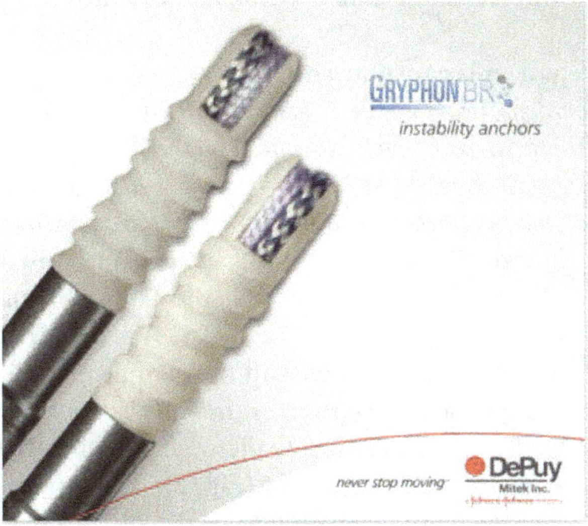

Fig. 6: The dual-loaded Gryphon anchor is usually used for the labral repair.

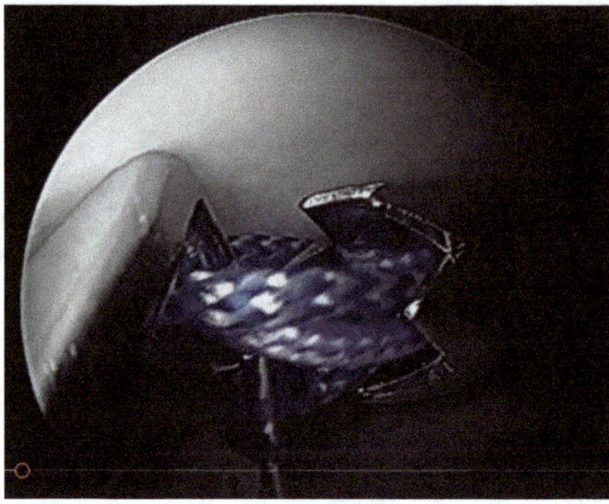

Fig. 7: One limb from each suture pair is retrieved to the antero-inferior portal.

retrieved to the antero-inferior cannula, separated and parked there (Fig. 7).

(3) **Labral repair and capsular shift**

Conceptually, one pair of sutures is tasked with tying the posterior labrum and shifting the posteroinferior capsule and the posterior IGHL superiorly. The other pair is used to tie the posterior labrum and to shift the lateral capsule medially, thereby closing the posterior portal.

(3.1) **First pair of sutures (shifting the capsule superiorly)**

- The cannula is withdrawn slightly to enable the soft tissue rim of the portal to be seen. The Acupass (70° straight) is then passed behind the soft tissue of the portal and directed along posterior labrum, *outside of the capsule*, from about the 8 o'clock position, to pierce and re-enter the joint space at the 6 o'clock position (Fig. 8). *It is important **NOT** to dive deep inferiorly blindly, as the nerves are nearby. Keep the Acupass suture passer just beneath the capsule. To further prevent nerve injury, apply a gentle traction on the arm inferiorly.*
- The monofilament delivered is retrieved from the anteroinferior portal, and one limb of the purple pair of sutures is then shuttled (Fig. 9). Tying the knot (outside of the

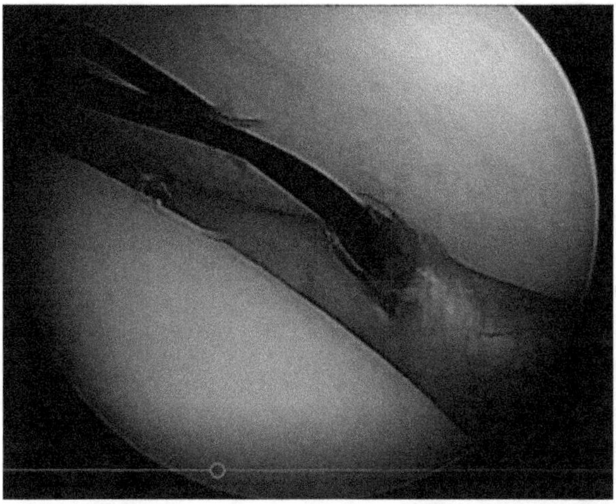

Fig. 8: A suture passer takes a bite of the labrum and the posteroinferior capsule.

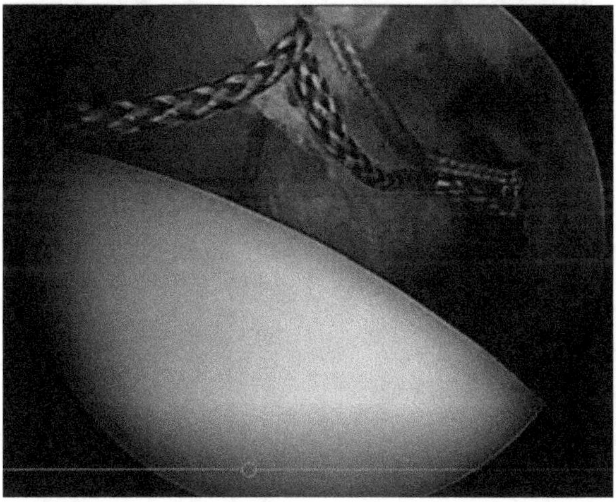

Fig. 9: The purple suture is shuttled through to tent and pull the inferior capsule upwards.

capsule) will hitch up the posteroinferior capsule and posterior IGHL superiorly, creating an inferior-superior shift (Fig. 10). This is done with the arm in neutral rotation, that is, facing forwards.

Note: tying this knot may partially occlude the posterior portal, but it is patent enough to complete the repair.

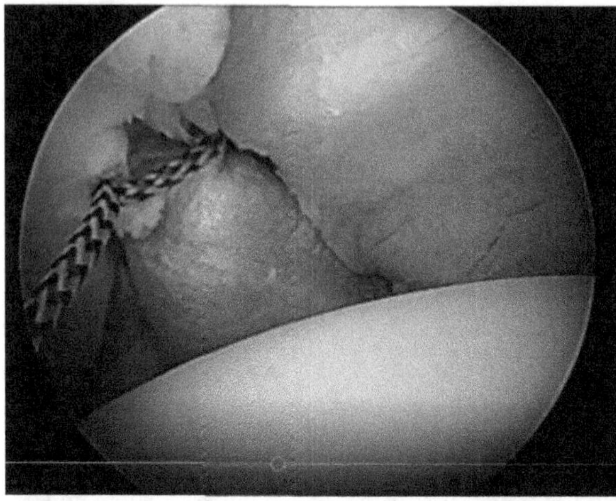

Fig. 10: Tying the purple suture achieves a significant inferior capsular shift upwards.

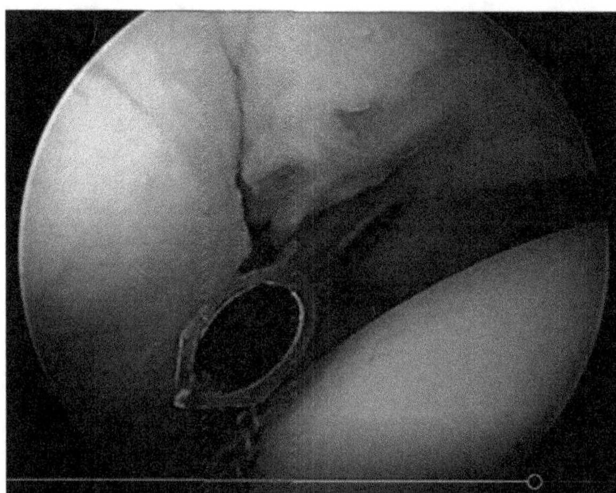

Fig. 11: The suture passer then takes a bite of the posterolateral capsule.

(3.2) **Second pair of sutures (shifting the capsule medially)**

- With the cannula partially withdrawn, the Acupass suture passer is now passed laterally, outside the capsule, to pierce and re-enter the joint space about 2–3 cm lateral to the portal (Fig. 11). The filament is then retrieved from the

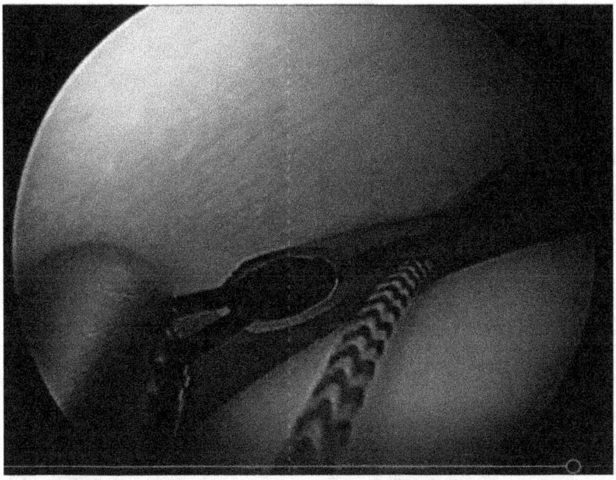

Fig. 12: The monofilament is retrieved to the anterosuperior portal.

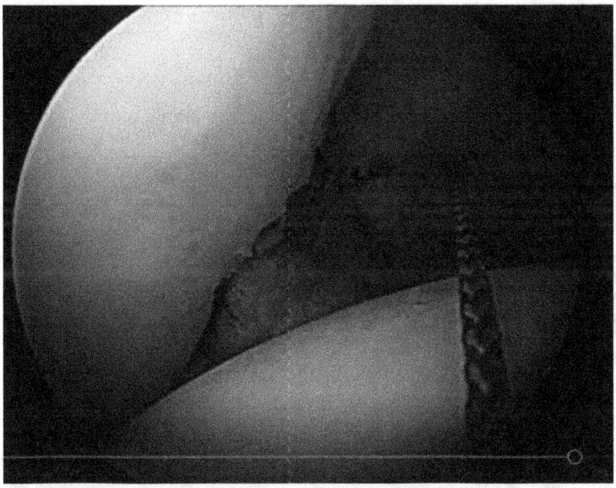

Fig. 13: The blue suture is then shuttled through.

anteroinferior portal and the limb of the blue pair of sutures shuttled (Figs. 12 and 13).

- The knot is tied with the arm in neutral rotation (Fig. 14). This will not only create a significant medial-lateral capsular shift, but will also close the posterior portal (Fig. 15).

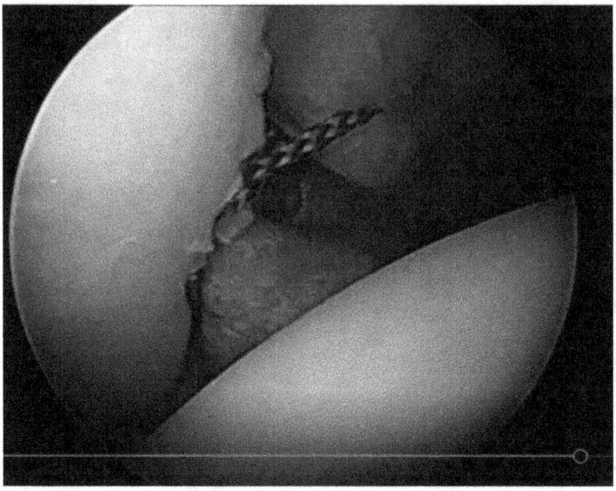

Fig. 14: Tying the blue suture tightens the posterolateral capsule medially, effecting a significant medial shift.

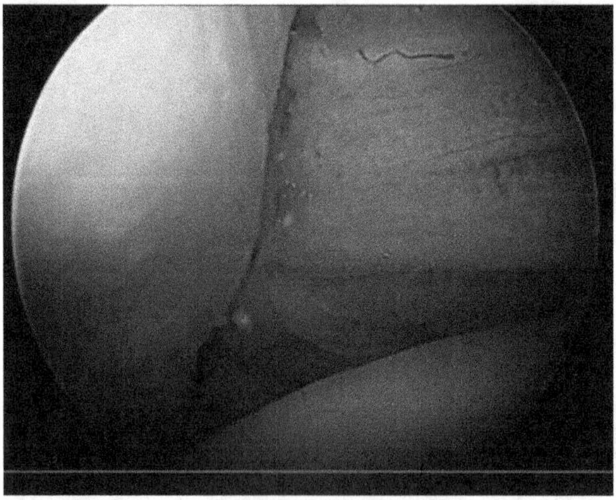

Fig. 15: The labral repair and a significant inferior and lateral capsular shift is achieved.

5.2.1 *The additional mid posterior anchor*

A second anchor can be used, delivered via the same posterior portal. In the author's opinion, this is seldom needed. The second anchor is positioned at the 9–10 o'clock position (right shoulder), a single-loaded 4 mm

Gryphon anchor is adequate. One limb of the suture is retrieved behind the labrum and the sutures tied over the labrum using a sliding knot or any knotting technique of choice.

5.3 *Arthroscopic Repair of Posterior Labral Tear in Lateral Decubitus Position*

The advantage of the lateral decubitus position for posterior labral repair is the increase in the posterior glenohumeral space working space with the traction on the shoulder. In addition, the lateral decubitus position also permit access to manage anterior and superior labral tears as well as cuff lesions.

- **Position:** The patient is placed on a lateral decubitus position and the shoulder is secured on a standard lateral traction kit with 10 lbs of traction. The shoulder joint is positioned at 15° of forward flexion and 30° of abduction.
- **Viewing portals:** Posterior portal and anterior superior portal.
- **Working portals:** Posterolateral portal and mid anterior portal.
  (1) **Visualisation and creation of portals**
    - The standard posterior viewing portal is created and the initial assessment of the glenohumeral joint is performed.
    - Once the lesion is localised, the anterior superior and mid anterior working portals are created. A 5 mm cannula is inserted over the anterior superior portal and an 8 mm cannula is inserted over the mid anterior portal.

  (2) **Preparation of the posterior labrum**
    - A switching stick is inserted into the posterior viewing portal and arthroscopy is switched to the anterior superior portal. The anterior superior portal allows the visualisation of the posterior labral lesion.
    - The intra-articular position of the posterolateral portal is located with a spinal needle. For surface marking, it is located 1 cm lateral and 1 cm inferior to the posterior tip of the acromion. The direction of the spinal needle should have mobility

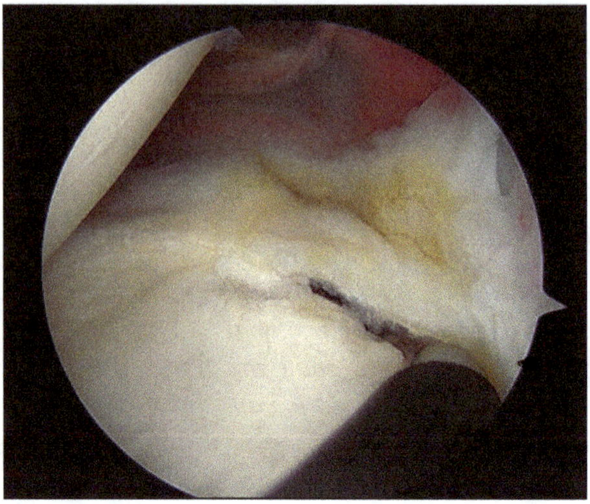

Fig. 16: Preparation of Posterior labral tear of the right shoulder in the lateral decubitus position (viewing portal: anterior superior, working portal: mid anterior).

to access the labral lesion and insertion of the suture anchor. The anchor must be directed at about 45° angle oblique to the plane of the glenoid.

- An 8 mm cannula is inserted over the posterolateral portal.
- The posterior labrum lesion is mobilised and debrided in preparation for repair (Fig. 16). Posterior labral tear is commonly associated with paralabral cyst. This should be decompressed as part of the debridement.

(3) **Choice of suture anchor**

- The posterior labrum has a lower volume compared to anterior labrum. The aim of the repair is to reattach the labrum and decompress associated paralabral cyst.
- Single loaded pre knotted anchor, e.g. Mitek Proknot or double loaded anchor, e.g. Mitek Gryphon may be used. The single loaded suture anchor is suitable for small tear. The double loaded anchor allows two points of repair.

(4) **Repair technique**

- Depending of the preference of the surgeon, suture passing may be achieved with the use of a bird peak passer or monofilament suture passer.

- **Bird Beak Passer:** Following insertion of the single loaded pre knotted suture anchor, a bird beak passer is inserted through the posterolateral portal to penetrate the labrum and retrieve the post limb of the suture to the posterior surface of the labrum. The knot is tied to complete the repair.
- **Monofilament suture passer:** After insertion of the suture anchor, the sutures are retrieved to the mid anterior portal with a suture retriever. The monofilament suture passer (45° right for right shoulder) is inserted into the posterolateral working portal to penetrate the posterior labrum. The monofilament loop is retrieved to the mid anterior portal and one limb of the post suture is shuttled though the posterior labrum. The corresponding limb of the suture is retrieved back through the posteolateral portal and the knot is tied to complete the repair. The second set of suture is similarly managed to enable repair with two sets of interrupted sutures (Fig. 17).

(5) **Extended labral repair**

- **SLAP repair:** The anterior superior portal and mid anterior portal are used as the working portals. The standard posterior portal is used as the viewing portal.

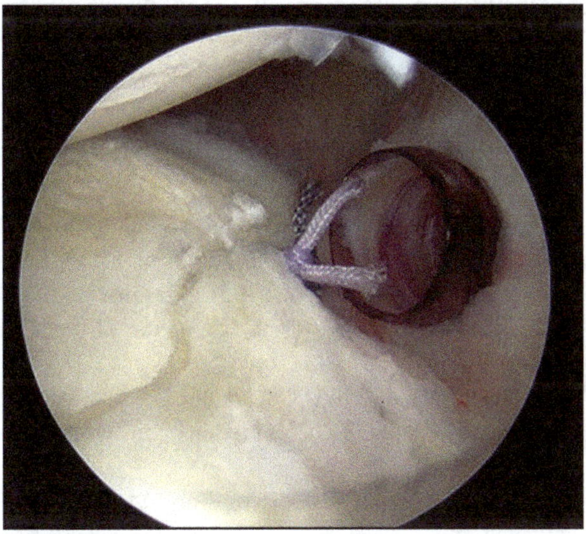

Fig. 17: Posterior labrum repair with a double loaded suture anchor.

- **Anterior labrum repair:** The anterior superior and mid anterior portals are used as the working portal. The standard posterior portal is used as the viewing portal.

6. Post-op Management and Rehabilitation

All patients are placed in a gunslinger brace and started on pendulum exercises in the immediate postoperative period. The brace is discontinued at 4 weeks and active shoulder ROM is started. Strengthening exercises are started at 2–3 months after surgery. Patients are permitted to return to sporting activities at 4–6 months of rehabilitation after they are achieved full ROM and enough strength.

7. Outcomes

In a mini-series review of nine shoulders with capsulolabral injury in eight patients, all patients underwent arthroscopic posterior capsulolabral reconstruction in the beach-chair position. There was significant improvement in UCLA scores (18.4 vs 29.8) ($P = 0.001$), Oxford Shoulder Score (37.8 vs 16.1) ($P < 0.001$) and VAS score (3.9 vs 1.3) ($P = 0.017$) at 2 years postoperatively. There was improvement in Range of motion (Forward flexion and abduction), Isometric strength and Constant Shoulder Scores, though not statistically significant.

References

1. Provencher MT, Bhatia S, Ghodadra NS, *et al.* Recurrent shoulder instability: Current concepts for evaluation and management of glenoid bone loss. *J Bone Joint Surg Am* 2010;92(Suppl) 2:133–151. doi:10.2106/JBJS.J.00906.
2. Boyd HB, Sisk TD. Recurrent posterior dislocation of the shoulder. *J Bone Joint Surg Am* 1972;54(4):779–786.
3. Lenart BA, Sherman SL, Mall NA, Gochanour E, Twigg SL, Nicholson GP. Arthroscopic repair for posterior shoulder instability. 2012. doi:10.1016/j.arthro.2012.03.011.
4. Owens BD, Duffey ML, Nelson BJ, DeBerardino TM, Taylor DC, Mountcastle SB. The incidence and characteristics of shoulder instability at the United

States Military Academy. *Am J Sports Med* 2007;35(7):1168–1173. doi:10.1177/0363546506295179.

5. Neer CS. Involuntary inferior and multidirectional instability of the shoulder: etiology, recognition, and treatment. *Instr Course Lect* 1985;34:232–238.
6. Kim SH, Park JC, Park JS, Oh I. Painful jerk test: A predictor of success in nonoperative treatment of posteroinferior instability of the shoulder. *Am J Sports Med* 2004;32(8):1849–1855. doi:10.1177/0363546504265263.
7. Kim SH, Park JS, Jeong WK, Shin SK. The Kim test: A novel test for posteroinferior labral lesion of the shoulder — A comparison to the Jerk test. *Am J Sports Med* 2005;33(8):1188–1192. doi:10.1177/0363546504272687.
8. Millett PJ, Clavert P, Hatch GFR, Warner JJP. Recurrent posterior shoulder instability. *J Am Acad Orthop Surg* 2006;14(8):464–476. doi:10.5435/00124635-200608000-00004.
9. Schwartz E, Warren RF, O'Brien SJ, Fronek J. Posterior shoulder instability. *Orthop Clin North Am* 1987;18(3):409–419.
10. Robinson CM, Aderinto J. Current concepts review: Recurrent posterior shoulder instability. *J Bone Jt Surg — Ser A* 2005;87(4):883–892. doi:10.2106/JBJS.D.02906.
11. Liu F, Cheng X, Dong J, *et al.* Imaging modality for measuring the presence and extent of the labral lesions of the shoulder: A systematic review and meta-analysis. *BMC Musculoskelet Disord* 2019;20(1):487. doi:10.1186/s12891-019-2876-2876.
12. Privitera DM, Siegel EJ, Miller LR, Sinz NJ, Higgins LD. Glenoid version and its relationship to glenohumeral instability and labral tears. *J Shoulder Elb Surg* 2016;25(7):1056–1063. doi:10.1016/j.jse.2015.11.013.
13. Gottschalk MB, Ghasem A, Todd D, Daruwalla J, Xerogeanes J, Karas S. Posterior shoulder instability: Does glenoid retroversion predict recurrence and contralateral instability? *Arthrosc — J Arthrosc Relat Surg* 2015;31(3):488–493. doi:10.1016/j.arthro.2014.10.009.

https://doi.org/10.1142/9789811249846_0010

Chapter 10

Arthroscopic Repairs of Superior Labral (SLAP) Tears

Denny T.T. Lie, Thomas Kuo and Zhu Meng

Summary of Chapter

1. Introduction and epidemiology of SLAP injuries
2. Clinical presentation of SLAP injuries
3. Pathophysiology of SLAP pathologies
4. Diagnosis and imaging, approach
5. Surgical technique of arthroscopic SLAP repair
6. Rehabilitation
7. Clinical outcomes

1. Introduction and Epidemiology of SLAP Tears

Andrew *et al.* [1] first described tears of the superior labrum in a series of 73 overhead athletes undergoing arthroscopy for shoulder pain. The first classification system of these lesions was established by Snyder *et al.* [2] in 1990, characterising SLAP lesions into Types I–IV; this system was further expanded in 1995 to include Types V–VII by Maffet *et al.* [3].

Superior labral tears tend to occur in the younger age groups, between 20–29-year-olds and 40–49-year-olds [4], and more often in overhead athletes [5]. SLAP tears account for about 6% of all shoulder arthroscopic procedures performed [2]. Out of 61 labral repairs performed in a study, 16 out of 61 (26%) were type 2 SLAP tears and 19 out of 61 (31%) were type 5 SLAP tears [6].

2. Clinical Presentation

Patients often describe a deep aching pain after a pull or jerk, usually with the arm in the overhead position. The persistent pain may be associated with a pop or clicking sensation. This injury may also occur in the athlete after repetitive overhead throws. Active range of motion of the shoulder is frequently preserved. Atrophy of the infraspinatus muscle can be found in patients who develop a spinoglenoid cyst in association with the SLAP tear. Overhead athletes with symptomatic SLAP lesions report loss of throwing velocity, control, and power during the late cocking and early acceleration phase; these patients also frequently have associated pain with the throwing motion.

On examination, tenderness may be elicited over the long head of the biceps tendon. Occasionally, subluxation of the biceps tendon may be provoked by internally and externally rotating the arm. Speed's and Yergason's tests may be sensitive but are not particularly specific for SLAP injuries. The O'Brien test (see Chapter 1) is usually used to clinically diagnose or suspect a SLAP injury, although the specificity is 61% [7].

3. Pathophysiology of Problem

SLAP injuries could be due to an acute trauma, chronic attrition or degenerative in origin. Acute traumatic mechanisms include direct compression injury to a forward flexed shoulder, for example when falling on outstretched arm; or traction injuries to the biceps when the humeral head is inferiorly subluxed, for example when attempting to lift a heavy load. The extent of the tear could be predominantly at the posterior part of the superior labrum (most common), anterior part, or equally, extending anterior to posterior.

Several mechanisms have been proposed to explain the aetiology of SLAP tears. Burkhart *et al.* [8] described dynamic peel-back of the posterosuperior labrum due to the increased torsional forces at the bicep root when the shoulder is in a maximum abduction-external rotated position. This is accompanied by posterior glenohumeral capsule contracture, which causes a biomechanical cascade in overhead athletes, resulting in peel-back SLAP tears. SLAP tears have also been proposed to result from repeated internal impingement — where the posterosuperior rotator cuff is pinched between the greater tuberosity and the posterosuperior glenoid labrum when the shoulder is in a position of 90 degrees abduction and 90 degrees external rotation. Tensile overload at the superior labral insertion due to eccentric bicep contraction in the follow through phase of pitching is also a suggested cause of SLAP tears.

4. Diagnosis and Imaging, Algorithm

MRI and MR arthrography (Fig. 1) are the imaging of choice to clearly visualise the SLAP injury. Variations in superior labral anatomy visible on the MRI in the asymptomatic overhead athlete are common enough that caution should be exercised before concluding that the SLAP injury is the sole cause of the shoulder pain [9]. Age-stratified approaches to treatment of SLAP tears are shown in Figs. 2 and 3.

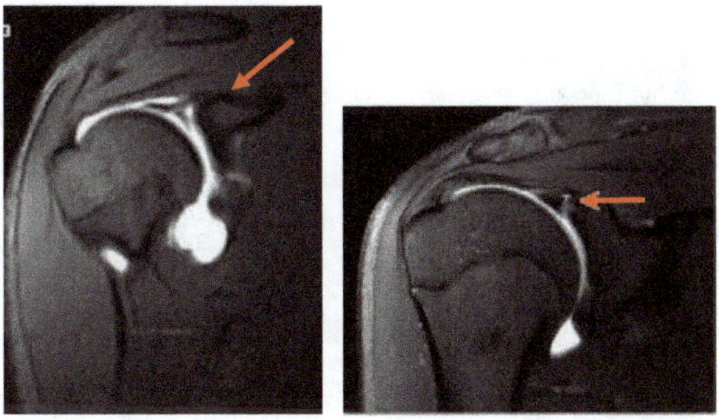

(a) (b)

Fig. 1: MRI images of SLAP tears. (a) An MR arthrogram which shows a SLAP tear possibly type 2. (b) Type 1 degenerate superior labrum.

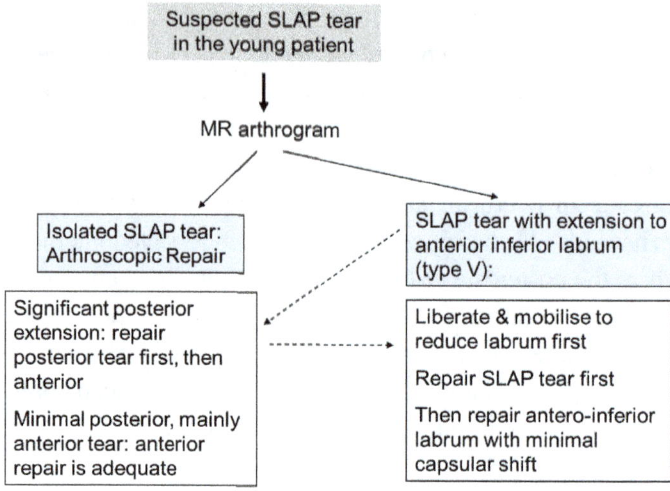

Fig. 2: Algorithm of treatment plan in the young patient. In isolated SLAP tears, the posterior part of the SLAP is repaired first, then anterior. In type V with extension to the anterior labrum, the SLAP tear is repaired first, then the anterior labrum.

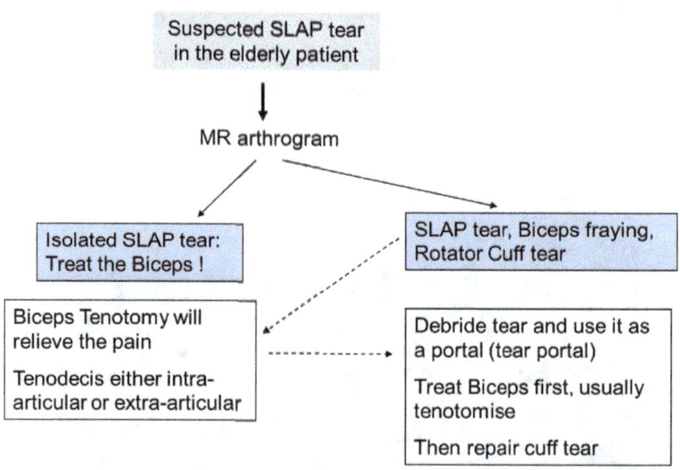

Fig. 3: Algorithm of treatment plan in the elderly patient. In isolated SLAP tears, the biceps tendon is either tenotomised or tenodesed. SLAP tears in the elderly usually occur with cuff tears.

5. Arthroscopic Repair of the Superior Labral (SLAP) Tears

(a) Position and Portals
Position: Beach chair
Portals:

- **Viewing/working portal:** Posterior.
- **Antero-superior portal:** This is placed high in the rotator interval, just beside the origin of the long head of the biceps tendon, at the junction of the biceps and superior labrum. Often the torn superior labrum may overhang and droop, or extensive fraying and inflammation may make visualisation difficult. *It is critical that this portal placement would permit the cannula (and hence instruments and anchors) to be positioned both anterior and posterior to the biceps tendon.* Then insert an 8.5 mm cannula.
- **Antero-inferior portal:** This is placed in the rotator interval to facilitate suture passing. An 8.mm cannula is also used here.
- **Alternative Nevaisier portal:** This is inserted from the junction of the inner borders of the spine of scapula and lateral acromion. The needle is directed inwards to the glenohumeral joint. This portal is useful to establish anchors at the superior edge of glenoid, and is often used during Superior Capsular Reconstruction rather than during SLAP repairs.
- **Optional Wilmington portal:** This portal is from the postero-lateral edge of the acromion directed to the joint and traverses the muscular portion of the supraspinatus-infraspinatus border. The author does not encourage its use as it may cause musculotendinous junction tears.

(b) **Inspection of biceps and superior labrum**
- The biceps tendon is immediately evident as the glenohumeral joint space is entered. Using a probe from the anterior portal, the insertion of the long head of the biceps at the superior labrum is lifted and checked.
- Assess for complete detachment of the superior labrum from the glenoid, look out for fraying, overhanging labrum and bucket-handle tears. Assess the extent of the tear from the base of the

biceps origin, and its progression anteriorly or posteriorly. Most SLAP tears have a posterior extension. Some extent anteriorly and then progresses inferiorly to become type V SLAP tears.

- It is recommended to place two anchors; one posterior and another anterior to the biceps tendon, unless the posterior extension is minimal. In type V tears it is the observation of the author that the posterior extension is usually limited, hence there is no need to stabilise the superior labrum posterior to the biceps origin in such cases.

(c) **Debriding the superior and anterior labrum (in type V)**

- The rasp is inserted from the antero-superior portal and the attachment of the superior labrum to the superior glenoid is then rasped and roughened (Fig. 4(a)). If the rasp does not easily enter this supra-glenoid space, re-consider the need for a repair as it may be a type 1 tear, in which case in the author's opinion, surgery may not be necessary.
- In type V tears, it is important to debride and mobilise the antero-inferior labrum prior to repairing the SLAP tear. *Failure to do so will limit the anatomical reduction and repair of the superior labrum, as the antero-inferior labrum is tethered down.*

(d) **The posterior anchor**

- Flip the antero-superior cannula over the biceps so that it is directed obliquely to the superior edge of the glenoid, *posterior to* the biceps tendon.

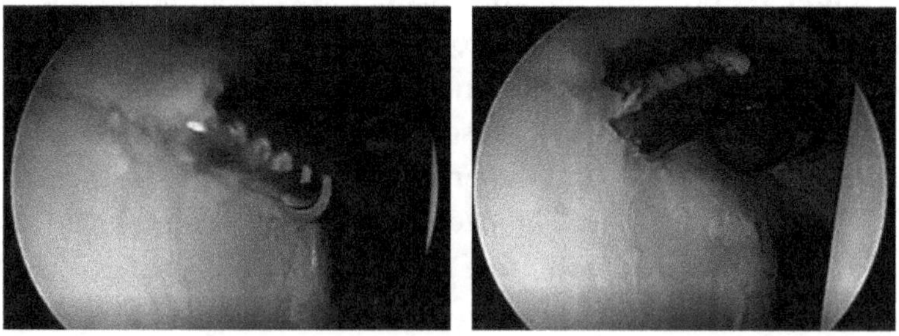

(a) (b)

Fig. 4: Preparation: (a) A shaver from the antero-superior portal debriding the superior labrum and roughening the surface. (b) Gryphon anchor is placed just posterior to the biceps origin.

- Use the cannula to sweep the labrum up to reduce it to its anatomical origins. The drill and awl should be directed about 45° to the plane of the glenoid, at the edge of the glenoid; then place an anchor (Gryphon ProKnot anchor) (Fig. 4(b)). *Be careful when inserting the anchor; if the guide is too horizontal the anchor will skive off the back of the glenoid as the vault of the glenoid slopes down. If the guide is too vertical, there is danger the anchor will be in the weak subchondral bone, it can be seen as a bulge beneath the cartilage and will easily break off when the suture is pulled.*
- Separate the sutures of the anchor, tug on the sutures first to identify the loose suture (the other suture limb being attached to the plastic suture board). Use a suture retriever from the antero-inferior portal to retrieve and bring the loose suture to the antero-inferior portal (Fig. 5(a)).

(e) **Securing the posterior SLAP**

- A suture passer (70° straight Acupass) is inserted from the antero-superior portal. Withdraw the cannula slightly without letting it slip into the soft tissues. A large bite of the superior labrum just posterior to the biceps tendon is taken by the Acupass (Fig. 5(b)) and the monofilament retrieved from the antero-inferior portal (Fig. 5(c)).
- The looped monofilament is then used to shuttle the loose suture from the Gryphon Pro-knot anchor, through the superior labrum and to the antero-superior portal.

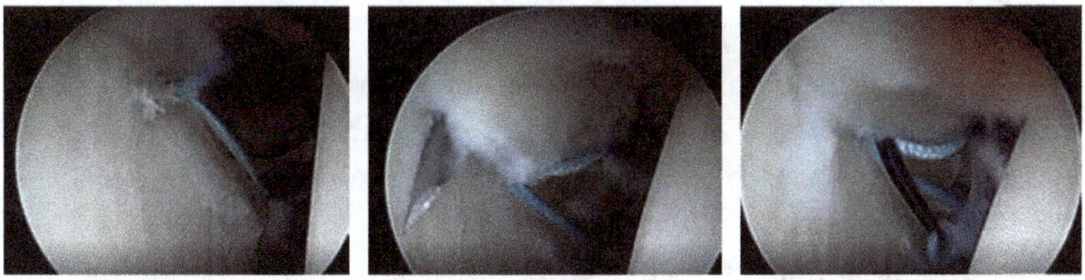

(a) (b) (c)

Fig. 5: The posterior SLAP: (a) Separation of the sutures, the loose limb being shuttled to the antero-inferior portal. (b) Acupass suture passer takes a bite of the posterior SLAP. (c) A monofilament is used to shuttle the loose suture limb from the Gryphon anchor through the posterior SLAP.

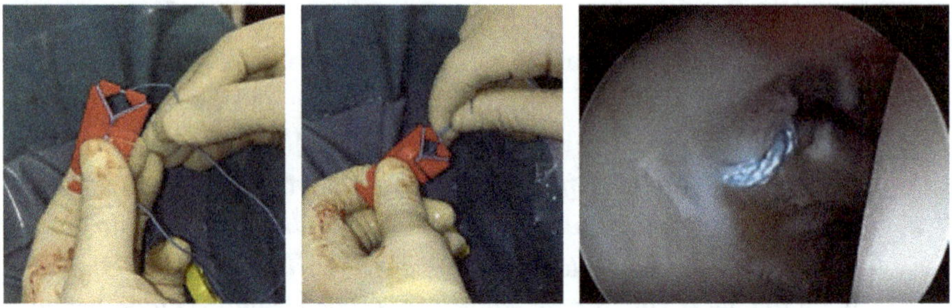

(a) (b) (c)

Fig. 6: The ProKnot sliding knot. Outside the shoulder the loose suture limb is passed through the kite of the suture board, shown in (a) and tugged sharply in (b), to create a sliding knot. This is then passed down and tied firmly onto the posterior SLAP. (c) The tied sutures just posterior to the biceps origin.

- The loose suture is then passed through the loop on the suture board outside the shoulder (Figs. 6(a) and 6(b)) and the ProKnot sliding knot passed down (Fig. 6(c)). As the knot is delivered in, direct the antero-superior cannula medially, above and medial to the superior labrum so that the knot is delivered away from the articulating surface of the glenoid.
- Separate the sutures of the anchor and tighten individually. Then secure the knot by delivering two half-hitch knots.

(f) **Repairing the anterior SLAP**

- Flip the antero-superior cannula back to its original position anterior to the biceps tendon. In a similar way, place an anchor about 7–10 mm anterior to the biceps tendon, at about 45° to the plane of the glenoid (Fig. 7(a)).
- Separate the sutures and retrieve the loose suture to the antero-inferior portal (Fig. 7(b)). Then use an Acupass from the antero-superior portal to take another bite of the superior labrum, anterior to the biceps (Fig. 8(a)).
- The monofilament is passed to the antero-inferior portal, there to shuttle the loose suture back to the antero-superior portal. Prepare the synch knot and deliver to the anterior SLAP, ensuring the knot stays away from the articulating glenoid surface (Fig. 8(b)). Secure it by passing two half-hitch sutures (Fig. 9).

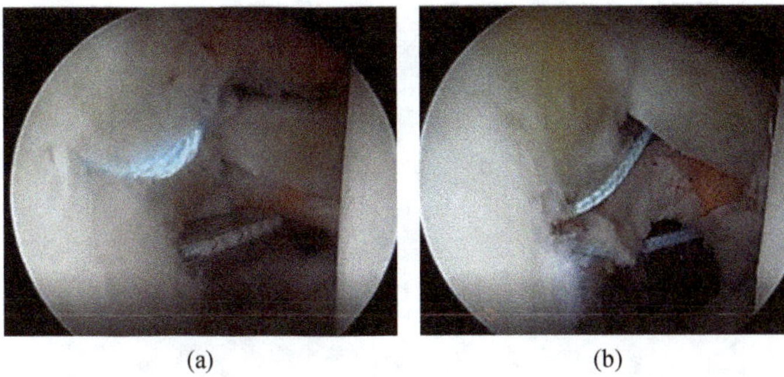

Fig. 7: The anterior SLAP. (a) Shows another Gryphon Pro-knot anchor being inserted about 7–10 mm anterior to the biceps origin. (b) The sutures are then separated and the loose suture limb passed to the antero-inferior portal.

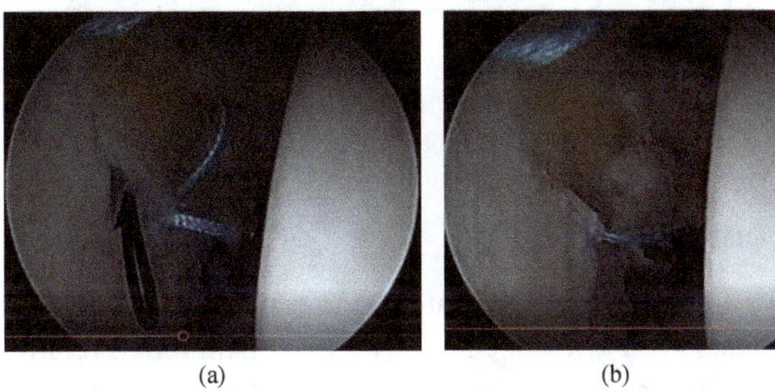

Fig. 8: Tying the anterior SLAP. (a) Acupass taking a bite of the superior labrum anterior to the biceps origin, to shuttle the loose suture limb. (b) A knot is prepared and passed down to secure and tie the anterior portion of the SLAP.

6. Post-op Management and Rehabilitation

Patients are kept in an arm-sling for the first 2 weeks only, during which they are permitted passive ROM as tolerated. From weeks 3 to 6, overhead movements like forward flexion and abduction are discouraged, only internal and external rotation are continued. This prevents excessive traction on the SLAP repair. From week 6 onwards, active ROM is gradually increased, and strengthening as well, till about week 12. Overhead sports is permitted usually between 4 and 6 months after surgery.

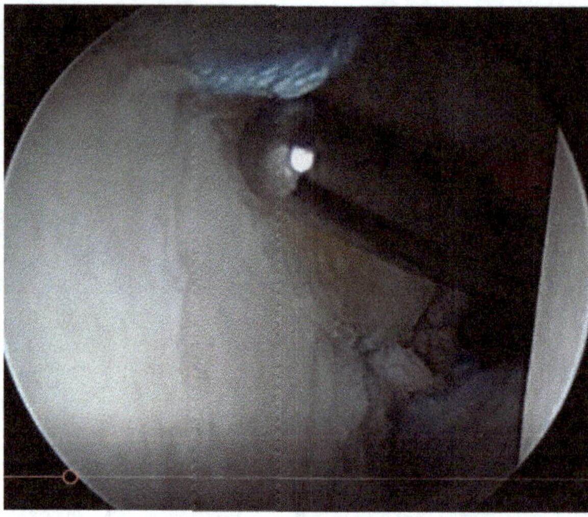

Fig. 9: Inspecting the superior labrum. The superior labrum is thus secured with Gryphon anchors anterior and posterior to the biceps anchor. It shows a probe from the antero-superior portal assessing the stability of the repair.

7. Outcomes

Overall, SLAP repair provides satisfactory clinical outcomes. Repair of the SLAP tears has been associated with good pain relief, return of function and high patient satisfaction. Prospective studies by Brockmeier [10] and Friel [11] reported favourable outcomes in 87% and 79% of patients, respectively. These results were similar to previous studies, reporting success rates of 90–98% [12–13]. However, the proportion of patients who were able to return-to-sports (RTS) at pre-injury level were lower — ranging from 22% to 84% in the same studies.

In our study, after a 2-year follow-up of 16 patients aged from 22 to 35 year-old who had undergone a SLAP repair [6], the majority (88%) had improvement of pain on the affected shoulder after the surgery. Shoulder ranges of motion improved from 129° (interquartile range, 113–140°) to 139° (125–144°) in forward flexion, and from 117° (86–137°) to 136° (96–147°) in abduction. Shoulder function scores such as UCLA shoulder score and Constant shoulder score improved significantly after surgery. Oxford Shoulder Instability Score, with a score range from 12 to 60 and lower score indicating a better outcome, is a widely employed self-reported outcome measurement for patients with shoulder instability. The median Oxford Shoulder Instability Score for those underwent the SLAP repair improved from 28 (24–39) to 14 (12–19), with one third of the patients achieved the best score. The SLAP repair surgery has met 81% of patients' expectations.

Similar results were observed for 19 patients who had a type V SLAP tear, in their re-dislocation rate, pain relief, as well as shoulder ranges of motion 2-year after arthroscopic repair. Oxford Shoulder Instability Score for these patients improved from 33 (29–42) to 18 (15–24), marginally higher in the absolute scores but similar in the improvement of scores, when compared to the previous group. This could be due to the more extensive tear of the labrum.

References

1. Andrews JR, Carson WG, Jr., McLeod WD. Glenoid labrum tears related to the long head of the biceps. *Am J Sports Med* 1985;13(5):337–341.
2. Snyder SJ, Karzel RP, Del Pizzo W, Ferkel RD, Friedman MJ. SLAP lesions of the shoulder. *Arthroscopy* 1990;6(4):274–279.
3. Maffet MW, Gartsman GM, Moseley B. Superior labrum-biceps tendon complex lesions of the shoulder. *Am J Sports Med* 1995;23(1):93–98.
4. Zhang AL, Kreulen C, Ngo SS, Hame SL, Wang JC, Gamradt SC. Demographic trends in arthroscopic SLAP repair in the United States. *Am J Sports Med* 2012 May;40(5):1144–1147.
5. Miniaci A, Mascia AT, Salonen DC, Becker EJ. Magnetic resonance imaging of the shoulder in asymptomatic professional baseball pitchers. *Am J Sports Med* 2002;30(1):66–73.
6. Meng Zhu, Jerry Yongqiang Chen, Hwei Chi Chong, Paul Chang Chee Cheng and Denny Lie Tijauw Tjoen. Comparative study on clinical results of arthroscopic repair of anteroinferior, superior, and combined glenoid labral tear. *J Orthop Surg* 2018;26(1):1–6.
7. Ben Kibler W, Sciascia AD, Hester P, Dome D, Jacobs C. Clinical utility of traditional and new tests in the diagnosis of biceps tendon injuries and superior labrum anterior and posterior lesions in the shoulder. *Am J Sports Med* 2009;37(9):1840–1847.
8. Burkhart SS, Morgan CD. The peel-back mechanism: its role in producing and extending posterior type II SLAP lesions and its effect on SLAP repair rehabilitation. *Arthroscopy* 1998;14(6):637–640.

9. Mathew CJ, Lintner DM. Superior labral anterior to posterior tear management in athletes. *Open Orthop J* 2018;12:303–313.
10. Brockmeier SF, Voos JE, Williams RJ, 3rd, Altchek DW, Cordasco FA, Allen AA. Outcomes after arthroscopic repair of type-II SLAP lesions. *J Bone Joint Surg Am* 2009;91(7):1595–1603.
11. Nicole A. Friel, Vasili Karas, Mark A. Slabaugh, Brian J. Cole. Outcomes of type II superior labrum, anterior to posterior (SLAP) repair: Prospective evaluation at a minimum two-year follow-up. *J Shoulder & Elbow Surg* 2010;19(6):859–867. doi.org/10.1016/j.jse.2010.03.004.
12. Ide J, Maeda S, Takagi K. Sports activity after arthroscopic superior labral repair using suture anchors in overhead-throwing athletes. *Am J Sports Med* 2005;33:507–514.
13. Kim SH, Ha KI, Kim SH, Choi HJ. Results of arthroscopic treatment of superior labral lesions. *JBJS Am* 2002;84:981–985.

https://doi.org/10.1142/9789811249846_0011

Chapter 11

Arthroscopic Biceps Tenotomy and Tenodesis

Denny T.T. Lie and Don Koh

Summary of Chapter

1. Introduction and epidemiology of LHBT pathologies
2. Clinical presentation of LHBT injuries
3. Pathophysiology of LHBT pathologies
4. Diagnosis and imaging, approach
5. Surgical technique of arthroscopic biceps tenotomy
6 Surgical technique of arthroscopic biceps tenodesis
7. Rehabilitation
8. Clinical outcomes

1. Introduction and Epidemiology

The long head of the biceps brachii tendon (LHBT) has been recognised as pain generator in the shoulder for almost three centuries. However, there has been inconsistent interest owing to uncertainty of its role around the shoulder. Recent advancements in imaging as well as a renewed interest in its function and histological changes have shed greater insight into LHBT tendinopathies. LHBT tendinopathies encompass a spectrum of pathologies — tenosynovitis, tendinosis, partial tear to complete ruptures.

LBHT pathologies rarely occur in isolation [1]. Isolated LHBT subluxation has been reported in a select group — mainly affecting the throwing arm of younger athletes participating in overhead throwing sports (for example javelin throwers, baseball pitchers, quarterbacks in football). 60% to 76% of rotator cuff tears have associated LHBT pathology [2]. More recently, Murthi and colleagues reported that in macroscopically degenerate LHBT, up to 91% of patients had concomitant rotator cuff tears [3].

2. Clinical Presentation

Anterior shoulder pain is a common complaint, due to the rich network of sensory sympathetic fibres that innervate the tendon [4]. The pain can be reproduced at the bicipital grove and may radiate down the bicep muscle belly. In patients with LHBT tenosynovitis, anterior shoulder pain can be provoked through shoulder extension or internal rotation and these patients often demonstrate positive signs of impingement. The common tests of LHBT tenosynovitis, the Speed's and Yergason tests, are described in Chapter 1.

In LBHT instability, a clicking sensation or snapping pain is a common symptom. Brought about through overhead activities, especially when attempting an overhead throw. In chronic cases, a LHBT rupture can ensue, leading to the muscle belly retracting to its distal attachments, resulting in a mass over the muscle belly — commonly referred to as the Popeye's sign.

3. Pathophysiology

An understanding of the anatomy of the LHBT will shed light on the complexity of its pathophysiology. The LHBT rises from the supraglenoid tubercle and the posterosuperior glenoid labrum. The proximal portion of the LHBT is intra-articular (within the glenohumeral joint) but extra-synovial. LHBT is encased within a synovial sheath that extends from the articular capsule to the inferior extent of the bicipital grove. The LHBT exits the glenohumeral joint running deep to the coracohumeral ligament entering the rotator interval before diving into the bicipital grove [5]. As the LHBT passes over the humeral head, it is at risk of impingement with the subacromial process. Within rotator interval, Werner and colleagues demonstrated a stabilising pulley sling encasing the LHBT consisting of structures form the coracohumeral ligament, superior glenohumeral ligament and subscapularis tendon [6]. The intimate association of the LHBT with the supraspinatus and subscapularis tendons within the rotator interval is the reason why LHBT tendinopathies also result in rotator cuff pathologies.

Within the bicipital groove, the transverse humeral ligament which spans the greater and lesser tuberosities forming a bridge over the LHBT. The morphology and depth of the groove as well as the above mention stabilising pulley are instrumental in ensuring stability of the LHBT. Due to its long course through the shoulder and evolving anatomy, the LHBT bears more on the medial wall of the bicipital groove and lesser tuberosity — thereby being vulnerable to medial subluxation [7].

Histologically, inflammation is rarely appreciated both macroscopically as well as microscopically in biceps tendinopathy. Instead, in tendinosis, degenerative changes predominate. Glait and colleagues reported that in the setting of concomitant rotator cuff tears, mucinous degenerative changes are found more along the proximal attachments as well as within the bicipital groove with the distal musculotendinous junctions being relatively spared [8]. Multiple theories have been proposed to explain LHBT tendinopathies — at present, like its management, remains inconclusive.

4. Diagnosis and Imaging, Algorithm

Ultrasonography is a useful imaging modality used in the diagnosis of LHBT pathologies (Fig. 1). Views of overlying the groove allows for appreciation of the anatomical characteristics of the bicipital groove. The tendon sheath can be easily traced from its origin down to the bicipital groove allowing for appreciation of tears, increased vascularity and impingement through the use of dynamic assessment. Ultrasonography

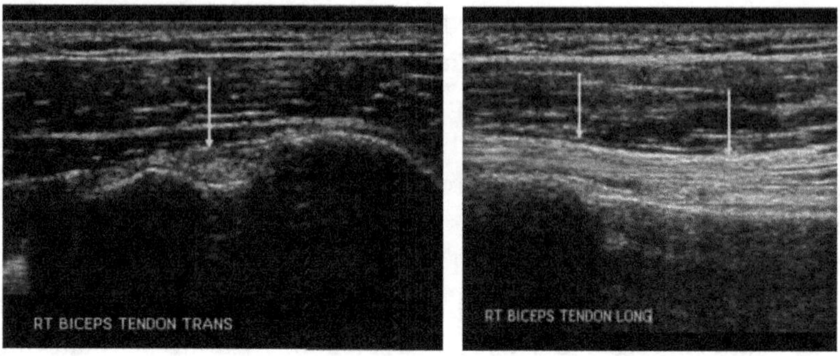

(a) (b)

Fig. 1: (a) Ultrasonographic transverse view of the biceps tendon, enlocated in the groove. (b) Ultrasonographic longitudinal view of the biceps tendon.

Table 1. Factors determining choice between tenotomy or tenodesis.

Factor	Tenotomy	Tenodesis
Age	Old	Young (<40 years)
Physical activity level	Sedentary	Active (athletes, labourers)
Physical demand needs	Low	High
Arm size	Fat, obese	Thin, normal
Cosmetic concerns	No	Yes
Workers compensation	No	Yes

Source: Adapted from Hsu and colleagues. *J Shoulder Elbow Surg* 2011; 20:326–332.

also allows for concomitant assessment of surrounding rotator cuff pathologies. Magnetic resonance imaging is increasingly more common, to provide a detailed assessment of surrounding structures and appreciation of the intra-articular structures. However, it does not offer dynamic assessment.

The management however remains widely debated. LHBT tenotomy or tenodesis are the two most common techniques used to manage LHBT pathologies (Table 1). However, there is a lack of consensus regarding the choice of procedure due to the lack of high levels of evidence. Most authors are guided by algorithms proposed by experts within literature. Hsu and colleagues advocate the use of tenotomy in elderly or high

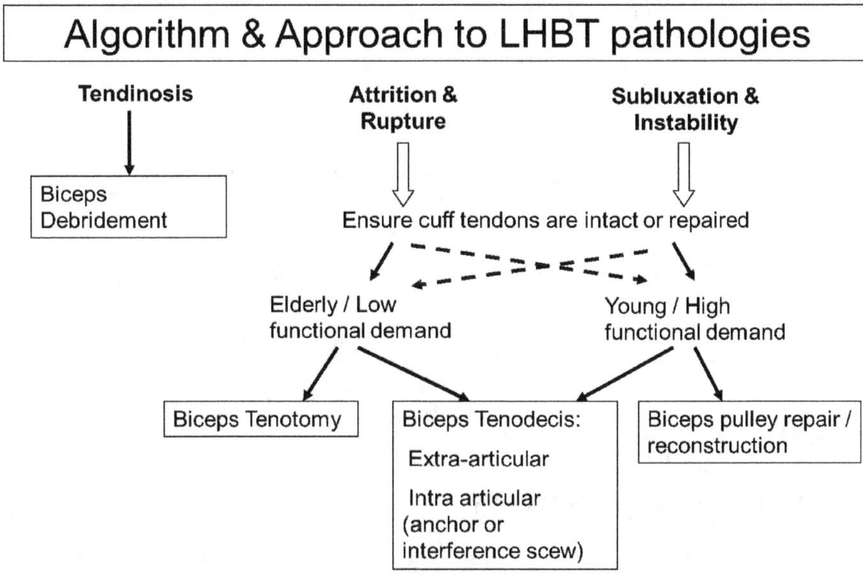

Fig. 2: Suggested algorithm and approach to pathologies of the long head of the biceps tendon (LHBT).

body-mass-index patients with sedentary lifestyle, whilst tenodesis is reserved for younger (less than 40 years of age), slimmer, active patients with high physical demands [1,9].

The decision can also be surgeon dependent (Fig. 2). Tenotomy of the LHBT is an effective technique as it requires shorter operative time, technically less demanding, requires less post-operative rehabilitation and therefore an earlier return to daily activities. It is also well tolerated by patients, with no significant loss of strength in forearm supination and elbow flexion or function. Tenodesis is technically more challenging, entailing longer operative time and requires a graduated rehabilitation for the patient following surgery (Table 2).

Literature reviews report comparable clinical outcomes, patient satisfaction as well as complication rates between tenotomy and tenodesis [9,10]. Careful patient selection and shrewd clinical judgement will be instrumental in ensuring good clinical outcomes as we await better evidence within literature to guide practice.

Table 2. Comparative survey between biceps tenotomy and tenodesis.

	Pros	**Cons**
Biceps Tenotomy	Shorter operating time Simpler Rehab Low surgical morbidity No implant complications	Cosmesis — Popeye sign Deep muscle ache Loss of power (minimal)
Biceps Tenodecis	Better cosmesis Maintenance of power	Longer surgical time Technically more challenging Bicipital pain Implant related issues

5. Arthroscopic Surgery

5.1 Indications for Surgery

- Biceps tenotomy or tenodesis as a stand-alone procedure is not common, it is usually done in conjunction with a cuff repair or subacromial decompression.
- Symptomatic biceps injury or when the biceps is torn, frayed or degenerate.

5.2 Positioning and Portals

- Standard posterior and anterior portals, and an additional antero-lateral portal as for cuff repair.

5.3 Arthroscopic Biceps Tenotomy

Arthroscopic biceps tenotomy should be considered for elderly patients with biceps pain or biceps fraying and injury shown on imaging. It can also be considered in patients with lower physical demands and in those with high BMI; in whom the (Popeye deformity) effects of biceps tenotomy will be less evident.

(a) **Inspection of the long head of biceps**
   - With the camera kept in the posterior portal, the insertion of the long head of the biceps tendon to the superior glenoid tubercle is immediately evident. It is the reference landmark in arthroscopy of

the glenohumeral joint and in the beach chair position, the camera should be turned so that the biceps tendon crosses the view horizontally.

- A probe is then inserted from the anterior portal, to probe the insertion of the long head of the biceps at the superior labrum. Assess for complete detachment of the superior labrum from the glenoid, look out for fraying, overhanging labrum and bucket-handle tears.
- Then turn the camera to look lateral as the long head of the biceps plunges into the groove. Use the probe to hook the biceps tendon up and thus pull the tendon into the shoulder joint. This allows inspection of biceps tendon as it curves over the humeral head. *Some inflammation is usually seen over the biceps as it makes the sharp bend.*
- Assess for stability of the biceps and ensure integrity of the biceps sling, at the base near the insertion of the subscapularis tendon.

(b) **Tenotomy of the long head of biceps**

- A radiofrequency (RF) probe is inserted from the anterior portal. The ablate mode is used to cut the biceps tendon as it widens and flares to insert to the superior labrum (Fig. 3(a)). *Do not cut the biceps at the tubular portion of the tendon; instead, cut it as it flares and widens at the insertion.*
- Ablate and cut from the under-surface of the tendon till half of the thickness is cut. Then flip the RF wand *over and above* the biceps tendon and complete the cut (Fig. 3(b)).

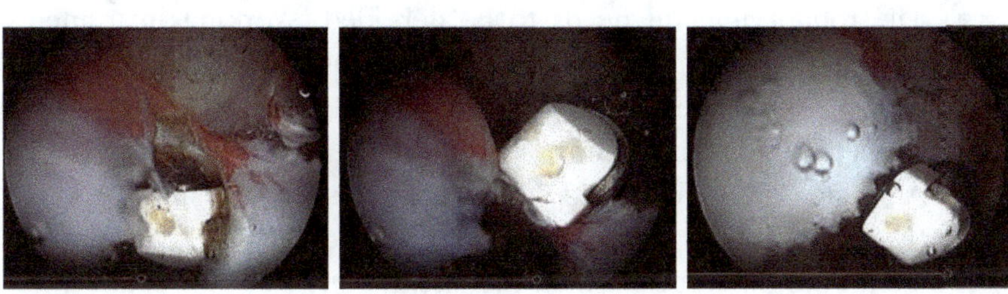

(a) (b) (c)

Fig. 3: Biceps tenotomy: (a) An RF wand performing a tenotomy by ablating from the undersurface. (b) The RF wand is then flipped over the biceps, to complete the tenotomy. (c) This prevents injury to the cuff tendons. The superior labrum is then debrided clean.

- The cut end of the biceps tendon should be a little bulbous and this prevents the tendon from slipping into the biceps groove, thus minimising the Popeye deformity. Any fraying of the superior labrum is then debrided clean (Fig. 3(c)). *Residual SLAP tears need not be repaired after biceps tenotomy as there is no more tension pulling on the torn superior labrum.*

5.4 Arthroscopic Biceps Tenodesis with Suture Anchor

Arthroscopic biceps tenodesis should be considered for younger patients with higher physical demands, and those whose arm girth are less or smaller. This will reduce the cosmetically deforming effects of biceps tenotomy, though the reduction of loss of strength is doubtful.

(a) **Inspection of the long head of biceps**
- The long head of the biceps is inspected as described above and indications for biceps tenodesis confirmed.

(b) **The antero-lateral portal**
- An antero-lateral (or biceps) portal is needed in addition to the anterior portal as the trajectory of the anterior portal is incorrect to place the tenodesis anchor or to tie the sutures. This portal is located over to or just medial to the long head of the biceps, and can be palpated as such. Alternatively, a portal can be created over the tear of the supraspinatus, and this tear portal can be used to perform the tenodesis.
- The rotator interval needs to be debrided. Working instruments from the antero-lateral portal can then access the biceps by tucking in at the lateral edge of the rotator interval.

(c) **The biceps tenodesis anchor**
- A single or double-loaded 4.5 mm suture anchor is strong enough (Fig. 4). The awl (and later the suture anchor) enters the antero-lateral portal, is tucked in at the lateral corner of the rotator interval, and pushes the biceps tendon away posteriorly (Fig. 5). It is directed perpendicular to the surface of the humeral head, beneath the biceps tendon as it plunges over the humeral head to enter the groove. The anchor is secured and sutures separated.

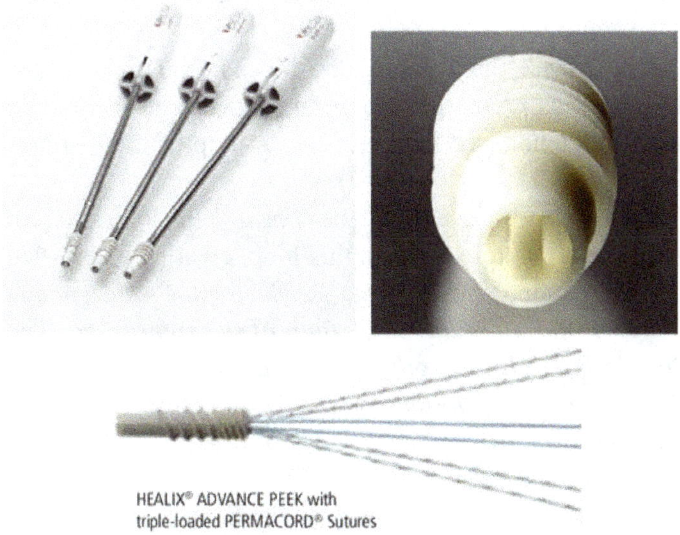

Fig. 4: The Healix advance anchor.

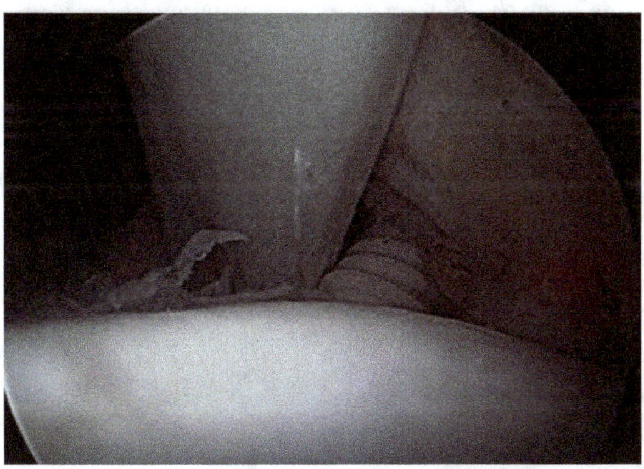

Fig. 5: Biceps tenodecis anchor. The Healix anchor is tucked at the biceps groove, just anterior to the supraspinatus tendon.

(d) **The lasso-loop suture through the tendon**

- A bird beak retriever is used either through the antero-lateral or tear portal. One limb of a suture from the anchor is picked up and placed away from the biceps *in the expected or anticipated location where the bird beak retriever is expected to emerge after penetrating the biceps tendon.*

- The bird beak then pierces the biceps tendon in mid-substance (Fig. 6(a)) as it emerges from the groove or at the location where it is to be tenodesed, and retrieves a loop of the displaced suture (Fig. 6(b)).
- The bird beak retriever then goes *through* the loop and retrieves the ***same*** limb of suture through this loop, creating a lasso-loop suture through the tendon (Fig. 6(c)). *Retrieving the same suture limb can be tricky and often the other limb of the suture is pulled instead. One tip is to clip the other loose suture limb with an artery and give it a gentle tug to identify the suture limps. Retrieve the suture limb that is not tugged.*

(e) **The encircling suture**

- A suture retriever is now used to pick up the other limp of suture, the loose limb not tied to the lasso-loop (Fig. 7(a)). Again, it is placed a distance away from the biceps tendon. The suture retriever then *goes over the biceps tendon to retrieve this suture, thus bringing the suture over and around the biceps tendon (encircling it)* (Fig. 7(b)).
- Pulling the encircling suture compresses the biceps tendon onto the anchor, whilst pulling on the lasso-loop suture actually lifts it off the anchor. The encircling suture is the suture post when tying the knot (Fig. 7(c)).

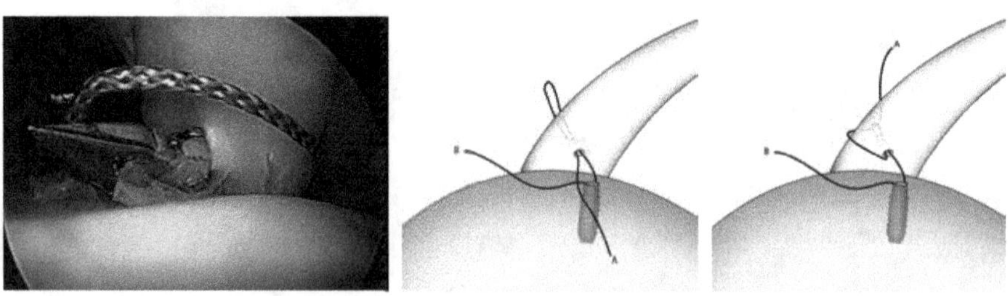

(a) (b) (c)

Fig. 6: The Lasso-Loop suture: (a) A bird beak retriever creating a loop by pulling on a suture limb, as shown in (b). The same limb is then retrieved through the loop, shown schematically in (c).

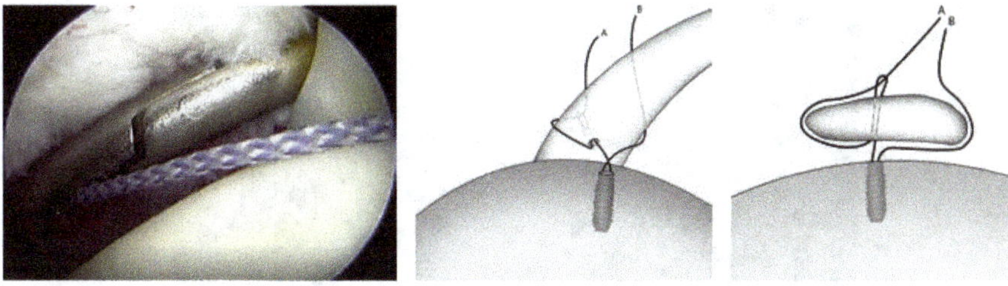

(a) (b) (c)

Fig. 7: The encircling suture: (a) A grasper retrieving the other suture limb to encircle the biceps tendon. This is shown schematically in (b) and a cross-section view of the biceps is shown in (c).

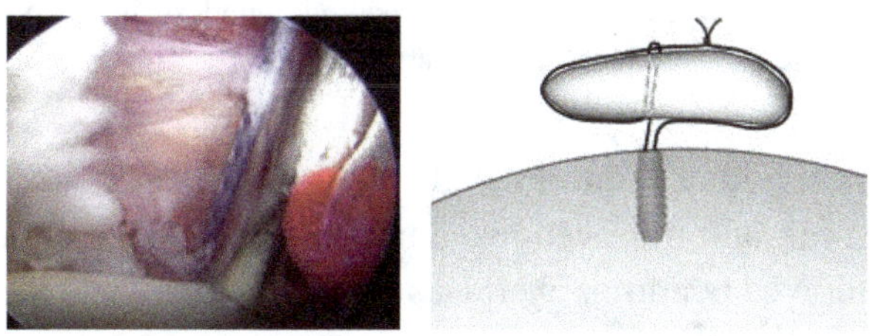

(a) (b)

Fig. 8: Securing the biceps tendon: (a) The sutures are then tied, with the encircling suture being the post as shown in (b).

- Complete the knot with six half-hitches (Fig. 8(a)). The first two half-hitches are in the same direction, before alternating directions for subsequent throws (Fig. 8(b)).

(f) **Biceps tenotomy — completing the task**

- The biceps tendon is then cut away from the tenodesis sutures, using arthroscopic scissors or an RF wand (Fig. 9). The cut end is then clamped using graspers from the antero-lateral or tear portal, from which it is then delivered out of the shoulders after the biceps tendon origin is cut at its insertion at the superior labrum.

6. Post-op Management and Rehabilitation

Post-operative management varies dependent on the concomitant procedures performed. In both tenotomy and tenodesis of the LHBT, the

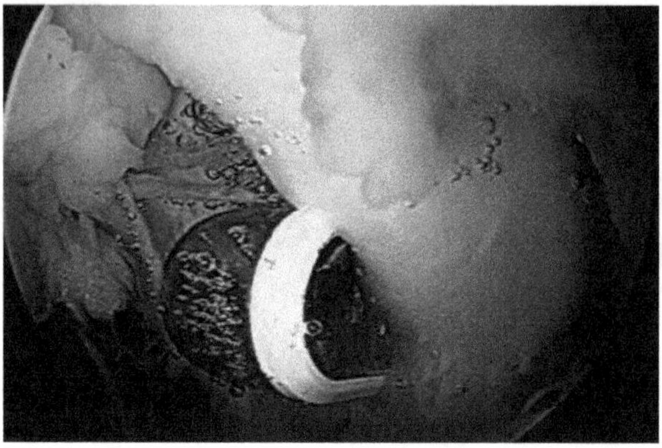

Fig. 9: Biceps tenotomy. After the biceps is secured, tenodesis is completed by cutting the biceps using an RF wand above the tied sutures.

shoulder joint is kept immobilised in an arm sling postoperatively. Appropriate oral and intravenous analgesia is used for pain control. Patients are allowed pendular exercises postoperatively and are discharged from the hospital on the first postoperative day.

After two weeks, the patients are assessed in the outpatient setting for would healing. The first 4 weeks of rehabilitation will entail pendular exercises and passive range of motion. The subsequent 6 weeks will involve improving active range of motion. Strength training will only commence after the first 4 weeks of rehabilitation. This allows for auto-tenodesis of the LHBT within the bicipital groove in the setting of tenotomy or for tenodesis repair to heal.

7. Outcomes

The outcomes between biceps tenotomy and tenodesis is comparable even when performed concomitantly with rotator cuff repair. Mak and Lie reported comparable clinical outcomes amongst patient with or without LHBT procedures [11]. Gurnani and colleagues reported comparable Constant-Murley shoulder outcome scores between both LHBT tenotomy and tenodesis [12]. Lee and colleagues conducted a prospective randomised control trial which reported no clinical difference in the American

Shoulder and Elbow Surgeons score, visual analogue pain score or range of motion postoperatively [13].

Each technique however has its own unique set of complications and side effects.

1. **Elbow flexion and supination strength**

In a systematic review by Gurnani and colleagues, five studies reporting postoperative elbow flexion strength showed no difference between either technique. In addition, 3 studies reported no difference with forearm supination as well [12].

2. **Popeye's deformity**

Popeye's deformity is the loss of the fusiform appearance of the biceps tendon after tenotomy. Popeye's deformity occurs in both tenotomy and tenodesis. However, the reported incidence of Popeye's deformity is 2 to 3 times more likely to occur after LHBT tenotomy [13]. This complication however is well tolerated by patients and has been proven to not affect clinical outcomes negatively.

3. **Biceps muscle cramping**

Biceps muscle camping was less common amongst patients with tenodesis. Patients with tenotomy occasionally complain of an aching, cramping sensation over the biceps belly.

4. **Persistent pain**

Hsu and colleagues in a systematic review reported persistent pain isolated to the bicipital groove more common amongst patients who underwent LHBT tenodesis [9].

References

1. Meeks BD, Meeks NM, Froehle AW, Wareing E, Bonner KF. Patient satisfaction after biceps tenotomy. *Orthop J Sports Med* 2017;5(5):2325967117707737.
2. Chen C-H, Hsu K-Y, Chen W-J, Shih C-H. Incidence and severity of biceps long head tendon lesion in patients with complete rotator cuff tears. *J Trauma* 2005;58(6):1189–1193.

3. Murthi AM, Vosburgh CL, Neviaser TJ. The incidence of pathologic changes of the long head of the biceps tendon. *J Shoulder Elbow Surg* 2000;9(5): 382–385.
4. Alpantaki K, McLaughlin D, Karagogeos D, Hadjipavlou A, Kontakis G. Sympathetic and sensory neural elements in the tendon of the long head of the biceps. *J Bone Joint Surg Am* 2005;87(7):1580–1583.
5. Elser F, Braun S, Dewing CB, Giphart JE, Millett PJ. Anatomy, function, injuries, and treatment of the long head of the biceps brachii tendon. *Arthroscopy* 2011;27(4):581–592.
6. Werner A, Mueller T, Boehm D, Gohlke F. The stabilizing sling for the long head of the biceps tendon in the rotator cuff interval. A histoanatomic study. *Am J Sports Med* 2000;28(1):28–31.
7. Walch G, Nové-Josserand L, Boileau P, Levigne C. Subluxations and dislocations of the tendon of the long head of the biceps. *J Shoulder Elb Surg* 1998;7(2):100–108.
8. Glait SA, Mahure S, Loomis CA, Cammer M, Pham H, Feldman A, *et al.* Regional histologic differences in the long head of the biceps tendon following subpectoral biceps tenodesis in patients with rotator cuff tears and SLAP lesions. *Knee Surg Sports Traumatol Arthrosc* 2018;26(8):2481–2489.
9. Hsu AR, Ghodadra NS, Provencher MT, Lewis PB, Bach BR. Biceps tenotomy versus tenodesis: a review of clinical outcomes and biomechanical results. *J Shoulder Elbow Surg* 2011;20(2):326–332.
10. Castricini R, Familiari F, De Gori M, Riccelli DA, De Benedetto M, Orlando N, *et al.* Tenodesis is not superior to tenotomy in the treatment of the long head of biceps tendon lesions. *Knee Surg Sports Traumatol Arthrosc Knee Surg Sports Traumatol Arthrosc* 2018;26(1):169–175. doi:10.1007/s00167-017-4609-4.
11. Keong MW, Tjoen DLT. Does bicep pathology affect rotator cuff repair outcomes? *J Orthop Surg (Hong Kong)* 2018;26(1):2309499018762852.
12. Gurnani N, van Deurzen DFP, Janmaat VT, van den Bekerom MPJ. Tenotomy or tenodesis for pathology of the long head of the biceps brachii: a systematic review and meta-analysis. *Knee Surg Sports Traumatol Arthrosc* 2016; 24(12):3765–3771.
13. Lee H-J, Jeong J-Y, Kim C-K, Kim Y-S. Surgical treatment of lesions of the long head of the biceps brachii tendon with rotator cuff tear: a prospective randomized clinical trial comparing the clinical results of tenotomy and tenodesis. *J Shoulder Elbow Surg* 2016;25(7):1107–1114.

https://doi.org/10.1142/9789811249846_0012

Chapter 12

Arthroscopic Repair of Subscapularis Tears

Denny T.T. Lie and Jeremy K.M. Goh

Summary of Chapter

1. Introduction and epidemiology of subscapularis tears
2. Clinical presentation of subscapularis injuries
3. Pathophysiology of problem
4. Diagnosis and imaging
5. Surgical technique of the arthroscopic dual-row subscapularis repairs
6. Rehabilitation
7. Clinical outcomes

1. Introduction and Epidemiology of Subscapularis Tears

The subscapularis tendon, part of the rotator cuff tendons, is one of the less commonly injured tendons. This may partly be due to the fact that it is difficult to diagnose clinically and has been less well studied than the other cuff tendons. Tears of the subscapularis most commonly occur in conjunction with tears of the rest of the cuff or the biceps tendon and its prevalence in patients needing rotator cuff repairs has been reported to be up to 31.4% [1]. Isolated subscapularis tears are even less common and likely to be post traumatic as studied by Gerber *et al.* [2]. Advances in imaging modalities and clinical suspicion have led to increasing awareness of the pathology and interests in its repair.

2. Clinical Presentation of Subscapularis Injuries

Subscapularis tears commonly occur with other rotator cuff tears and patients may present with anterior shoulder pain or difficulties with activities that involve internal rotation of the shoulder. There may also have been a preceding event of forced external rotation, especially in the younger population.

Examination may reveal pain over the anterior shoulder on palpation, increased passive external rotation of the shoulder compared to the normal side (in cases of full thickness tears) and decreased shoulder internal rotation strength [3]. Many tests have been described for diagnosing subscapularis tears and these include: Lift off test, Belly press test, Napoleon test, Bear hug test, Positive internal rotation lag sign [2]. These signs are described in Chapter 1. A systemic review by Rigsby *et al.* found internal rotation lag sign (98%), Napoleon sign (98%) and lift off (94%) with the highest sensitivities in full thickness tears [4]. However, for partial thickness tears, pooled sensitivities for all the tests were low to moderate, with the highest sensitivity being the belly (69%) off test [4].

3. Pathophysiology of Problem, Classification

Subscapularis tears in older adults are thought to be due to degenerative processes similar to that of the supraspinatus and infraspinatus tendons. Impingement by the coracoid process and propagation of anterior tears of the supraspinatus to the subscapularis may also result in subscapularis tears. In some cases, an acute event such as a traumatic shoulder dislocation may be the cause. In the younger patient, tears may be due to a high energy forced external rotation to the shoulder. In Gerber's series of isolated subscapularis tears, most presented with a history of violent external rotation of the adducted arm or violent hyperextension and to a

Table 1. Lafosse subscapularis tear classification [5].

Type	Subscapularis Tendon
1	Upper 1/3 of tendon, partial tear
2	Upper 1/3 of tendon, complete tear
3	Upper 2/3 of tendon, complete tear
4	Entire tendon, full thickness tear
5	Entire tear irreparable, anterosuperior subluxation

lesser extent, motor vehicle accidents or traumatic anterior shoulder dislocation [2].

There have been many proposed classification systems of subscapularis tears, one commonly used is by Lafosse *et al.* [5]. This was based on the anatomical footprint of the tendon and guides reparability (Table 1).

4. Diagnosis and Imaging

Ultrasound is cost effective and allows for dynamic assessment, however, it may not be as sensitive as MRI in picking up smaller tears. MRI offers more information on the rotator cuff and amount of fatty infiltration which may prove useful in surgical planning. Having said that, occasionally imaging modalities may not pick up tears of the subscapularis and instead they are identified during surgery, especially with arthroscopy.

5. Arthroscopic Surgery

1. **Indications for surgery**
   - Symptomatic tears (pain, weakness on belly press and external lag sign positive) proven on imaging (LaFosse types 2–4).
   - Tears detected during arthroscopic repair of other cuff tendons, type 2 or worse (Figs. 1(a) and 1(b)).
2. **Positioning & portals**
   - **Position:** Beach chair.
   - **Posterior:** Standard posterior for viewing.

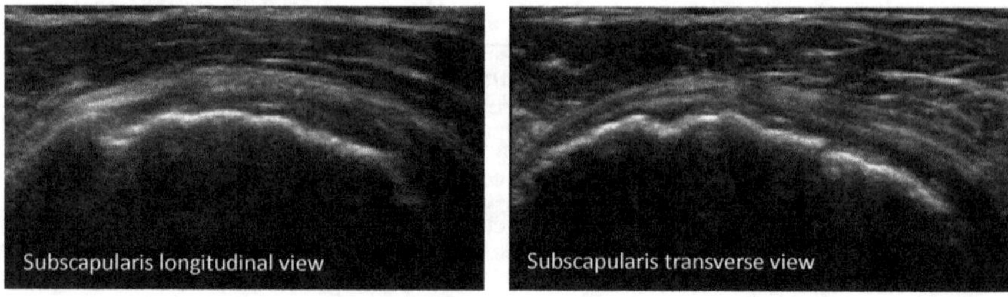

(a) (b)

Fig. 1: Ultrasound images of subscapularis tear. The longitudinal (a) and transverse (b) views, as marked by the radiologist, show a thin sliver of fascia, and absence of normal thick tendon and muscle belly.

- **Antero-superior:** This portal is surface-marked just lateral to the tip of the coracoid, and enters the joint in the middle of the rotator interval, *as medial as possible.* This trajectory, when pointed laterally, brings it over the lesser tuberosity. A 5mm cannula is inserted in this portal, used for anchor placement and suture management.
- **Antero-lateral:** This portal is surface-marked about 1 cm below the antero-lateral corner of the acromion, and enters the joint at the lateral corner of the rotator interval, just anterior to the biceps tendon and above the insertion of the subscapularis. If desired, an 8mm cannula can be used in this portal, which is used for tendon suturing (Fig. 2(a)).
- **Tear portal:** If the subscapularis repair is done together with repair of the supraspinatus tendon, then a lateral portal is created over the supraspinatus tear, *hence labelled tear portal.* This portal is the widened and is used for the subscapularis tendon suturing, instead of the antero-lateral portal.

5.1 *Arthroscopic repair of Subscapularis tears (type I and II tears)*

(a) **Mobilisation of the subscapularis tendon**

- In type I and II tears of the subscapularis, a significant portion of the lower muscular part of the tendon is usually intact. The tear is

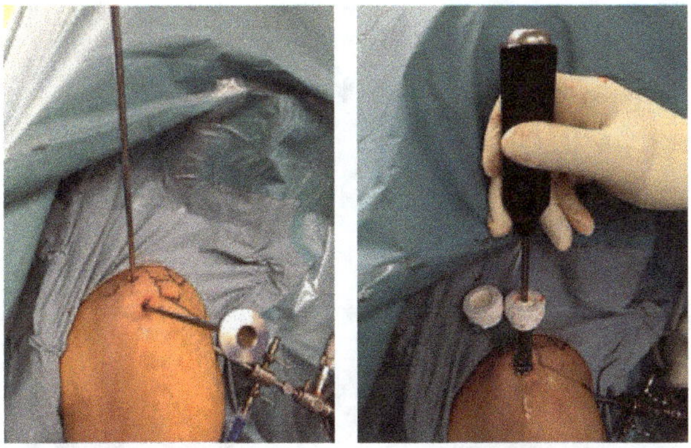

(a) (b)

Fig. 2: Portal and Anchor Placement. (a) Shows the antero-lateral portal created to access the subscapularis. (b) Shows the angle at which the awl is positioned, to place the anchor at the insertion of the subscapularis.

often missed, leading to the question: ***How do we identify a tear of the subscapularis tendon?*** The key is to identify the MGHL, which slopes 45 degree obliquely down from the labrum to the humeral head. If the MGHL is not seen, the upper portion of the subscapularis is torn and retracted medially.

- A grasper from the antero-lateral portal is used to pull the torn tendon laterally, to reduce the torn upper edge of the subscapularis to its insertion. The tendon is adequately reduced when the MGHL is bought to view **(*the MGHL sign*)**.
- Debride the plane between the glenoid and the subscapularis, inadequate debridement of the adhesions in this plane will prevent good reduction of the torn tendon. *It is not safe to blindly debride the plane external to the subscapularis.*

(b) **Placement of the suture anchor**

- A shaver from the antero-superior portal is used to debride and decorticate the insertion of the subscapularis tendon, that is, the **lesser tuberosity and the facet** just above it. The facet and insertion area are better seen by **flexing the arm forward and internally rotating the arm**, this movement will bring it directly in the trajectory of the antero-superior portal (Fig. 2(b)).

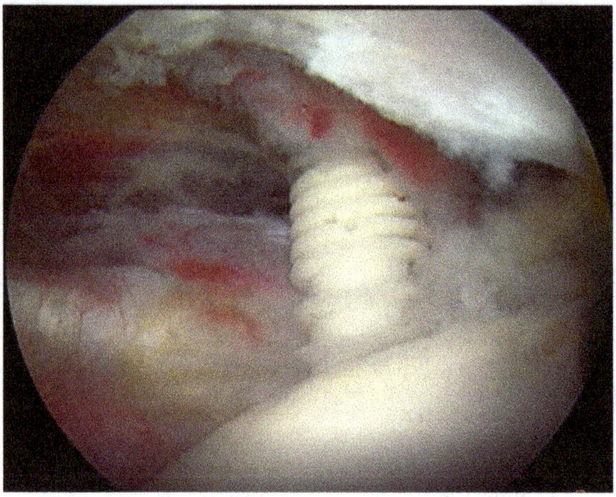

Fig. 3: Angle of Anchor Placement. In this example of right shoulder, the anchor is positioned almost vertically near the insertion of the subscapularis.

- From the same portal, a dual-loaded anchor (4 mm Gryphon BR anchor) is placed just above the lesser tuberosity (Fig. 3). Retrieve both limbs from suture (A) and one limb from suture (B) from the antero-lateral (or tear) portal. Leave the remaining limb of suture (B) in the antero-superior portal.

(c) **Suturing the tendon with modified Mason-Allen suture configuration**

- A grasper from the antero-superior portal is used to hold the tendon in the reduced position.
- Using a suture passer (Express Sew III) or an Acupass suture retriever from the antero-lateral portal, retrieve a limb from suture (A) through the upper part of the subscapularis tendon, from the articular surface outwards (Fig. 4(a)). The first suture is placed **medial but with a shallow pass** (biting only the superior aspect) of the tendon (Fig. 4(b)).
- The other limb of suture (A) is then retrieved **more lateral with a deep pass** (often at the inferior muscular portion) (Fig. 5(a)). Both sutures are kept in the antero-lateral portal (Fig. 5(b)).
- One suture limb from suture (B) is then passed **in between the suture limbs** of suture (A), and retrieved to the antero-superior portal (Fig. 6). The other suture limb still arises from the anchor.

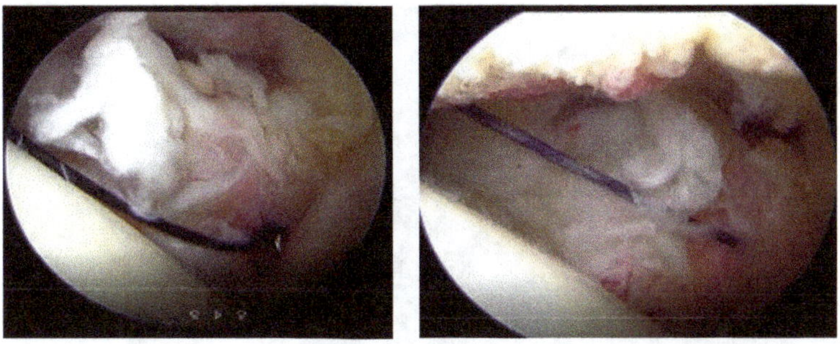

(a) (b)

Fig. 4: The mattress stitch — upper stitch. (a) shows an Acupass piercing the superficial and medial part of the LEFT subscapularis. A filament is passed to shuttle the striped blue suture from the anchor, shown in (b).

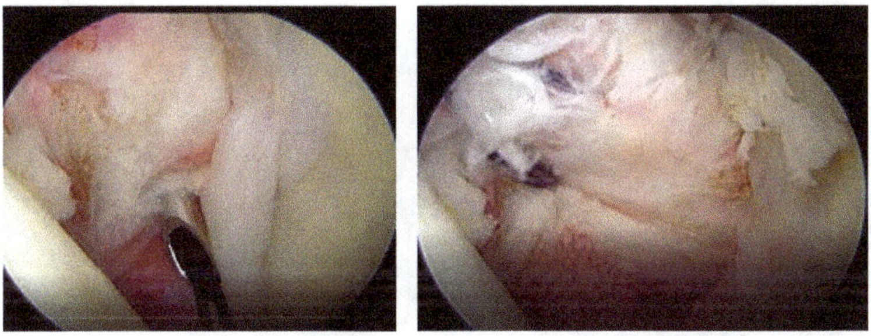

(a) (b)

Fig. 5: The mattress stitch — lower stitch. In (a) the Acupass pierces the deeper part of the LEFT subscapularis to shuttle the other limb of the striped blue suture. This creates a mattress stitch configuration as shown in (b).

- Both limbs of suture (a) are then tied with the arm in internal rotation, creating an oblique mattress suture (Fig. 7). Both sutures are then cut.
- Suture limbs from suture (b) are then tied, creating a simple stitch configuration, over the tendon and across the mattress stitch, thus creating a modified Mason-Allen configuration (Fig. 7). *This technique provides a strong compression repair of the tendon but often does not lateralise the tendon adequately to cover the insertion footprint.*

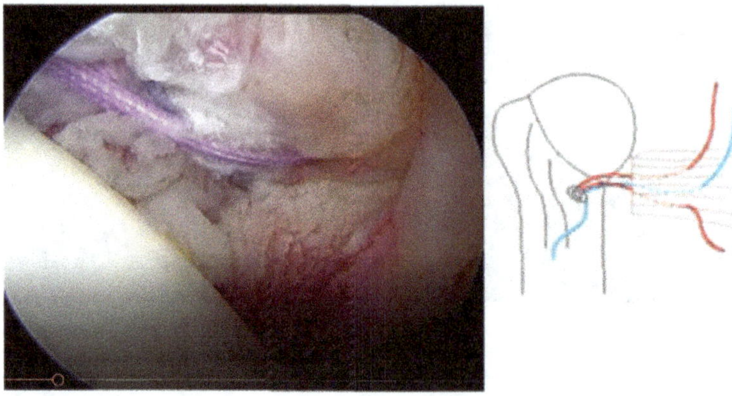

Fig. 6: The Simple Stitch. The purple stitch is passed in between the blue sutures, to cross perpendicular to the mattress suture configuration.

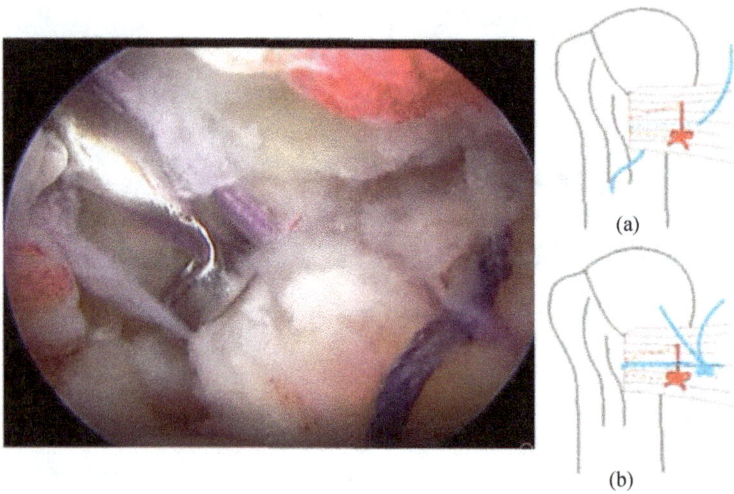

Fig. 7: The Mason-Allen suture configuration. After the blue sutures are tied to create the mattress configuration, the purple stitch is stitched perpendicular to the mattress suture, creating the Mason-Allen configuration. (a) Mattress suture configuration and (b) simple stitch configuration.

(d) The optional additional whip stitch and lateral row

- To lateralise the tendon further, it is necessary to add a lateral row. One suture limb from suture (B), already tied over the tendon, is passed over the upper edge of the subscapularis tendon once again, creating a loop whipstitch. This is done by a suture passer (Express Sew III) or an Acupass suture retriever from the antero-lateral portal (Figs. 8(a) and 8(b)).

- The whipstitch suture is retrieved in the subacromial space and together with sutures from the supraspinatus repair, is then tied to a lateral row anchor (Versalok PEEK) (Fig. 9). The subscapularis would thus be compressed and lateralised onto its insertion

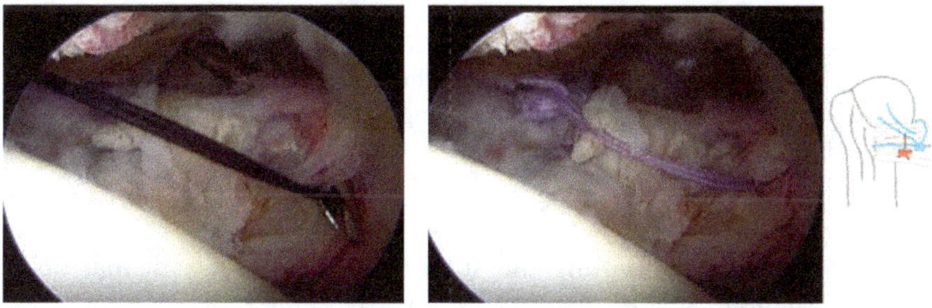

(a) (b)

Fig. 8: The whip stitch. In (a) the Acupass is passed again over the superficial part of the LEFT subscapularis, (b) shows how the purple suture, having tied the simple stitch, is shuttled through, creating a whip stitch to grip the tightly the superficial part of the tendon.

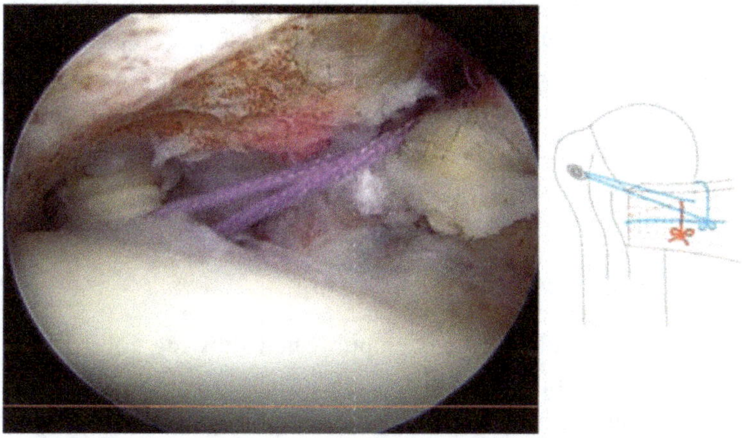

Fig. 9: The dual-row repair. The purple sutures, gripping the upper part of the subscapularis tendon, is then secured to a lateral anchor to create the dual-row repair.

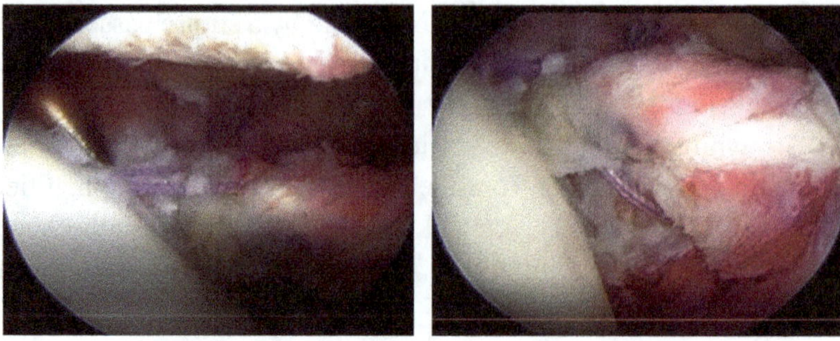

(a) (b)

Fig. 10: The final check: (a) An obturator used to probe the purple sutures tied to the lateral row. (b) The effect of the whip stitch tenting up and gripping the upper part of the subscapularis.

footprint, incorporating the subscapularis repair with that of the supraspinatus (Fig. 10(a) and 10(b)). *Note that this additional suture bridge repair from the subscapularis can only be done if the biceps tendon is tenotomised or tenodesed.*

6. Post-op Management and Rehabilitation

The arm is immobilised in an arm sling for 2 weeks, though passive range of motion (ROM) exercises immediately post-surgery is tolerated. The patient is seen by the physiotherapist to be educated on pendular ROM exercises before discharge. Active ROM and gradual strengthening exercises is only commenced 6 weeks post-operatively as recommended by the American Society of Shoulder and Elbow Therapists [6].

7. Outcomes

A good number of studies have been published showing good clinical and functional outcomes post-operatively at short and medium term follow up [7–11]. Significant improvement in patient reported outcomes, pain scores and strength can be expected compared to pre-operative scores. However, these patients should be monitored closely as re-rupture rates have been reported to be up to 11% in one study [8]. In our own series of 40 cases there was good overall improvement in pain and functional scores at 2 years post-operatively and a low re-tear rate (2.5%) [7]. These included isolated subscapularis repairs and also in conjunction with other cuff tears (e.g. supraspinatus) which both resulted in good outcomes post-operatively.

Previously repairs of the subscapularis were performed open, however with the advancement of arthroscopic techniques, more studies have been published showing comparable outcomes [12]. Debates persist whether single or double row techniques are superior, as with repairs of the other rotator cuff tendons. One study has shown no difference in outcomes between the two techniques for subscapularis repairs [13].

References

1. Narasimhan R, Shamse K, Nash C, *et al.* Prevalence of subscapularis tears and accuracy of shoulder ultrasound in pre-operative diagnosis. *Int Orthop* 2016;40(5):975–979. doi:10.1007/s00264-015-3043-9.
2. Gerber C, Krushell RJ. Isolated rupture of the tendon of the subscapularis muscle. Clinical features in 16 cases. *J Bone Joint Surg Br* 1991;73(3): 389–394. doi:10.1302/0301-620X.73B3.1670434. PMID: 1670434.
3. Lenart BA, Ticker JB. Subscapularis tendon tears: Management and arthroscopic repair. *EFORT Open Rev* 2017;2(12):484–495. doi: 10.1302/2058-5241.2.170015. PMID: 29387471; PMCID: PMC5765990.
4. Rigsby R, Sitler M, Kelly JD. Subscapularis tendon integrity: an examination of shoulder index tests. *J Athl Train* 2010;45(4):404–406. doi: 10.4085/1062-6050-45.4.404. PMID: 20617916; PMCID: PMC2902035.
5. Lafosse L, Lanz U, Saintmard B, *et al.* Arthroscopic repair of subscapularis tear: Surgical technique and results. *Orthop Traumatol Surg Res* 2010;96. Epub ahead of print 2010. doi:10.1016/j.otsr.2010.09.009.
6. Thigpen CA, Shaffer MA, Gaunt BW, Leggin BG, Williams GR, Wilcox RB. The American Society of Shoulder and Elbow Therapists consensus statement on rehabilitation following arthroscopic rotator cuff repair. *J Shoulder Elb Surg* 2016;25(4):521–535. doi:10.1016/j.jse.2015.12.018.
7. Meng JGK, Chen JYQ, Lie DTT. A new technique of arthroscopic subscapularis repair with 2-year clinical outcomes in an Asian population. *J Orthop Surg* 2017;25(3):230949901772790. doi:10.1177/2309499017727902.

8. Lanz U, Fullick R, Bongiorno V, *et al.* Arthroscopic repair of large subscapularis tendon tears: 2- to 4-year clinical and radiographic outcomes. *Arthroscopy* 2013;29(9):1471–1478. doi:10.1016/j.arthro.2013.06.004.
9. Lafosse L, Jost B, Reiland Y, *et al.* Structural integrity and clinical outcomes after arthroscopic repair of isolated subscapularis tears. *J Bone Joint Surg Am* 2007;89(6):1184–1193. doi:10.2106/JBJS.F.00007.
10. Nové-Josserand L, Hardy M, Leandro Nunes Ogassawara R, *et al.* Clinical and structural results of arthroscopic repair of isolated subscapularis tear. *J Bone Joint Surg Am* 2012;94(17):e125. doi:10.2106/JBJS.K.00008.
11. Toussaint B, Audebert S, Barth J, *et al.* Arthroscopic repair of subscapularis tears: preliminary data from a prospective multicentre study. *Orthop Traumatol Surg Res* 2012;98(8):S193–S200. doi:10.1016/j.otsr.2012.10.004.
12. Saltzman BM, Collins MJ, Leroux T, Arns TA, Griffin JW, Romeo AA, … Forsythe B. Arthroscopic repair of isolated subscapularis tears: a systematic review of technique-specific outcomes. *Arthroscopy* 2017;33(4): 849–860. doi:10.1016/j.arthro.2016.10.020.
13. Yoon J.-S, Kim S.-J, Choi Y.-R, Kim S.-H, Chun Y.-M. Arthroscopic repair of the isolated subscapularis full-thickness tear: single-versus double-row suture-bridge technique. *Am J Sports Med* 2019;47(6):1427–1433. doi: 10.1177/0363546519838281.

https://doi.org/10.1142/9789811249846_0013

Chapter 13

Arthroscopic Subacromial Decompression and Acromioplasty Arthroscopic Mumford's Procedure

Denny T.T. Lie and Punn Kuhataparuks

Summary of Chapter

1. Introduction and epidemiology of subacromial pain
2. Pathophysiology and causes of impingement
3. Clinical presentation and examination
4. Diagnosis and imaging
5. Surgical technique of arthroscopic subacromial decompression Surgical technique of arthroscopic Mumford's procedure
6. Rehabilitation
7. Clinical outcomes

1. Introduction and Epidemiology

(a) Shoulder pain is the third most common musculoskeletal complaint seen in primary care with an estimated prevalence of 7–34% among the general population [1].

(b) Subacromial impingement syndrome (SIS) is the most common cause of shoulder complaints and it comprises 44–65% those cases [2].

(c) Risk factors for developing SIS include occupational or sports related repetitive activities, age, instability of glenohumeral joint, and congenital/acquired skeletal anatomy.

2. Pathophysiology

(a) SIS is caused by the compression of the rotator cuff, subacromial bursa, and other soft tissues between the humeral head and the under surface of the acromion, acromioclavicular joint or the coracoacromial arch.
(b) Classically described into three stages according to the Neer Classification, 1983:
   (i) **Stage I:** Reversible inflammation, oedema and haemorrhage, age less than 25 years old.
   (ii) **Stage II:** Fibrosis and tendinitis, age 25–40 years old.
   (iii) **Stage III:** Rotator cuff tear, biceps tendon rupture, bony change, age more than 40 years old.
(c) **Primary external impingement** is caused by mechanical narrowing of the subacromial space due to structural changes such osteophytes formation, bony malposition following a fracture, or enlargement of subacromial soft tissues (i.e. bursitis or tendon calcifications).
(d) **Secondary external impingement** is a result of functional abnormality in centring of the humeral head leading to displaced centre of rotation during elevation and soft tissue entrapment. Generally, it is caused by muscle imbalance and loose glenohumeral joint capsule and ligaments.
(e) **Internal impingement** is mostly seen in throwing or overhead athlete resulting in posterior shoulder pain. This is due to the impingement of articular surface of rotator cuff against the posterior-superior-glenoi and glenoid labrum.

3. Clinical Presentation

3.1 *History of Symptoms*

(a) Patient should be assessed for the progression, duration, characteristic of pain, radiation, precipitating trauma, and analgesic use.

SIGNS SUGGESTIVE OF SUBACROMIAL IMPINGEMENT
1. PAINFUL ARC 2. EXT ROTATION TEST 3. JOBE'S TEST

(b) Common symptoms include anterolateral arm pain, pain on elevation of the arm between 70 and 120°, pain on forced arm elevation above the head, and pain while lying on the affected side.

3.2 *Physical Examination*

(a) No single test is sufficient to diagnose SIS and a combination of multiple tests help to increase the accuracy of diagnosis.
(b) In addition to the standard shoulder examination, the Dutch Orthopaedic Association Guideline recommends a combination of **Hawkins-Kennedy test, the painful arc test, and the infraspinatus muscle strength test**. Furthermore, drop-arm test, infraspinatus and supraspinatus muscle strength test should be used to assess for rotator cuff tear.
(c) Michener *et al.* studied the result of the five physical examination tests for impingement (Neer, Hawkins–Kennedy, painful arc, Jobe's and external rotation resistance tests) in relations to the surgical findings [5]. The study suggested that single tests of painful arc, external rotation resistance and Neer's test help to rule out SIS, while single tests of **painful arc, external rotation resistance, and Jobe's test** are helpful in confirming SIS. The authors concluded that three or more positive tests confirm SIS and less than three positive tests rules out SIS.

4. Imaging

1. **Plain film radiographs**
   (a) **Anterior-posterior (AP) view** for assessing glenohumeral joint, osteophytes and sclerosis of the greater tuberosity:

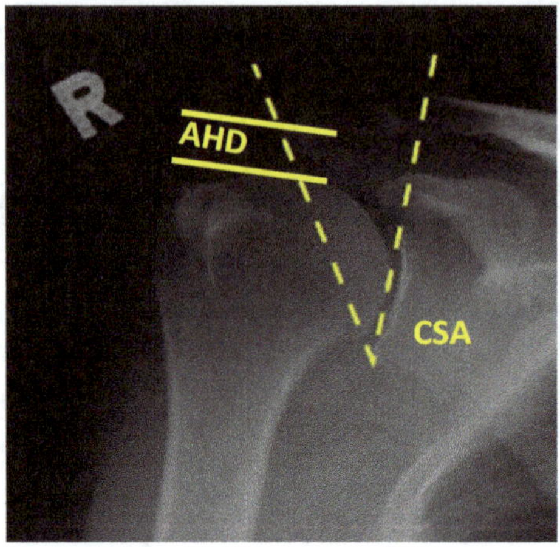

Fig. 1: The critical shoulder angle and acromio-humeral distance. CSA formed by a line connecting the inferior with the superior border of the glenoid fossa and another line connecting the inferior border of the glenoid with the most inferolateral point of the acromion. AHD is the distance between the acromion and humeral head.

(i) **Critical shoulder angle (CSA)** of more the 35° increase the risk of developing rotator cuff lesion (Fig. 1) [6].

(ii) **Acromio-humeral index (AI)** quantifies the lateral extension of the acromion. A high AI indicates increase lateral extension and significantly associated with rotator cuff tears (Fig. 2) [7].

(iii) **Acromio-humeral distance (AHD)** typical measures 7–14 mm in men and 7–12 mm in women. Abnormally low AHD suggests a defect of more than one rotator cuff tendon [8].

(b) **Scapular Y view** for assessing subacromial space and classifying the acromion type (Bigliani and Morrison classification) (Fig. 3).

(c) **Axillary view** for evidence of os acromiale, a potential cause of secondary. impingement (Fig. 4).

2. **Ultrasonography (US)** can show bursitis and tendon changes or ruptures. The US sensitivity and specificity is equivalent to those of MRI for diagnosis complete rotator cuff injuries [4]. However, it is largely

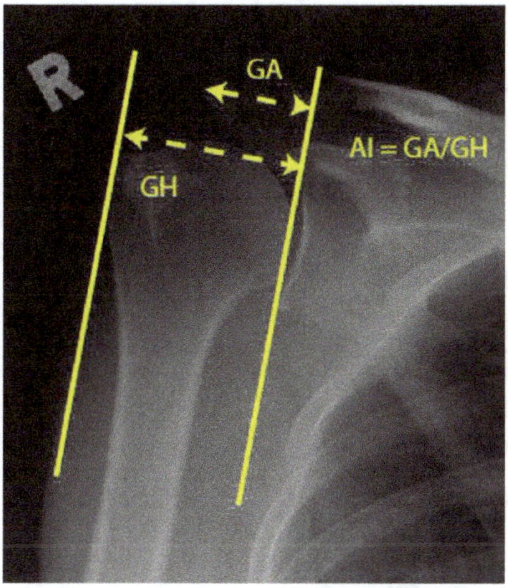

Fig. 2: Acromial index. The AI is the distance from the glenoid plane to the lateral border of the acromion (GA) divided by the distance from the glenoid plane to the most lateral aspect of the humeral head (GH) [9].

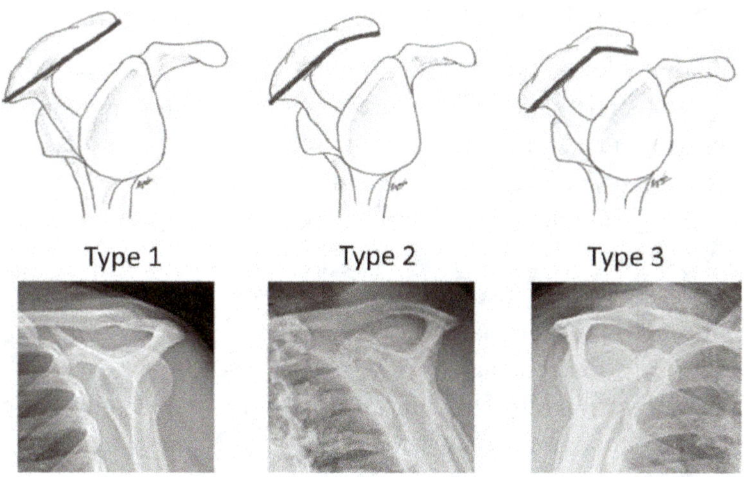

Fig. 3: Bigliani classification. Bigliani's classification of acromial morphology with corresponding X-rays outlet views [1].

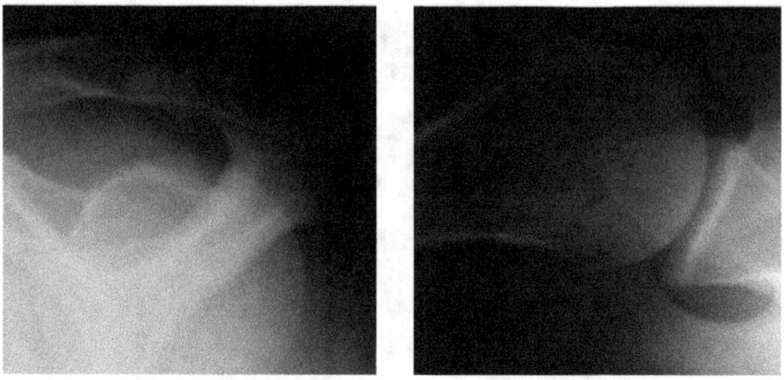

Fig. 4: Os Acromiale. It is not obvious on the outlet view but the os acromiale can be seen on the axillary view.

dependent on the operator and the anatomy of the lesion cannot be fully appreciated.

3. **Magnetic resonance imaging (MRI)** for assessing soft tissues, degree of muscle atrophy, and fatty infiltration with a sensitivity of 92% and specificity of 93% in detecting rotator cuff tears [10].

5. Arthroscopic Surgery

1. **Indications for surgery:**
    - symptomatic patients with tendinosis proven on imaging, presenting with recalcitrant pain and impingement test positive;
    - failed physiotherapy and H&L injection attempted;
    - anterior overhanging spur proven on imaging and typical symptoms;
    - ACJ OA seen on X-rays and pain on cross-body adduction.
2. **Positioning and portals:**
    - **Position:** Beach chair.
    - **Posterior portal:** This portal is used for initial viewing of the subacromial space, and surface marked 2 cm medial and about 1 cm inferior to the postero-lateral corner of the acromion. Run the obturator beneath the bony acromion, at all times the bony acromion must be felt as a solid roof of the subacromial space. The trajectory is pointing superiorly. A direct horizontal trajectory runs the risk of the obturator piercing/penetrating through the muscle of the supraspinatus. Once the obturator is in the subacromial space,

make brisk sweeping movements to clear the bursa. If this is difficult, consider re-entering the space.

- **Antero-superior:** Visualisation in the subacromial space filled with inflamed bursa would be challenging, if this portal is created directly from the outside in. An easier way would be inside-out. The camera from the posterior portal is pushed anteriorly, to a point just lateral to the coracoid tip. A small skin incision is made to allow the camera to spear out, over which a 5 mm cannula is threaded in. As the camera is receded back into the subacromial space, a shaver or RF wand is inserted into the cannula. Keep the instruments within visualisation, but be careful not to damage the lens as the RF is used. In a very densely inflamed bursa, the instruments can get easily blocked by the inflammed tissues.
- **Lateral:** This is surface marked in the middle of the lateral edge of the acromion, about 2 cm from the bone edge. A needle pointing 30° to 45° superiorly will lead to the subacromial space. Both these portals, lateral and antero-superior provide orthogonal views to debride the bursa and shave the acromion.
- **Acromio-clavicular joint (ACJ) portal:** This portal is made through the AC joint, from the superior capsule of the joint a needle is inserted about 20–30° obliquely medial. It is widened using an obturator and can fit a shaver to perform the Mumford's procedure.

CONTROLLING BLEEDING:
1. INCREASE FLUID PRESSURE 2. ADD EPINEPHRINE IN SALINE 3. USE RADIOFREQUENCY WANDS

3. **Arthroscopic Subacromial Decompression and Acromioplasty**
   (a) **Debriding the space**
   - Begin by shaving away the bursa with the shaver tip under direct visualisation. Create a space, then slowly debride away the bursa (Figs. 5(a)–5(c)).
   - Use the RF wand in ablate mode to clear the bursa from the acromion superiorly, to skeletonise the acromion free of soft tissues.

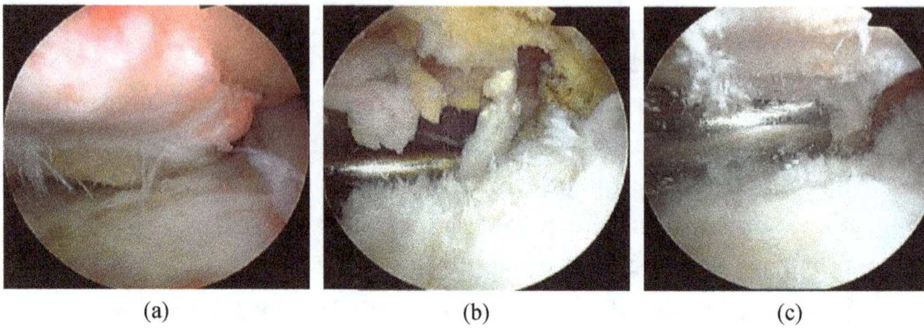

Fig. 5 (a), (b), (c): Subacromial Decompression and Acromioplasty. The bursa can be thickened (a) as in this example. A shaver from the lateral portal (b) clears the bursa and a burr can be used to flatten the overhanging acromion (c).

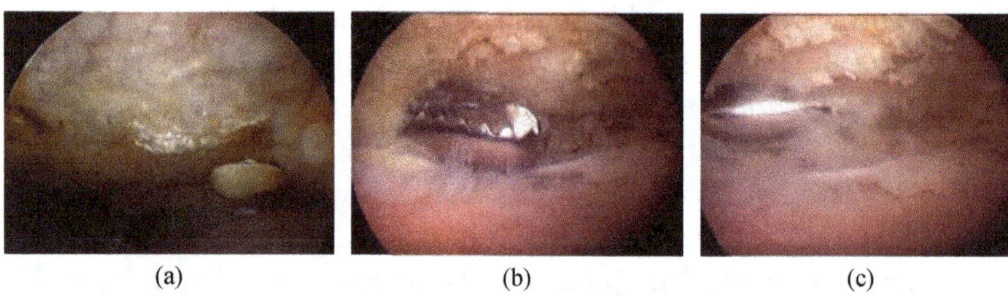

Fig. 6 (a), (b), (c): Acromioplasty. The shape of the acromion can only be ascertained after clearing the acromion of soft tissues (a). In this case, a shaver is used to perform the acromioplasty (b). The acromion is shaved till flat, viewed from posterior (c) and lateral portals.

- Inflammed bursa tends to bleed easily. To minimise bleeding, measures include:
  i. Increasing the fluid pressure to at least 90 mm Hg.
  ii. Addition of 1 mL epinephrine every 3 L of arthroscopic saline.
  iii. Use of radiofrequency to cauterise bleeding bursa.

(b) **Anterior limits of the subacromial space**

- Anteriorly, debride the bursa till the **anterior edge of the acromion**, which is covered by the **CA ligament**. Detach the CA ligament completely, from anterior to mid-lateral acromion (Fig. 6(a)). Beyond this the muscle fibres of the anterior deltoid come into view, be careful when shaving this layer as the muscle layer bleeds easily. *Only after detaching the CAL can the morphology of the acromion be appreciated.*

- Medial to the acromion, the inferior aspects of **the ACJ and lateral end of the clavicle** can be debrided.

(c) **Lateral limits**

- Superiorly the deltoid muscles are attached to the **lateral edge of the acromion**. Be careful not to cause muscular bleeding as the bursa is being debrided.

  Using a shaver, make brisk sweeping movements to clear the bursa over the rounded convex humeral head till the normal whitish tendon is seen. *Be careful not to debride the capsule about 4 cm below the tuberosity of the humeral head, below this the axillary nerve is at risk. It is difficult to access the capsule this low.*

(d) **Medial limits**

- The straight trajectory from the posterior portal lies over the muscular portion of the supraspinatus. Medial to this is **fat pad**, which hides a rich vascular supply and the supraclavicular nerve. Debride the fat pad limitedly and slowly, and only if needed.
- An accompanying vessel usually follows the nerve as it curls around the spine of the scapula, at the postero-medial corner of the subacromial space. Be careful when shaving this region.

(e) **Posterior decompression**

- Posteriorly the bursa is limited by a soft tissue curtain. By switching the camera to view from the lateral portal, a shaver from the posterior portal is used to clear the posterior bursa.

LIMITS OF SUBACROMIAL DECOMPRESSION
Anterior: acromion, CA ligament, anterior deltoid, ACJ, clavicle Lateral: acromion with attachment of deltoid Medial: the fat pad overlying the muscles of the supraspinatus Posterior: bursa ends like a curtain

(f) **Acromioplasty**

- A 3.5 mm burr or the shaver (in forward unidirectional mode, at max speed of 2600 rpm) can be used from the lateral portal to debride and shave away the overhanging osteophytes (Fig. 6(b)). Decorticate the acromion till bleeding cancellous bone is visible.
  (*The author's preference is NOT to use the burr, as it causes scalloping of the acromion under-surface. A shaver creates a more even debriding.*)
- *When is adequate acromioplasty done, how much bone should be debrided away?* A guide would be the following criteria:
  i. The acromion must appear flat in both orthogonal views. From the posterior view, it must be flat medial-laterally (Fig. 6(c)). Switch the camera to the lateral view, the acromion must be flat postero-anteriorly. Create a slope anteriorly and laterally, so that the superior edge of the acromion does not end abruptly but slopes away antero-laterally.
  ii. Minimise the thickness of the acromion by 3–5 mm, more if needed.
  iii. Ensure the subacromial space is widened to 7–10 mm with the fluid at 90 mm Hg pressure.

4. Arthroscopic Mumford's procedure

This procedure, if indicated, is done at the same time as SAD. It is not done routinely.

- Establish the ACJ portal as described above. A needle is used to pierce the ACJ from superior and the inferior penetration viewed in the subacromial space. It is widened to fit in a shaver (Fig. 7(a)).
- The ACJ is debrided by sweeping the shaver in the ACJ in the anterior-posterior direction. Do not shave the anterior and posterior ligaments of the ACJ. The lateral end of the clavicle can also be debrided to further widen the ACJ (Fig. 7(b)).

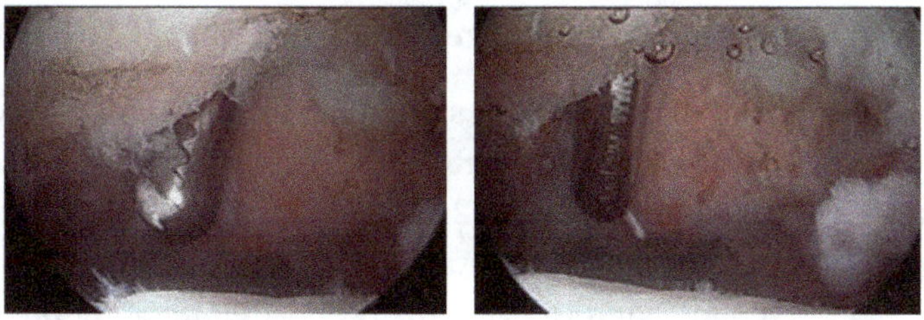

(a) (b)

Fig. 7: (a), (b): Mumford's procedure. An ACJ portal is created in the joint, then widened with an obturator. A shaver is used to debride the acromion (a) and the lateral end of the clavicle (b) to widen the ACJ joint space.

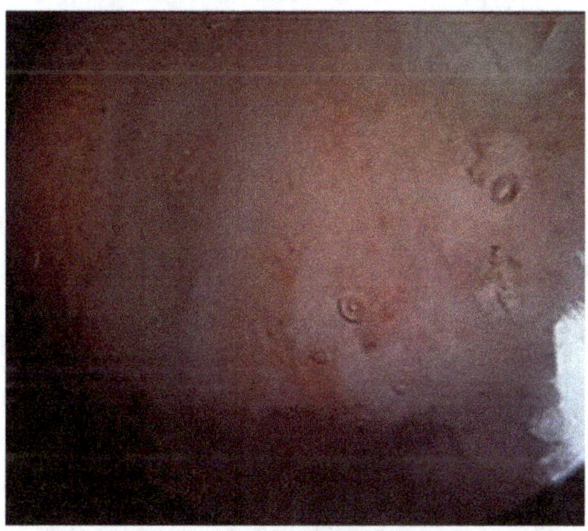

Fig. 8: The widened AC joint space. After the Mumford's procedure and the ACJ is completely debrided and widened, it is seen from beneath. A space between the acromion and clavicle must admit at least the shaver (7–10 mm wide).

- The shaver is then employed from the antero-superior portal to debride and minimise the inferior surface of the lateral clavicle. At the end of the procedure, the widened ACJ must be clearly visible (Fig. 8).
- This technique of Mumford's procedure compromises the superior and inferior capsule of the ACJ but preserves the anterior and posterior ligaments. *It does not destabilise the ACJ nor cause subluxation after the procedure.*

6. Post-operative Management and Rehabilitation

(a) Arm sling for initial comfort but should be encouraged to remove and begin active ROM and passive ROM exercises. Abduction exercises should be avoided in the initial 2 weeks as to minimise unnecessary compression of subacromial structures.
(b) Once pain is reduced and ROM is restored, strengthening physiotherapy exercises should be initiated.
(c) Sports-specific activity should wait until patients regain full ROM and normal strength (approximately 3–4 months).
(d) Post-operative plain X-rays should be obtained to assess for adequate subacromial decompression, which would be seen as a type I acromial arch without any residual spurring.

7. Outcomes of SAD

(a) With the current published evidence, the opinion on the outcome of SAD remains inconclusive. Some of the studies suggested that there is no difference in outcome between conservative and surgical management of Impingement Syndrome, while other studies noted a significant difference in favour of SAD especially for RCT studies with more than 10 years of follow up [11–13].
(b) Bjornsson *et al*. showed a reduction in prevalence of rotator cuff tears among SAD patient compared with asymptomatic adult of the same age [14].

References

1. Vivek P, Jaap WW. Rotator cuff tear: A detailed update; *Asia-Pacific J Sports Med* 2015;11(1). doi: 10.1016/j.asmart.2014.11.003.
2. Consigliere P, Haddo O, Levy O, Sforza G. Subacromial impingement syndrome: management challenges. *Orthop Res Rev* 2018;10:83–91.
3. Neer CS 2nd. Impingement lesions. *Clin Orthop Relat Res* 1983 Mar; (173):70–77.
4. Diercks R, Bron C, Dorrestijn O, *et al*. Guideline for diagnosis and treatment of subacromial pain syndrome: a multidisciplinary review by the Dutch

Orthopaedic Association. *Acta Orthop* 2014;85(3):314–322. doi:10.3109/17453674.2014.920991.

5. Michener LA, Walsworth MK, Doukas WC, Murphy KP. Reliability and diagnostic accuracy of 5 physical examination tests and combination of tests for subacromial impingement. *Arch Phys Med Rehab* 2009;90:1898–1903.
6. Katthagen JC, Marchetti DC, Tahal DS, Turnbull TL, Millett PJ: The effects of arthroscopic lateral acromioplasty on the critical shoulder angle and the anterolateral deltoid origin: an anatomic cadaveric study. *Arthroscopy* 2016;32:569–575.
7. Nyffeler RW, Werner CM, Sukthankar A, Schmid MR, Gerber C. Association of a large lateral extension of the acromion with rotator cuff tears. *J Bone Joint Surg Am* 2006;88:800–805.
8. Saupe N, Pfirrmann CW, Schmid MR, Jost B, Werner CM, Zanetti M: Association between rotator cuff abnormalities and reduced acromiohumeral distance. *Am J Roentgenol* 2006;187:376–382.
9. Merrill Lee, Jerry Yongqian Chen, Ming Han Lincoln Liow, Hwei Chi Chong, Paul Chang, Denny Lie. Critical shoulder angle and acromial index do not influence 24-month functional outcome after arthroscopic rotator cuff repair. *Am J Sports Med* 2017;45(13). doi: 10.1177/0363546517717947.
10. de Jesus JO, Parker L, Frangos AJ, Nazarian LN. Accuracy of MRI, MR arthrography, and ultrasound in the diagnosis of rotator cuff tears: a meta-analysis. *Am J Roentgenol* 2009;192:1701–1707.
11. Brox JI, Gjengedal E, Uppheim G, *et al.* Arthroscopic surgery versus supervised exercises in patients with rotator cuff disease (stage II impingement syndrome): a prospective, randomized, controlled study in 125 patients with a 2½-year follow-up. *J Shoulder Elbow Surg* 1999;8:102–111.
12. Magaji SA, Singh HP, Pandey RK. Arthroscopic subacromial decompression is effective in selected patients with shoulder impingement syndrome. *J Bone Joint Surg Br* 2012; 94B:1086–1089.
13. Farfaras S, Sernert N, Rostgard Christensen L, Hallström EK, Kartus JT. Subacromial decompression yields a better clinical outcome than therapy alone: a prospective randomized study of patients with a minimum of 10-year follow-up. *Am J Sports Med* 2018; 46:1397–1407.
14. Björnsson H, Norlin R, Knutsson A, Adolfson L. Fewer rotator cuff tears fifteen years after arthroscopic subacromial decompression. *J Shoulder Elbow Surg* 2010;19:111–115.

https://doi.org/10.1142/9789811249846_0014

Chapter 14

Arthroscopic Repair of Partial Tears

Denny T.T. Lie and Cheow Xunqi

Summary of Chapter

1. Introduction and epidemiology of partial tears
2. Pathophysiology and causes
3. Clinical presentation and examination
4. Diagnosis and imaging
5. Surgical technique of arthroscopic repair of PASTA lesions using TransTend system
6. Surgical technique of arthroscopic repair of bursal-sided tears
7. Rehabilitation
8. Clinical outcomes

1. Introduction and Epidemiology of Partial Tears

Partial thickness rotator cuff tears are a common cause of shoulder pain and loss of function in adult patients [1,2], and are more prevalent than full thickness tears [3,4]. The prevalence of partial thickness rotator cuff tears are thought to be about 20% in the general population [5], with marked increase in prevalence after 50 years of age [6]. Articular-sided partial thickness rotator cuff tears are thought to be about twice as common as bursal-sided tears [7].

Small tears can be treated conservatively without surgery [8,9], or with surgery [10–12]. However tear progression is a problem for patients who are treated non-surgically [13–16]. Arthroscopic repair has recently emerged as the surgical technique of choice, over open or mini-open repairs [17–19], with evidence favourable results in the short, medium [2,20], and long term [21–23].

2. Clinical Presentation

The patient typically complains of pain in the shoulder especially during overhead activities, and this could be worse during night time, in particular when sleeping on the affected shoulder. The patient may also complain of weakness in shoulder range of motion. Physical examination of the affected shoulder usually reveals a painful arc of motion between 60° and 120° of abduction in supraspinatus tears. Special tests as described in Chapter 1 can be done but signs are equivocal.

3. Pathophysiology of Problem

Partial thickness rotator cuff tears could have a variety of aetiology and pathogenesis, and these are contributed by both intrinsic and extrinsic factors. Articular-sided tears are believed to be mainly associated with intrinsic factors, while bursal-sided tears are mostly associated with extrinsic factors [24]. Intrinsic factors predispose the rotator cuff tendon to attrition, and these include age-related changes in the histological characteristics and vascularity of the tendon [3,6,25]. On the other hand, extrinsic factors can be contributed by subacromial impingement [26], as well as internal impingement [27]. Acute avulsion injuries of the rotator cuff have also been observed in patients following a fall or trauma to the shoulder [28,29].

4. Diagnosis and Imaging, Algorithm

4.1 *Ultrasound*

Ultrasound imaging is both effective and cost-efficient in the diagnosis of partial thickness rotator cuff tears (Fig. 1). However, its diagnostic

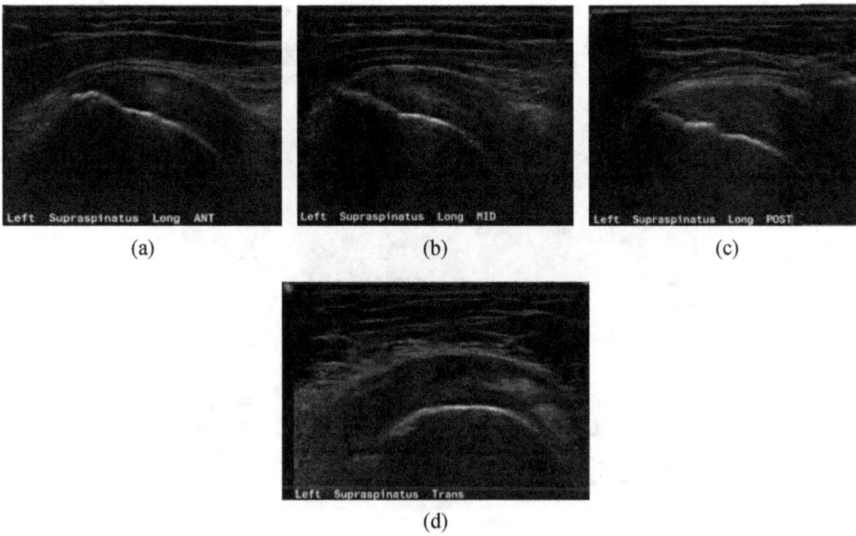

Fig. 1: Ultrasound images of partial thickness tear. (a) The ultrasound longitudinal view of an articular-sided partial thickness tear of the anterior supraspinatus tendon. (b) and (c): The tear diminishing in size. (d) The transverse view of the tendon showing the lift-off at the anterior edge of the tendon.

accuracy is highly user-dependent. It has been shown to be equal to MRI in terms of diagnostic accuracy in the hands of an experienced ultrasonographer [30,31]. In addition, it also allows for dynamic testing, and is widely available and accessible at most institutions.

4.2 *Magnetic Resonance Imaging*

Magnetic resonance imaging (MRI) remains the diagnostic standard for rotator cuff tears, with excellent sensitivity and specificity (Fig. 2). Compared to ultrasound imaging, it allows for evaluation of muscle quality and the degree of muscle fatty atrophy, and provides better characterisation of soft tissue structures in the shoulder joint [30].

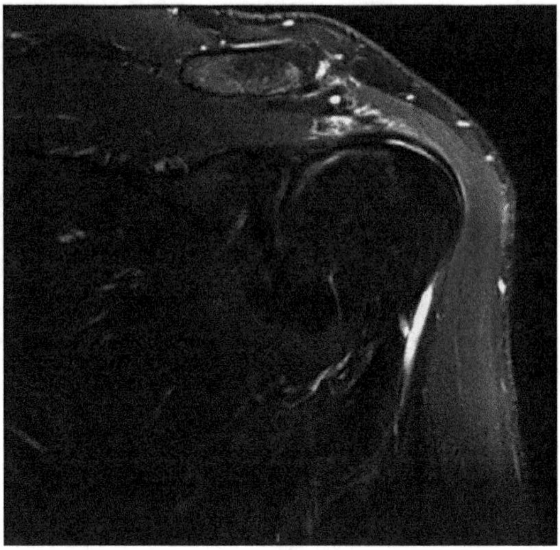

Fig. 2: MRI image of partial thickness tear. This MRI coronal view of shows the thinning out of the lateral of the supraspinatus tendon, suggesting an articular-sided partial tear.

4.3 *Treatment Algorithm for Partial Thickness Rotator Cuff Tears*

(a) **Tears <10 mm (AP direction)**
Such tears could be managed with a trial of conservative therapy, which entails analgesia, physiotherapy, activity modifications, as well as injections (e.g. steroid injections, platelet-rich plasma injections). The patient should be followed up subsequently and a repeat ultrasound at around 6–12 months could be considered to look for progression of the tear. Patients who fail conservative treatment after a period of at least 6 weeks should be counselled to consider surgical repair.

(b) **Tears >10 mm (AP direction)**
Patients with tears more than 10 mm should be counselled for surgical repair, see algorithm (Fig. 3), as the risk of tear progression without surgery is significant. Should the patient decide for conservative management, a repeat ultrasound should be performed at 6–12 months to look for progression of the tear.

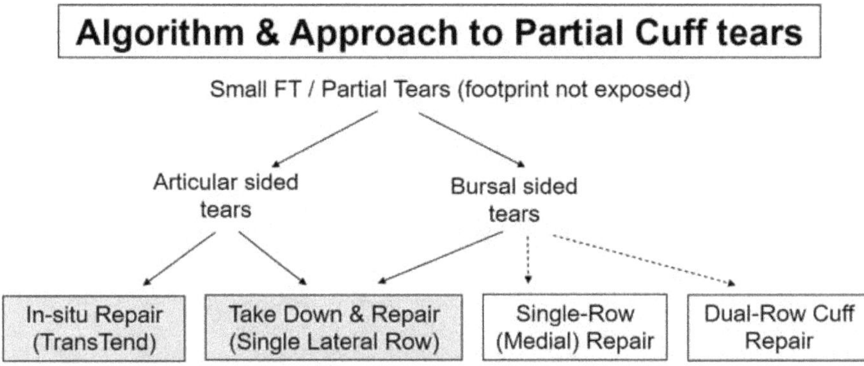

Fig. 3: Approach to partial thickness tears. Partial thickness tears are either articular or bursal-sided. Articular-sided tears are either repaired *in-situ* or taken down and repaired, as are bursal-sided tears. Repair is usually done by a single lateral-row technique described below.

5. Arthroscopic Surgery

5.1 *Arthroscopic Repair of Partial Articular-Sided Tears*

(a) **Indications for surgery**
- symptomatic partial articular-sided tears of the supraspinatus;
- >50% thickness involved;
- failed physiotherapy and medications;
- younger patients.

(b) **Special instruments**
- the TransTend anchor system (Figs. 4 and 5).

(c) **Positioning and portals**
- standard posterior, anterior and lateral portals.

5.2 *Arthroscopic Repair of Partial Articular-Sided Tears Using TransTend System and Dual-Pulley Compression Configuration*

This technique is useful for small partial-thickness articular-sided tears. The tear is first identified from the glenohumeral joint and two TransTend

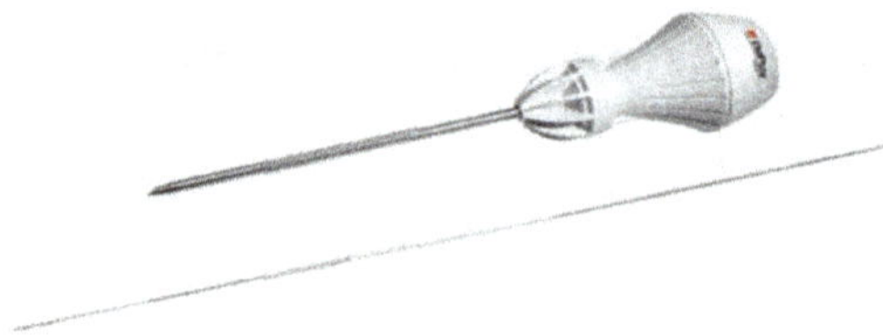

Fig. 4: TransTend wire and cannula.

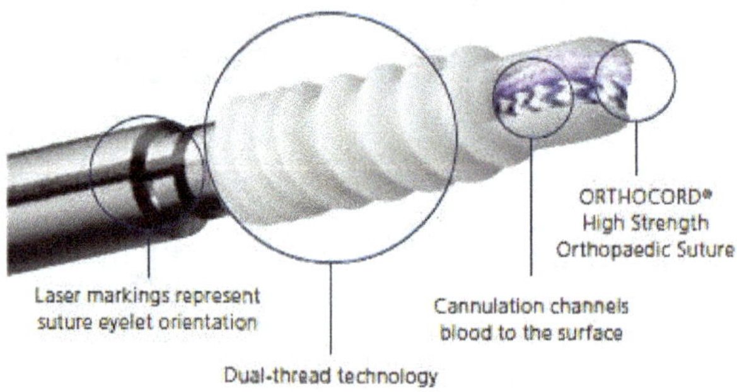

Fig. 5: TransTend anchor. The anchor design is similar to the Healix family of anchors.

anchors deployed. The sutures are then tied from the subacromial space and compression achieved. This technique involves several steps:

(a) **Identification, debridement and preparation of the tear from the glenohumeral**

- With the camera from the posterior portal, inspection begins in the glenohumeral joint and the partial tear on the under-surface of the supraspinatus tendon is identified.
- Visualisation is improved by bringing the arm to abduction and external rotation. If possible, debride and shave the frayed edges of the tear using a shaver from the anterior portal (Fig. 6).

(b) **Anterior anchor**

- A wire is used to pierce the tendon at the anterior edge of the tear, medial to the tear. It is critical the wire should pierce *normal and healthy tendon* ***medial*** to the tear and not the partial-thickness tear itself (Figs. 7(a) and 7(b)).

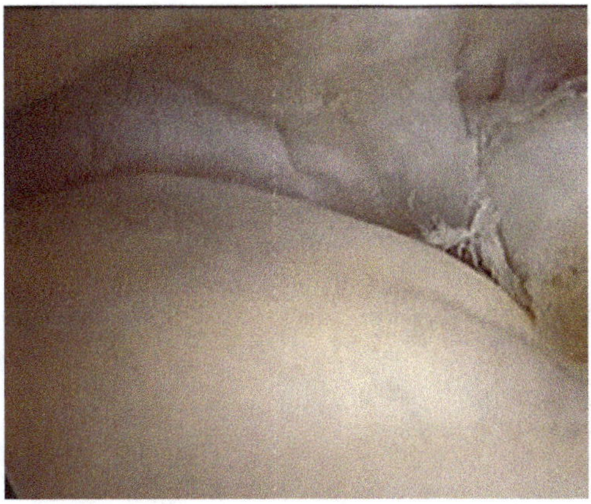

Fig. 6: PASTA lesion. By abducting and externally rotating the arm, the partial articular-sided tear is seen.

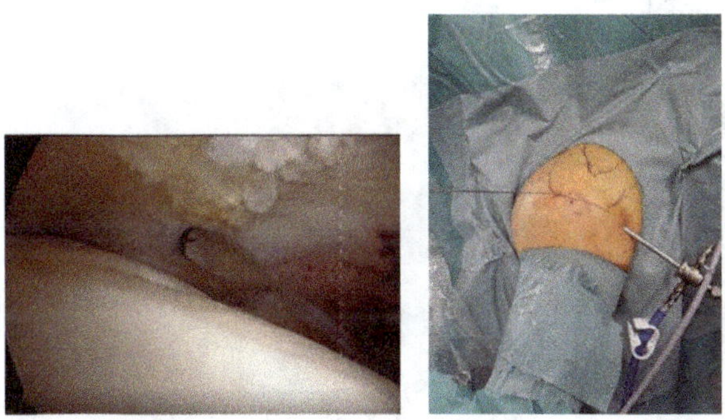

(a) (b)

Fig. 7: The anterior wire. (a) The wire piercing the healthy tendon medial to the tear, at the anterior edge of the tear. (b) The horizontal orientation of the wire, at the antero-lateral edge of the acromion.

- The cannula is then inserted over the wire (Fig. 8(a)) and holding the cannula over the exposed footprint at the anterior edge of the tear, an awl (Fig. 8(b)) is used before the anchor is inserted (Fig. 9).

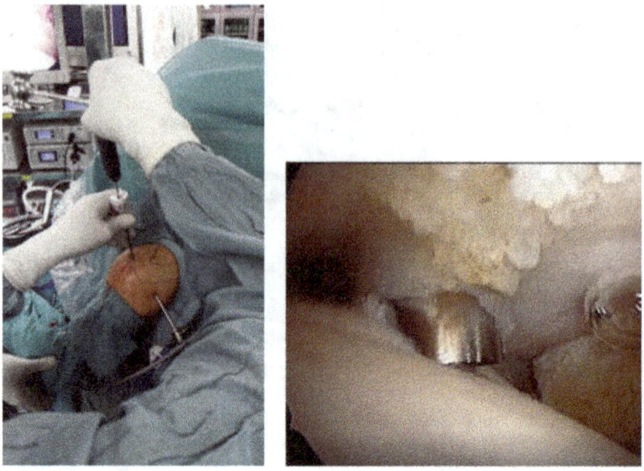

(a) (b)

Fig. 8: The cannula insertion. The cannula is then inserted over the wire and angled as shown in (a). (b) shows the position of the cannula, just medial to the footprint, where the anchor is to be placed.

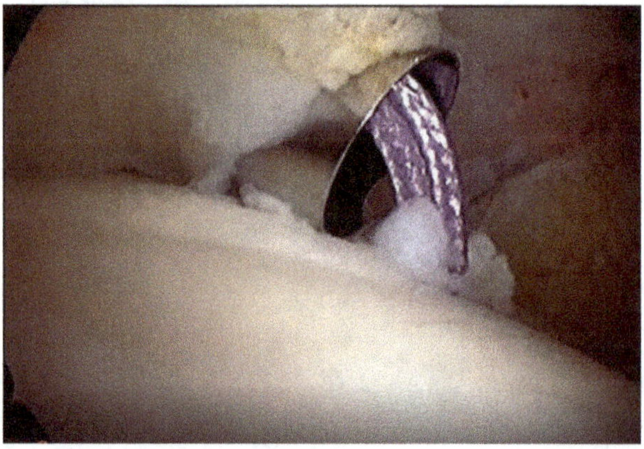

Fig. 9: The anterior anchor. It shows the sutures from the anterior anchor thus deployed.

(c) **Posterior anchor**

- In a similar way, a wire is used to pierce the posterior edge of the tear, in healthy tendon medial to the tear. The cannula is inserted over the wire and the posterior anchor is positioned at the posterior end of the footprint and inserted (Fig. 10).

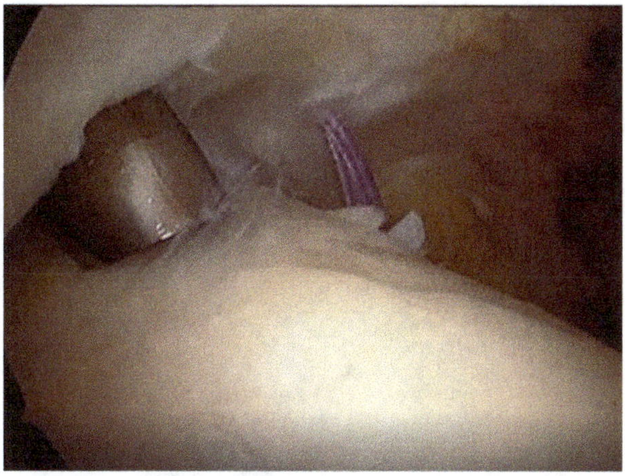

Fig. 10: The posterior anchor. In a similar a wire is positioned at the posterior end of the tear, over which the cannula is inserted and anchor deployed.

(d) **The transverse suture**

- The subacromial space is entered and carefully debrided. It is important to protect the four sutures from both anchors. An easy way is to insert knot-pushers into the sutures, hence localising them and protecting them at the same time. Keep these sutures taut and debride the bursa carefully to have a clear view of the four sutures (Fig. 11).
- Then retrieve all four sutures from the same soft tissue portal.
- Tie one suture limb from each anchor together thus creating a transverse suture between the anchors. This is the suture that will compress and thus repair the partial tear (PASTA) onto the original footprint (Fig. 12(a)).
- By pulling on the free suture limbs, the transverse suture is thus compressed by this dual-pulley technique (Fig. 12(b)).

(e) **Compression with a Versalok anchor**

- The key to healing of the PASTA repair is compression of the transverse tie. Tying the free suture limbs alone will not achieve adequate nor continual compression.
- Hence both free suture limbs are threaded into a Versalok anchor (Fig. 13(a)), which is then deployed over the greater tuberosity, equidistant from both anchors (Fig. 13(b)). *This dual-pulley*

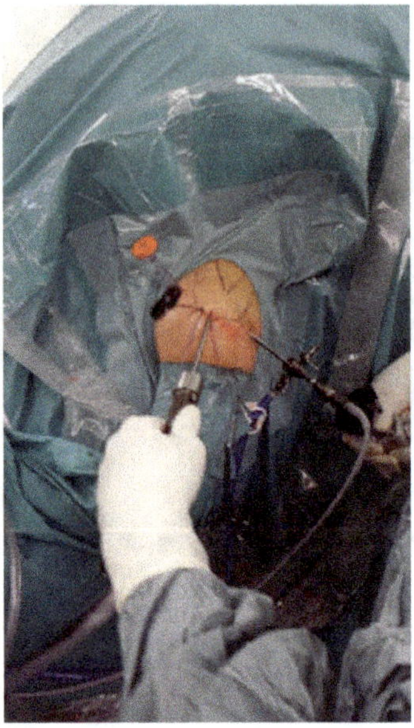

Fig. 11: Debriding the subacromial space. It shows a knot pusher is threaded into the suture to locate and protect it.

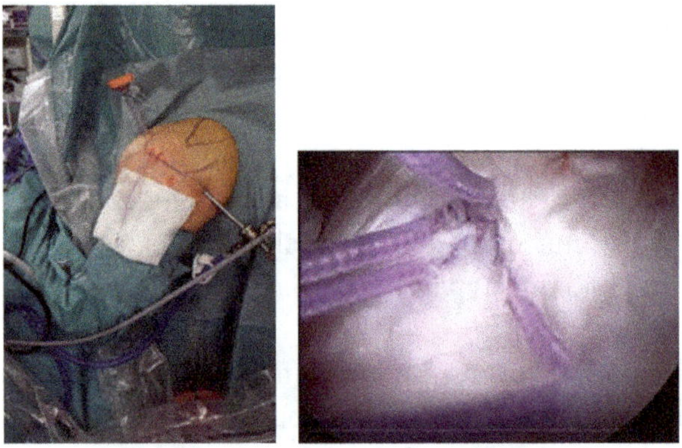

(a) (b)

Fig. 12: The horizontal tie. One suture limb from each anchor is retrieved and tied to each other, shown in (a). As the free suture limbs are pulled, the horizontal tie is delivered and compressed the partial tear, shown in (b).

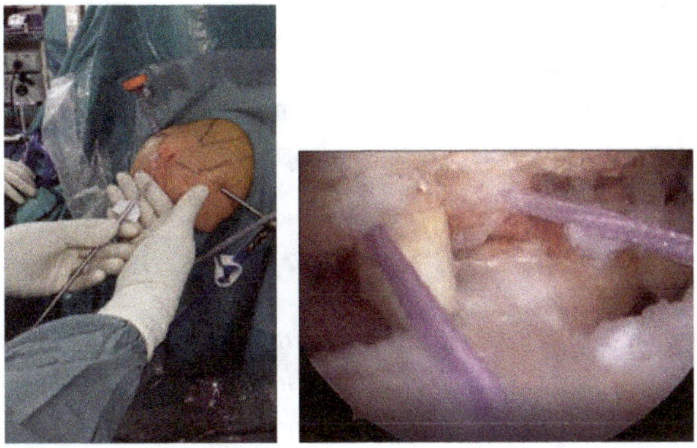

(a) (b)

Fig. 13: The lateral row. The free suture limbs are then threaded into a Versalok anchor shown in (a), which is then deployed over the greater tuberosity as shown in (b).

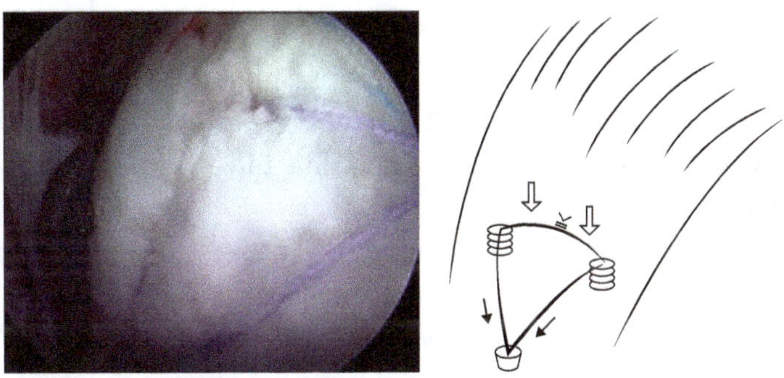

(a) (b)

Fig. 14: The double-pulley compression system. As the free suture limbs are pulled tightly by the Versalok anchor, the horizontal tie compresses the partial tear firmly onto its footprint, shown in (a) and schematically in (b).

technique thus restores and repairs PASTA tears on the original footprint, and achieves good compression by securing the free sutures to a Versalok anchor (Figs. 14(a) and 14(b)).

5.3 *Arthroscopic Repair of Articular or Bursal-Sided Tears by Single Lateral-Row Repair*

(a) **Indications for surgery:**

- symptomatic partial articular or bursal-sided tears of the supraspinatus;

- >50% thickness involved;
- failed physiotherapy and medications;
- older patients whose tendons are more degenerate.

(b) **Positioning and portals:** Standard portals used.

5.4 *Arthroscopic Single Lateral-Row Technique*

This technique is useful for small full-thickness tears, bursal-sided and articular-sided tears. In all these tears, the bony footprint of the tendon is small, not visible at all or covered with remnant tendon; hence medial row anchors are not required. This technique involves several steps:

(a) **Identification, debridement and preparation of the tear from the glenohumeral**
- From the glenohumeral joint with the camera from the posterior portal, the under-surface of the supraspinatus tendon is identified. *Visualisation is improved by bringing the arm to abduction and external rotation.* Articular-sided and full-thickness tears may be obvious.
- For bursal-sided tears, reference is made with the pre-operative MRI or ultrasound to geographically locate the tear; it usually is at the anterior edge of the supraspinatus tendon.
- A spinal needle is then inserted from the outside to locate the tear. It usually is from the antero-lateral portal, at the edge of the acromion lateral to the long head of the biceps (Fig. 15).
- A small skin incision is then made, the muscle and fascial layers dilated using a pair of forceps. Penetrate the partial tear/small full-thickness tear with the forceps then dilate the tear. Degenerate tendons easily fall away, while normal tendons offer a firm resistance.
- Shave the degenerate tendon at the rim of the small tear, degenerate tendons are soft and are shaved away easily. Avoid using RF at this stage to avoid charring the tissues. Any punctate bleeding from the tendon is a sign of healthy tendon.

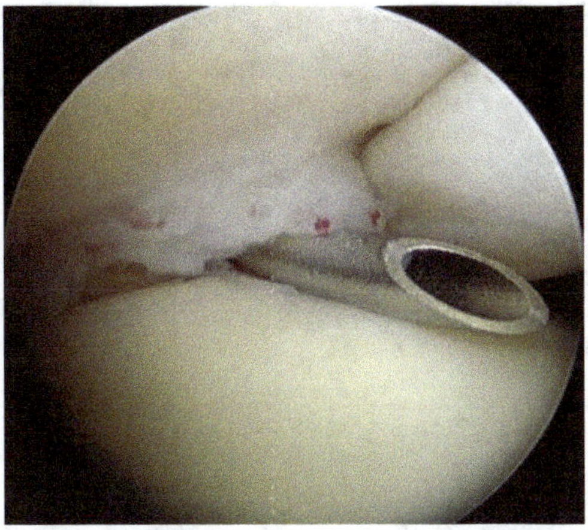

Fig. 15: Marking the partial tear. It shows the articular-sided tear clearly and this will be marked by a suture threaded through the needle.

(b) **Subacromial space preparation**

- The subacromial space is entered the usual way. Often the tear is not easily visualised in the subacromial space if the bursa is not adequately cleared. A guide is the antero-lateral portal created earlier to locate the tear.
- Use the obturator to probe the tendon and hence locate the tear (Fig. 16).
- Shave the edges of the tear till firm healthy-looking tendon is seen.

(c) **The anterior suture**

- A loose Orthocord© suture is loaded onto a suture passer (Express Sew© III). The camera is kept at the posterior portal with the arm in slight external rotation. The Express Sew suture passer is inserted via the antero-lateral portal, and its lower jaw is inserted into the tear at about 45° anterior to the axis of the tear (Fig. 17).
- The suture bite is made as deep/anterior as possible (length of the suture passer, at least 16 mm long). Be careful to avoid the biceps tendon just anterior to the tear, keep the lower jaw close to the under-surface of the tendon.

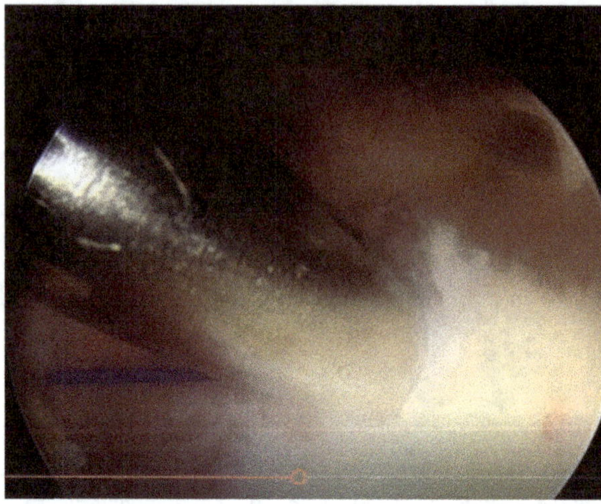

Fig. 16: Completing the partial tear. After a good subacromial decompression, the tear is localised and completed using an obturator, and shaved clean.

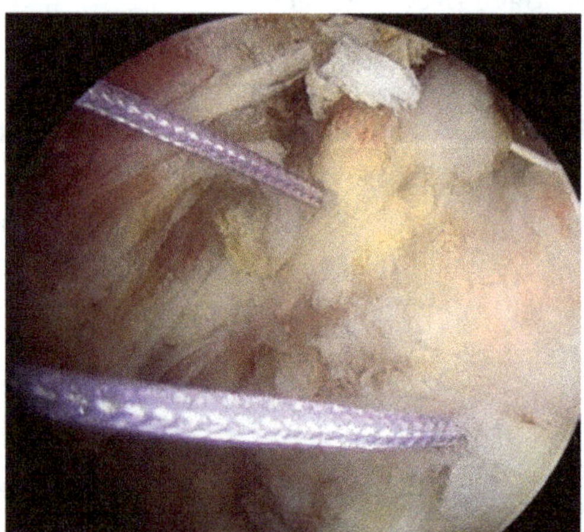

Fig. 17: The anterior suture. A loose Orthocord suture is passed antegrade using an Express Sew passer, anterior to the tear.

- The suture is then retrieved, passed to the anterior portal and clipped with an artery forceps. The middle of the loose suture is also clipped to maintain the loop.

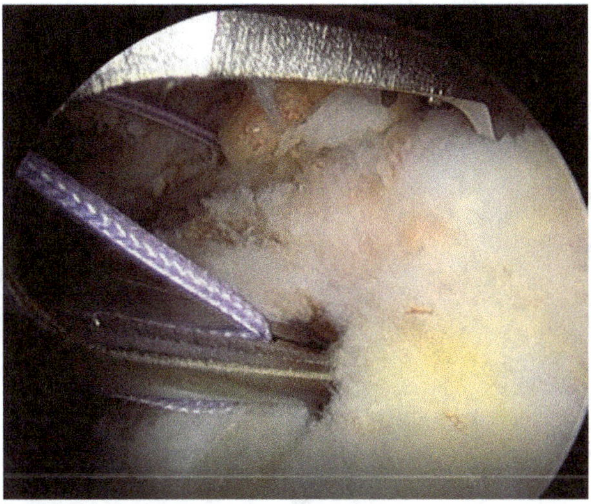

Fig. 18: The middle suture. The other limb of the loose suture is then passed directly medial to the tear. The bite is smaller than the previous, but the suture is not pulled through.

(d) **The looped middle suture**

- The other end of the suture is then loaded to the suture passer and the suture is passed in the middle of the tear, or along the axis of the tear at the centre (Fig. 18).
- The bite is made small; about half the length of the suture passer (about 8–10 mm long).
- It is retrieved from the same antero-lateral portal as the rest of the suture with an artery clipped in the middle loop (Fig. 19). *If a cannula is not used, ensure these sutures are in the same soft tissue portal. Retrieve all three sutures with a retriever to be safe!*
- On the outside of the shoulder joint, pass the suture limp into the loop. Then pull on both ends of the suture (the looped suture from the antero-lateral portal and the anterior suture from the anterior portal). The tear will close when the anterior suture is pulled tight (Fig. 20).

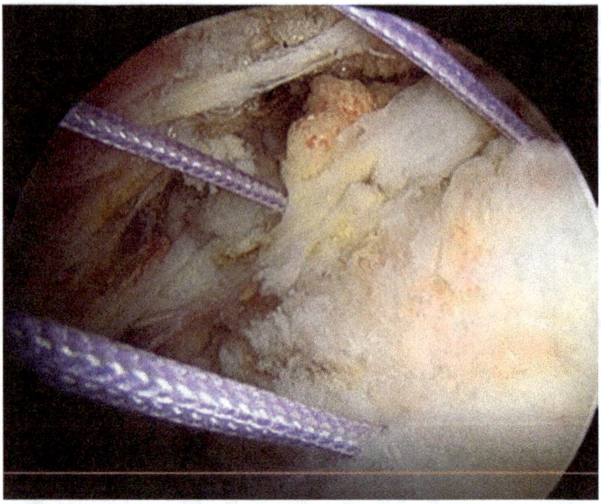

Fig. 19: Retaining the loop. The middle suture is NOT pulled through, to retain the loop.

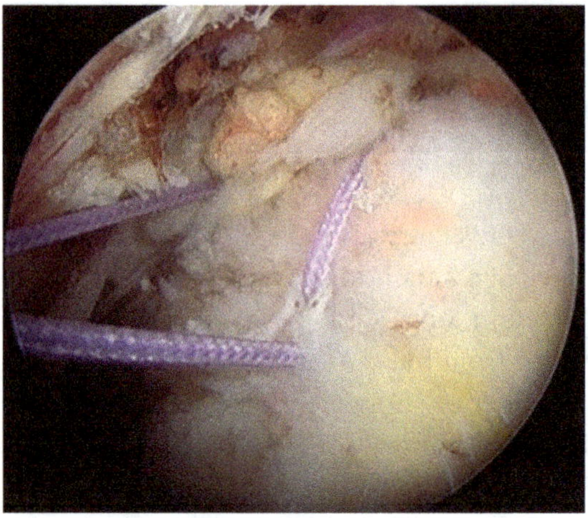

Fig. 20: The looped suture. The middle suture is passed through the loop. The tighter the anterior suture is pulled, the more compressed the looped suture will be.

(e) **The posterior suture**

- The end of the suture that was looped is then passed into the tendon posterior to the tear (Fig. 21). This can be done either antegrade or retrograde.

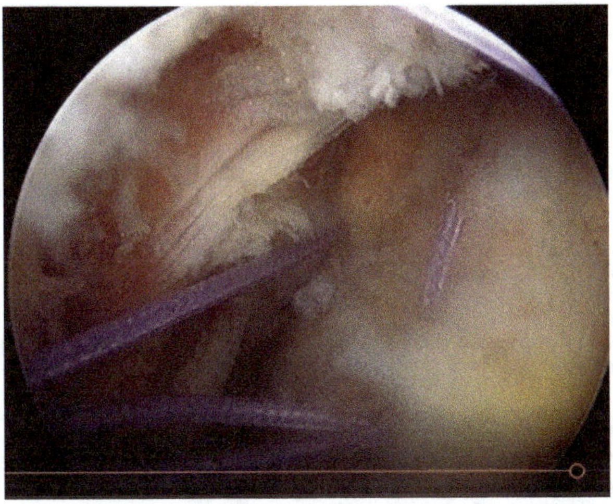

Fig. 21: The posterior suture. The middle-looped suture is then retrieved retrograde by a bird beak retriever, to become the posterior suture.

- Antegrade passing uses the suture passer angled at 45° posterior to the axis of the tear. The angle of approach may be difficult even after bringing the arm to internal rotation and the bite is limited to the length of the suture passer.
- A recommended way is retrograde passing using a bird beak retriever. The camera is shifted to the anterolateral portal, directly looking at the tear. A bird beak retriever is inserted from the posterior portal and pierces the tendon far posterior from the tear (usually at the infraspinatus, at least 20–25 mm posterior to the tear) to retrieve the suture.
- The suture is then retrieved from the anterior portal, where the anterior suture is parked. The camera is then transferred back to the posterior portal.

(f) **Securing the tear with a lateral row anchor**

- The two limbs of the loose suture are then retrieved from the antero-lateral portal, and secured to a lateral row anchor (Versalok anchor). *The tighter the anterior suture is pulled, the more compressed the tear will be. The tighter the posterior suture is pulled;*

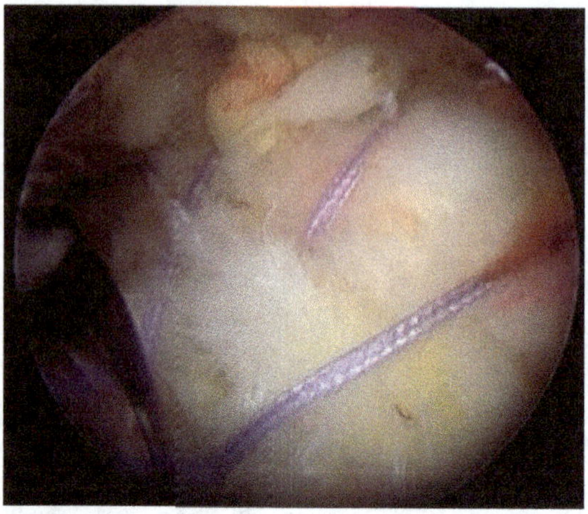

Fig. 22: The final check. Both ends of the suture are then secured to a Versalok anchor in the lateral row. The tighter the anterior suture is pulled, the more compressed the loop will become. The posterior suture lateralises the tendon, thus closing the tear.

the more approximated the anterior and posterior edges of the tear will become.

- The end result is thus a wide (about 20–30 mm apart) V-shaped suture configuration tied to a single lateral row anchor; in the middle of the which the tear is localised by the suture loop usually buried in (Fig. 22).
- The anterior suture compresses the tear, the posterior suture approximates and closes the tear.

6. Post-op Management and Rehabilitation

Post-operatively, the arm is supported in a universal arm-sling for 4 weeks. The patient is referred to the physiotherapist, and passive range of motion exercises are commenced 1 week post-operatively. Active range of motion exercises are only permitted from 6 weeks post-operatively, and progressive strengthening exercises are then introduced.

7. Outcomes

Arthroscopic repair of partial thickness rotator cuff tears has been shown in the literature to produce favourable functional outcome scores in the short, medium [2,20], and long term [21–23]. A meta-analysis of 347 athletes who underwent arthroscopic repair of rotator cuff tears showed an overall rate of return to sport of 70.2% at a mean follow-up of 40.1 months, with a higher rate of return to sports amongst recreational sports participants (73.3%) as compared to competitive sports (61.5%) and overhead sports (38%) participation [32].

There have been a few studies discussing the comparative outcomes of arthroscopic repair of articular-sided versus bursal-sided partial rotator cuff tears, with most agreeing that the location of the tears did not seem to affect the outcomes significantly [21,23,33]. Possible complications of arthroscopic repair of partial thickness rotator cuff tears include tear recurrence, failure to heal, infection, suprascapular nerve injury, shoulder stiffness, as well as pneumothorax.

In a study conducted in our institution evaluating and comparing the functional outcomes following arthroscopic repair of articular-sided versus bursal-sided partial thickness rotator cuff tears amongst 104 patients (65 patients with articular-sided tears and 39 patients with bursal-sided tears), we found that the patients in each group achieved statistically significant improvement in terms of pain relief and functional outcomes at 2 years. We also concluded that there was no statistically significant difference between the two groups in terms of improvement in range of motion, pain score, and functional outcome scores (Constant-Murley Shoulder Score, UCLA Shoulder Score, and Oxford Shoulder Score) at 2 years [34,35].

References

1. Ellman H. Diagnosis and treatment of incomplete rotator cuff tears. *Clin Orthop Relat Res* 1990;(254):64–74. doi:10.1097/00003086-199005000-00010.
2. Matthewson G, Beach CJ, Nelson AA, *et al.* Partial thickness rotator cuff tears: current concepts. *Adv Orthop* 2015;2015:458786. Epub 2015 Jun 11.
3. Lohr J, Uhthoff H. The pathogenesis of degenerative rotator cuff tears. *Orthop Trans* 1987;11:237–238.

4. Gartsman GM, Milne JC. Articular surface partial-thickness rotator cuff tears. *J Shoulder Elbow Surg* 1995;4(6):409–415. doi:10.1016/s1058-2746(05)80031-x.
5. Sher JS, Uribe JW, Posada A, Murphy BJ, Zlatkin MB. Abnormal findings on magnetic resonance images of asymptomatic shoulders. *J Bone Joint Surg Am* 1995;77(1):10–15. doi:10.2106/00004623-199501000-00002.
6. Milgrom C, Schaffler M, Gilbert S, van Holsbeeck M. Rotator-cuff changes in asymptomatic adults. The effect of age, hand dominance and gender. *J Bone Joint Surg Br* 1995;77(2):296–298.
7. Connor PM, Banks DM Tyson AB, Coumas JS, D'Alessandro DF. Magnetic resonance imaging of the asymptomatic shoulder of overhead athletes: A 5-year follow-up study. *Am J Sports Med* 2003;31(5):724–727. doi:10.1177/03635465030310051501.
8. Holmgren T, Björnsson Hallgren H, Öberg B, Adolfsson L, Johansson K. Effect of specific exercise strategy on need for surgery in patients with subacromial impingement syndrome: Randomised controlled study. *BMJ* 2012;344:e787. doi:10.1136/bmj.e787.
9. Ranebo MC, Björnsson Hallgren HC, Holmgren T, Adolfsson LE. Surgery and physiotherapy were both successful in the treatment of small, acute, traumatic rotator cuff tears: A prospective randomized trial. *J Shoulder Elbow Surg* 2020:459–470. Epub 2020 Jan 7. doi:10.1016/j.jse.2019.10.013.
10. Moosmayer S, Lund G, Seljom US, *et al.* At a 10-year follow-up, tendon repair is superior to physiotherapy in the treatment of small and medium-sized rotator cuff tears. *J Bone Joint Surg Am* 2019;101(12):1050–1060. doi:10.2106/JBJS.18.01373.
11. Kukkonen J, Joukainen A, Lehtinen J, *et al.* Treatment of nontraumatic rotator cuff tears: A randomized controlled trial with two years of clinical and imaging follow-up. *J Bone Joint Surg Am* 2015;97(21):1729–1737. doi:10.2106/JBJS.N.01051.
12. Lambers Heerspink FO, van Raay JJ, Koorevaar RC, *et al.* Comparing surgical repair with conservative treatment for degenerative rotator cuff tears: Arandomized controlled trial. *J Shoulder Elbow Surg* 2015;24(8):1274–1281. doi:10.1016/j.jse.2015.05.040.
13. Keener JD, Galatz LM, Teefey SA, *et al.* A prospective evaluation of survivorship of asymptomatic degenerative rotator cuff tears. *J Bone Joint Surg Am* 2015;97(2):89–98. doi:10.2106/JBJS.N.00099.
14. Maman E, Harris C, White L, Tomlinson G, Shashank M, Boynton E. Outcome of nonoperative treatment of symptomatic rotator cuff tears

monitored by magnetic resonance imaging. *J Bone Joint Surg Am* 2009;91(8):1898–1906. doi:10.2106/JBJS.G.01335.

15. Moosmayer S, Tariq R, Stiris M, Smith HJ. The natural history of asymptomatic rotator cuff tears: A three-year follow-up of fifty cases. *J Bone Joint Surg Am* 2013;95(14):1249–1255. doi:10.2106/JBJS.L.00185.
16. Ranebo MC, Björnsson Hallgren HC, Norlin R, Adolfsson LE. Clinical and structural outcome 22 years after acromioplasty without tendon repair in patients with subacromial pain and cuff tears. *J Shoulder Elbow Surg* 2017;26(7):1262–1270. Epub 2017 Jan 25. doi:10.1016/j.jse.2016.11.012.
17. Huang R, Wang S, Wang Y, Qin X, Sun Y. Systematic review of all-arthroscopic versus mini-open repair of rotator cuff tears: A meta-analysis. *Sci Rep* 2016;7;6:22857. Epub 2016 Mar 7. doi:10.1038/srep22857.
18. Yamaguchi K, Levine WN, Marra G, Galatz LM, Klepps S, Flatow EL. Transitioning to arthroscopic rotator cuff repair: The pros and cons. *Instr Course Lect* 2003;52:81–92.
19. Dunn WR, Schackman BR, Walsh C, *et al*. Variation in orthopaedic surgeons' perceptions about the indications for rotator cuff surgery. *J Bone Joint Surg Am* 2005;87(9):1978–1984. doi:10.2106/JBJS.D.02944.
20. Deutsch A. Arthroscopic repair of partial-thickness tears of the rotator cuff. *J Shoulder Elbow Surg* 2007;16(2):193–201. Epub 2006 Nov 16. doi:10.1016/j.jse.2006.07.001.
21. Vap AR, Mannava S, Katthagen JC, *et al*. Five-year outcomes after arthroscopic repair of partial-thickness supraspinatus tears. *Arthroscopy* 2018; 34(1):75–81. doi:10.1016/j.arthro.2017.07.028.
22. Plachel F, Korn G, Traweger A, Ortmaier R, Resch H, Moroder P. Long-term results after arthroscopic treatment of symptomatic Ellman grade 2 PASTA lesions. *J Shoulder Elbow Surg* 2019;28(7):1356–1362. Epub 2019 Mar 20. doi:10.1016/j.jse.2018.12.002.
23. Rossi LA, Atala NA, Bertona A, *et al*. Long-term outcomes after in situ arthroscopic repair of partial rotator cuff tears. *Arthroscopy* 2019; 35(3):698–702. Epub 2019 Jan 10. doi:10.1016/j.arthro.2018.09.026.
24. Ko JY, Huang CC, Chen WJ, Chen CE, Chen SH, Wang CJ. Pathogenesis of partial tear of the rotator cuff: A clinical and pathologic study. *J Shoulder Elbow Surg* 2006;15(3):271–278. doi:10.1016/j.jse.2005.10.013.
25. Sano H, Ishii H, Trudel G, Uhthoff HK. Histologic evidence of degeneration at the insertion of 3 rotator cuff tendons: A comparative study with human cadaveric shoulders. *J Shoulder Elbow Surg* 1999;8(6):574–579. doi:10.1016/s1058-2746(99)90092-7.

26. Neer CS 2nd. Impingement lesions. *Clin Orthop Relat Res* 1983;(173): 70–77.
27. Davidson PA, Elattrache NS, Jobe CM, Jobe FW. Rotator cuff and posterior-superior glenoid labrum injury associated with increased glenohumeral motion: A new site of impingement. *J Shoulder Elbow Surg* 1995;4(5):384–390. doi:10.1016/s1058-2746(95)80023-9.
28. Simank H, Dauer G, Schneider S, Loew M. Incidence of rotator cuff tears in shoulder dislocations and results of therapy in older patients. *Arch Orthop Trauma Surg* 2006;126(4):235–240. Epub 2005 Sep 8. doi:10.1007/s00402-005-0034-0.
29. Stayner LR, Cummings J, Andersen J, Jobe CM. Shoulder dislocations in patients older than 40 years of age. *Orthop Clin North Am* 2000;31(2): 231–239. doi:10.1016/s0030-5898(05)70143-7.
30. de Jesus JO, Parker L, Frangos AJ, Nazarian LN. Accuracy of MRI, MR arthrography, and ultrasound in the diagnosis of rotator cuff tears: A meta-analysis. *AJR Am J Roentgenol* 2009;192(6):1701–1707. doi:10.2214/AJR.08.1241.
31. Teefey SA, Rubin DA, Middleton WD, Hildebolt CF, Leibold RA, Yamaguchi K. Detection and quantification of rotator cuff tears. Comparison of ultrasonographic, magnetic resonance imaging, and arthroscopic findings in seventy-one consecutive cases. *J Bone Joint Surg Am* 2004;86(4):708–716.
32. Altintas B, Anderson N, Dornan GJ, Boykin RE, Logan C, Millett PJ. Return to Sport After Arthroscopic Rotator Cuff Repair: Is There a Difference Between the Recreational and the Competitive Athlete? *Am J Sport Med* 2020;48(1):252–261. doi:10.1177/0363546519825624.
33. Kanatlı U, Ayanoğlu T, Ataoğlu MB, Özer M, Çetinkaya M, Eren TK. Midterm outcomes after arthroscopic repair of partial rotator cuff tears: A retrospective study of correlation between partial tear types and surgical technique. *Acta Orthop Traumatol Turc* 2020;54(2):196–201. doi:10.5152/j.aott.2020.02.486.
34. Xunqi Cheow, Andy Yew, Benjamin Fu Hong Ang, Denny Lie. No difference in outcome between articular-sided and bursal-sided tears: Comparative study with minimum 2-year follow-up of arthroscopic repairs of 104 patients in a single surgeon series. *Arthroscopy* 2021. doi: 10.1016/j.arthro.2020.12.226.
35. Xunqi Cheow, Denny Lie. Arthroscopic single lateral row repair technique for small rotator cuff tears. *Arthrosc Tech* 2021;10(3):e775–780. doi: 10.1016/j.eats.2020.10.067.

https://doi.org/10.1142/9789811249846_0015

Chapter 15

Arthroscopic Dual-Row Cuff Repairs for Small to Mid-sized Full Thickness Tears

Denny T.T. Lie, Merrill Lee and Eileen Tay

Summary of Chapter

1. Introduction and epidemiology of mid-sized full thickness tears
2. Clinical presentation and examination
3. Pathophysiology of full thickness tears
4. Imaging and approach
5. Surgical technique of arthroscopic dual-row cuff repairs (with six different suture variations)
6. Rehabilitation
7. Clinical outcomes

1. Introduction and Epidemiology of Full-thickness Cuff Tears

Rotator cuff tears are among the most common disorders of the shoulder girdle requiring surgical management. The epidemiology of rotator cuff tears has been described in both cadaveric and clinical studies. Cadaveric dissections by Neer [1] reported an incidence of less than 5% of full-thickness tears in more than 500 cadavers, whereas Lehman *et al.* [2] reported an incidence of 17% in 235 cadavers, with increased incidence of full thickness tears in specimens older than 60 years. On the other hand, population-based studies such as that by Yamamoto *et al.* [3] have described approximately 25% of individuals in their 60s having full-thickness rotator cuff tears, and 50% of individuals in their 80s having full-thickness tears. Yamaguchi *et al.* [4] reported that if a patient had symptomatic rotator cuff tear, there was a 35% chance of a cuff tear on the contralateral shoulder, which increased to 50% if the patient as 66 years or older.

The common finding is that rotator cuff tears are more prevalent with increased age — suggesting that trauma and degeneration play key roles in cuff tear development. Other risk factors include smoking and dyslipidemia, as well as newer radiological parameters such as the Acromial Index (AI) and Critical Shoulder Angle (CSA) [5,6].

2. Clinical Presentation

Patients with rotator cuff tears often present with shoulder pain. Classically, shoulder pain is felt over the anterolateral aspect of the shoulder, and exacerbated by overhead activities such as placing objects onto a high shelf. Patients also typically complain of night pain when lying on the affected shoulder. Repetitive motion can also exacerbate the shoulder pain.

On physical examination, the surgeon usually examines both the active and passive range of motion (ROM) of the shoulder — due to a combination of pain and weakness, patients demonstrate loss of active ROM with greater or intact passive ROM. The surgeon can also perform specific tests for localisation of the rotator cuff tear, such as the Jobe test for a supraspinatus tear, the external rotation lag sign (ERLS) for an infraspinatus tear, the Hornblower's sign for a teres minor tear, and the Gerber lift-off test for a subscapularis tear.

3. Pathophysiology of Rotator Cuff Tears

The pathogenesis of rotator cuff tears remains poorly understood, and has been attributed to multiple factors which have been categorised into intrinsic, extrinsic, and traumatic causes. Intrinsic degeneration of the tendon is associated with age, reduced vascularity of the tissue, and fatty atrophy of the muscle. Extrinsic factors resulting in mechanical compression of the rotator cuff can be attributed to acromial morphology, and altered scapulothoracic kinematics [7]. Finally, traumatic causes would include shoulder dislocation or proximal humerus fractures.

4. Imaging and Algorithm of Treatment Options

Often the diagnosis of a rotator cuff tear can be made clinically. In our institution, the surgeon attending to the patient will typically order a standard anteroposterior shoulder radiograph, followed by either an ultrasonography of the shoulder, or a magnetic resonance imaging (MRI) scan of the shoulder (Fig. 1). The surgeon looks for radiological clues pointing towards a rotator cuff tear such as superior migration of the proximal humeral head, but more importantly, the presence of cuff arthropathy, which may dissuade the surgeon from arthroscopic cuff repair. Both ultrasonography and MRI allow the surgeon to localise the rotator cuff tear, as well as to quantify its size and depth. These variables are taken into account during surgical planning and intervention (Fig. 2).

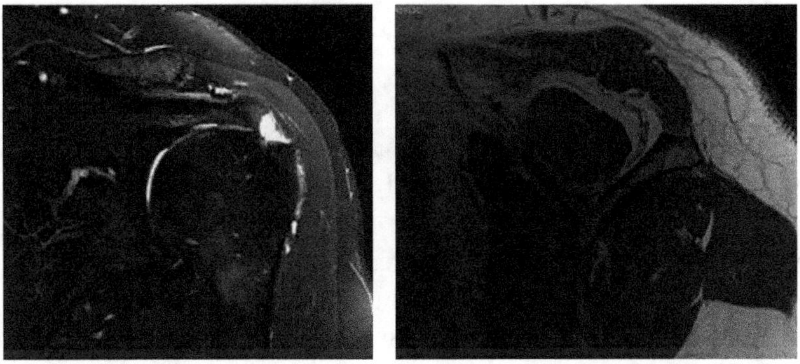

(a) (b)

Fig. 1: MRI images of full-thickness cuff tear. A 63-year old man presented with left shoulder pain of 1 year's duration. He was initially treated for tendinosis. (a) The coronal MRI view of full-thickness tear of the supraspinatus, reported measuring 2.3 cm with 1.8 cm retraction. (b) The sagittal view which shows Goutallier stage 1 of mild atrophy.

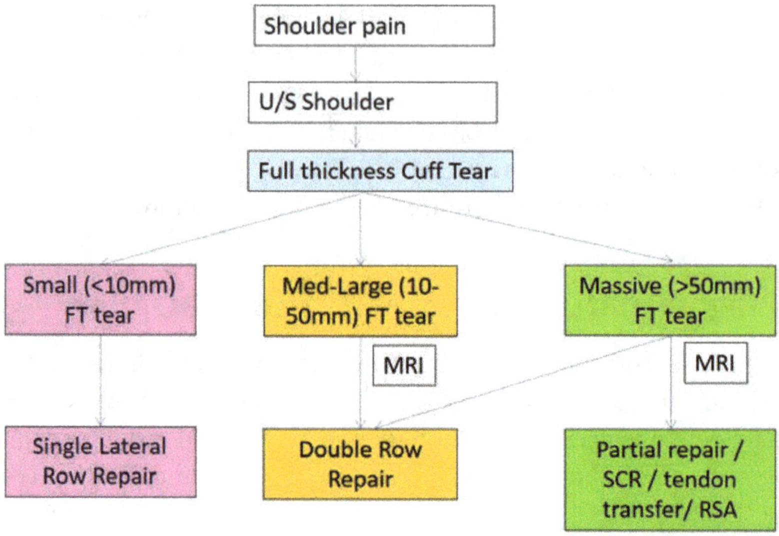

Fig. 2: Algorithm for full-thickness cuff tears. The type of surgical cuff repair is dependant on the size of the tear. Small full-thickness tears can be repaired by the single lateral row technique (Chapter 14). Most tears are mid-sized to large, and repaired with double-row technique. The various suture configurations in the double row technique are described below. Massive tears can be addressed by double-row repair where possible, otherwise a partial repair, superior capsular reconstruction or tendon transfer (the latter two described in Chapter 16) may be required. Often a reverse shoulder arthroplasty (RSA), described in Chapter 22, may be needed.

5. Arthroscopic Surgery

1. **Indications for surgery:**
   - Symptomatic (pain and mild weakness) tears proven on any imaging.
   - Tear that is proven to be progressively enlarging.
   - Traumatic tears, which tend to progress.
   - Degenerate tears in the elderly, as surrounding tissues tend to be unhealthy.
2. **Special instruments:**
   - Mitek rotator cuff instrument tray.
3. **Positioning and portals:**
   - **Position:** Beach chair.

- **Posterior portal:** Standard viewing portal for initial glenohumeral work, but may be difficult to see small anterior tears in the subacromial space.
- **Antero-superior portal:** For cuff repairs, this portal enters in the middle, not high in the interval. Useful mainly for glenohumeral debridement, limited use during cuff repairs except anterior tears and suture management.
- **Antero-lateral/tear portal:** This portal is created from the outside-in, preferably directly at the supraspinatus tear. A guide to this portal placement: project a line from the inner border of the spine of the scapula to the acromion. This portal is roughly along this line about 2 cm below the lateral edge of the acromion. This is the main working portal for anchor placement and suture management.
- **Postero-lateral portal:** Provides a good view of the entire cuff landscape. Project a line from the inner border of the clavicle to the acromion; a position about 1 cm from the edge of the acromion is the postero-lateral portal.
- **Lateral portal (optional):** This portal lies between the antero- and postero-lateral portals. Useful as adjunct working portal for large tears that includes the infraspinatus, and for suture management.

5.1 *Arthroscopic Dual-row Cuff Repairs (Incorporating Six Suture Variations) Principles of Suture Management*

Arthroscopic cuff repair is more of an art than a routine surgical manual. It is often unpredictable because each tear is unique and requires unique suture configurations. A description of the number of anchors alone does no justice to the complex and various suture configurations that each tear demands. What is predictable are guidelines described below:

(a) **Glenohumeral debridement and thorough inspection**
- With the camera in the posterior portal, a thorough inspection of the glenohumeral joint is performed. A shaver is employed from

the antero-superior portal to debride the **synovitis** and partially torn structures.

- Cuff tear pathologies do not occur in isolation and are usually associated with other pathologies; these include:
  - (i) **Capsulitis** to varying degrees, which can be seen by the contraction of the volume of the rotator interval. Debride the rotator interval completely as this will improve the external rotation of the arm. Perform a capsular release if needed (Chapter 3).
  - (ii) **Biceps tendinosis and partial tears**, degenerative SLAP tears: this occurs in about 30% of cuff repairs and a biceps tenotomy or tenodecis should be done (Chapter 11).
  - (iii) **Anterior or posterior degenerative labral tears:** only debridement is needed, it is in the author's opinion that co-existing labral tears in the elderly in whom the cuff repair is being performed, does not need repair.
  - (iv) **Cartilage** eburnation, fissures and ulcers: cartilage injuries to varying extents do occur in cuff tears, debride them and perform microfracture if needed.

(b) **Identification of tear, preparation of the footprint**

- A mid-sized to large full thickness tear of the tendon is evident from the glenohumeral joint. But a small tear may be difficult to visualise. *Keep the arm in slight abduction and external rotation*, small tears of the anterior supraspinatus can be seen from the articular aspect.
- Create the tear portal and debride the tear with a shaver, enlarging the tear as it is being debrided (Fig. 3(a)). *Degenerate tissues fall away easily when debrided, normal healthy tendons have a firm feel and are not easily debrided away.*
- Use a shaver to decorticate the footprint insertion of the (supraspinatus) tendon, till bleeding points are seen. *Do not decorticate too much*, loss of the cortical layer leaving only the cancellous bone will weaken the bone significantly and risk an anchor pull-out.
- Medialise the footprint by about 5–7 mm, shaving away the cartilage. This will increase the surface area on which the tendon will be repaired.

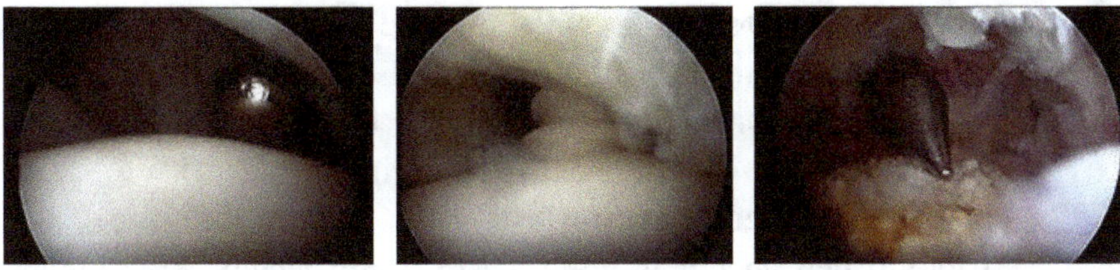

(a) (b) (c)

Fig. 3: View from Glenohumeral joint. (a) A shaver inserted through the tear in this right shoulder, to debride the edges and prepare the footprint. (b) A Healix anchor inserted, often the footprint is medialised. (c) Another example of a left shoulder, the footprint is visible and prepared. Microfracture can be done using the awl to create a *crimson duvet* for better healing.

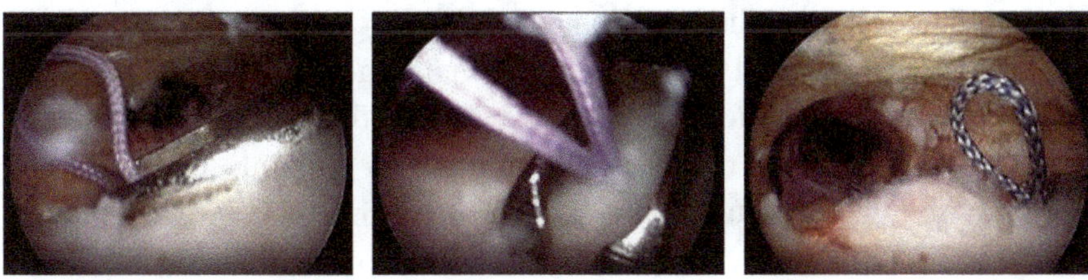

(a) (b) (c)

Fig. 4: Antegrade passing of the sutures. After debriding the subacromial space, the purple sutures from the Healix anchor is passed antegrade by an Express Sew passer as shown in (a) and (b). (c) Similarly shows the blue sutures from the medial row anchor passed antegrade.

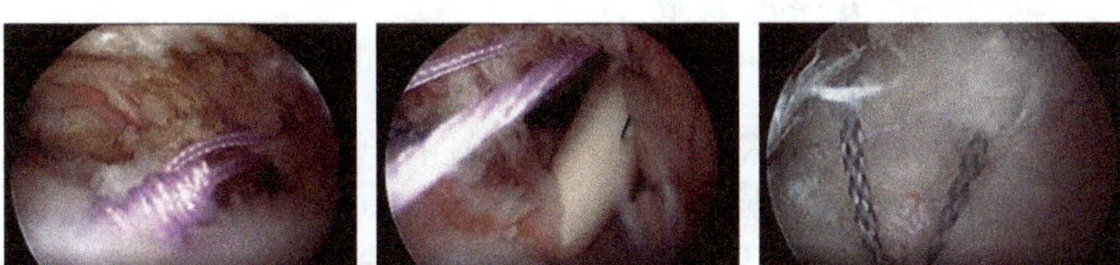

(a) (b) (c)

Fig. 5: Tying and the lateral row anchor. (a) The purple sutures being tied; this is optional. In fact, current practice is not to tie the knot, in order to ensure a better spread of the suture tension and compression. (b) The sutures retrieved and secured to a Versalok anchor in the lateral row. The final check is shown in (c); notice the blue and purple suture bridges diverge to achieve the wider spread of compression.

- In large exposed footprints with sclerotic bones, microfracture is performed using the awl and tapping it to a depth of 3–5 mm. These microfracture perforations should be about 5–7 mm apart and should evenly cover the entire footprint (Fig. 3(c)).

(c) **Placement of the medial anchor(s)**

- A triple-loaded anchor is preferred (5.5 mm Healix BR anchor). Viewed from the articular side, the awl followed by the anchor is negotiated from the tear portal and inserted at **about 30°– 45°** to the horizontal surface of the humeral head. **Medialise** the insertion of the anchor, to increase the surface area of tendon healing (Fig. 3(b)).
- *How many medial anchors should be deployed?* In general, one medial row anchor is needed for every 20–30 mm detachment of the tendon from the insertion (AP length of tear, not the retraction). Hence most small, mid-sized and even large tears need one medial row anchor. Some large tears involving the entire supraspinatus tendon (4 cm or more in AP length) and certainly massive tears involving both supraspinatus and infraspinatus tendons, require more than one anchor (usually 2 medial row anchors).

(d) **Subacromial decompression**

- Subacromial decompression is performed to clear away the inflammed bursa, and visualise the tear and normal healthy tendons. The sutures from the medial row anchors are parked in the antero-lateral portal. These should be clipped and held down during the decompression. *Remember to be mindful of the sutures as the shaver is being used!*
- Perform an acromioplasty to increase the subacromial space (Chapter 13).
- The Mumford's procedure is performed only if the patient exhibits pain over the ACJ and has pain during cross-body adduction.

(e) **Describing the tear morphology, trial reduction**

- Viewing from the postero-lateral portal, observe the tear and describe it under these parameters:
  (a) Location of tears: Most tears begin at the anterior supraspinatus, and usually progressively involve the rest of the tendon.

(b) Size of tears: Both in AP (antero-posterior) and ML (medial-lateral) retraction.

(c) Morphology: Describe the shape of the tear and whether it is symmetrical. Symmetrical tears are balanced; hence patients are less symptomatic. Asymmetric tears tend to cause more symptoms of pain and weakness, due to the abnormal kinematics.

- Attempt to mobilise the tendon and reduce the torn edge to the insertional footprint. Reduction is not always in the medial-lateral direction. It may need a more posterior-anterior shift of the tendon, mobilising the infraspinatus to achieve tear reduction and repair. Sometimes a combination of maneuvers may be needed.

(f) **Some theoretical considerations**

- **Functional unit of tendon repair**

  How many anchors are required to repair a cuff tear of a certain size? This vexing question has been raised many times yet the correct question should be *How many sutures traversing the tear are optimally required?* Too few sutures would compromise the strength and stiffness of the repair, and may cause gap formation which in turn, leads to failure to heal. It may be unnecessary to have too many sutures crossing the tear; suture tension and compression that is excessive may strangulate the blood supply of the tendon. Our study on gap formation [8] suggests that a pair of sutures traversing every 8–10 mm wide of cuff tear is adequate to limit gap formation and makes the repair very strong (Fig. 6). Thus, an axiom that is easy to remember is **a pair of sutures for every centimeter of cuff tear**.

- **Understanding the tear, the apex of the tear**

  Every tear is unique with its characteristic morphology, pathophysiology and propensity to propagate. Every tear has a *tear apex*, the lead point at which the tear initiated and continues to propagate. It is the point most retracted (Fig. 7(a)). Thus, it is the part of the tendon that must be addressed first (Fig. 7(b)), either to be tied to the medial anchor where possible or attached with

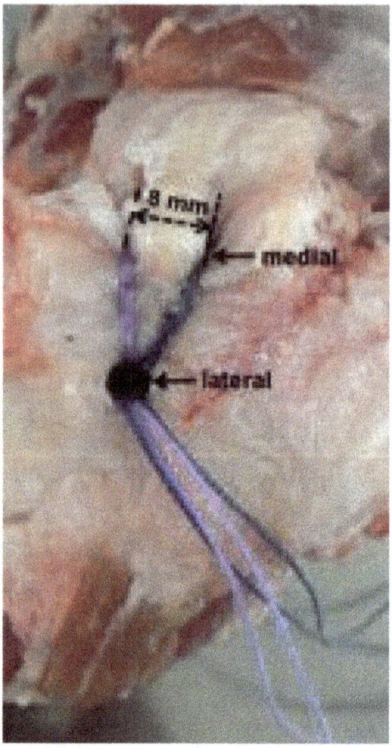

Fig. 6: Functional unit of tendon repair. A pair of sutures is needed to traverse a tear of length 8–10 mm wide, to achieve strong repair with minimal gap.

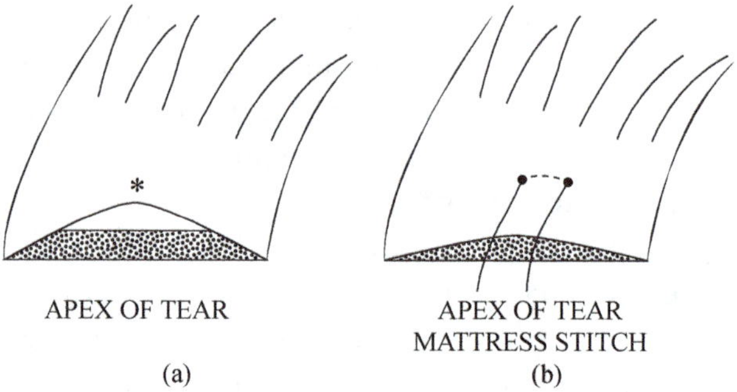

Fig. 7: Apex of the tear. The apex is the leading point of the tear and most retracted. It needs to be tagged with sutures and incorporated as part of the repair.

sutures to be fixed to the lateral row. **Controlling the tear apex** is critical for proper repair.

- **Suture spread: Divergent sutures, depth of bite, inter-suture distance**

  Sutures should be evenly spread over the area of tendon (the real estate) to be repaired, that is, lateralised and compressed. Some principles include:

  The **first principle** is that sutures must be deployed in a **divergent pattern** (Figs. 8(a) and 8(b)). From the anterior limit of the tear, the suture passer (Express Sew III) should be pointing either straight medially or **divergent about 30° anteriorly**. Sutures cannot be passed too anteriorly for fear of trapping the biceps tendon that runs close by. Along the length of the tear, sutures are passed either straight medially or slightly divergent from each other. At the posterior limit of the tear, sutures can be passed about **45°–60° divergent posteriorly**. This can be achieved antegrade with a suture passer (Express Sew III) (Figs. 4(a)–(c)) or retrograde by a bird-beak retriever from the posterior portal.

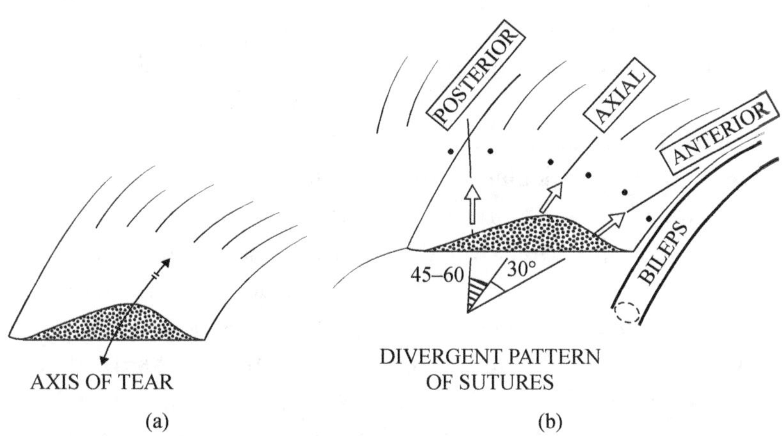

Fig. 8: Axis of the tear and Divergence of sutures. Every tear is unique and has its axis, illustrated in (a). (b) Shows how sutures should be placed along the axis of the tear, then 30° anterior to the axis and about 45°–60° posterior to the axis, to create a wide spread of sutures.

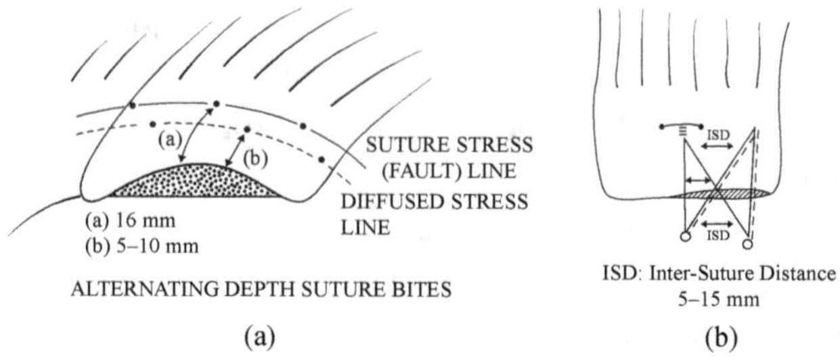

Fig. 9: The concepts of depth of suture bites and inter-suture distance. (a) Shows sutures should be passed at alternating depths to prevent concentration of stresses at the tendon which can cause secondary tears. (b) Illustrates inter-suture distance is recommended to be 5–15 mm apart to evenly spread out the suture stresses.

The **second principle** relates to the **depth of the suture bites/** passes. It would be tempting to pass the suture as deep as the suture passer would permit. For the Express Sew III passer, the depth of the bite is about 16 mm. Yet if all the sutures are passed about 16 mm deep, and these sutures are tied, it would create a line or a band of high tension and pressure (Fig. 9(a)). This is detrimental to the blood supply and may behave like a fault-line, from where secondary tears may develop. It is therefore recommended to take **alternating deep (16 mm) and shallow (5–10 mm)** bites to pass the sutures. This diffuses the high tension and pressure. Even if these sutures are tied, the tension lines would be diagonal and not perpendicular to the blood supply.

How close or far apart should these sutures be? The **third principle** attempts to answer this. Bunching up sutures and allowing them to overlap would create excessive pressure on the tendon and waste suture resources that is needed to spread out and cover the wide area of tendon to be repaired. Yet if the **inter-suture distance** is too far, there would be inadequate compression for tendon healing. The inter-suture distance should not be less than 5 mm nor greater than 15 mm (Fig. 9(b)). Hence the ideal distance between sutures should be **about 10 mm (5–15 mm).**

- **Near and Far sutures, recruiting more tendons**
  When repairing tendons, is taking the deepest possible bite with a suture passer (about 16 mm) adequate? If one is used to taking

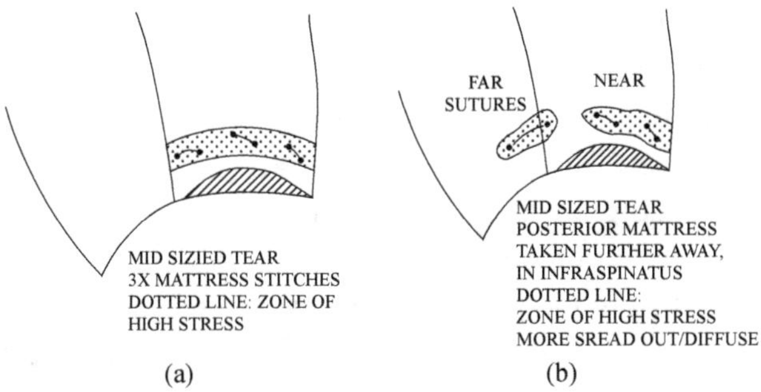

Fig. 10: Near and far sutures. (a) Shows if sutures are applied only in the vicinity of the tear, there is high concentration of stresses near the tear. (b) Shows the concept of tendon recruitment. If the posterior "far" sutures are passed through tendons further away to recruit them in the repair, the concentration of the stresses are better distributed.

retrograde bites, one is tempted to pass sutures deep, especially posteriorly into the infraspinatus, thus recruiting and incorporating more tendon surface into the repair, rather than limiting to a 16 mm rim around the tear. Passing sutures to the depth of the suture passers, called "near" sutures, increases the stiffness of the tendon-suture complex around the tear (Fig. 10(a)). By taking retrograde bites and passing the sutures "far", this area of increased stiffness is thus diffused and the area of higher tension spread out. More tendon material is recruited into the repair. In the author's opinion, this will help reduce the tension across the tear, thus increasing the chances of healing.

The concept of **near and far sutures**, recruiting more tendon into the repair to reduce the tension across the tear, is thus proposed (Fig. 10(b)). For the **anterior** part of the tear, antegrade suture passing is done with divergent suture placement, as described above. Suture passing in the **posterior** part of the tear is best done retrogradely, using a bird-beak retriever from the posterior portal.

- **To tie or not to tie: The lead suture technique**
  In general, it is not necessary to tie every suture in the cuff repair, lest the risk of compromising the blood supply. The author's preference is not to tie, only the apex of the tear needs to be tied (Fig. 5(a)).

For sutures that are not tied, they can be passed individually to achieve a better spread of sutures or passed together to create a fixed suture point. Passing sutures together can be done retrograde or antegrade. The **lead suture technique** uses any loose suture (e.g. Orthocord suture). It is passed antegrade to any desired position, then a pair of sutures to be delivered to that spot is tied using simple half-hitch knot. The loose suture will lead both sutures to be passed into the tendon, after which the lead suture can be pulled free and re-used. This technique is useful in large tears, to pass many sutures quickly without tying.

- **Dealing with the Dog-ear corners**

  Dog-ear corners of a repair suggest an uneven tension in the repair. The central portion of a tear (the apex of the tear) is pulled, reduced and repaired, at a higher tension than the surrounding normal intact tendon, creating a redundancy of the tissues (the dog-ear corners). The less than ideal appearance aside, dog-ear corners allow fluid to leak, causing a gap to form and potentially may affect healing (Fig. 11(a)).

  To even out dog-ear corners, a technique is to evenly spread out the suture distribution. Sutures from the medial row anchors, thus passed through the tendon and tied, before they are secured to the lateral row, are passed once again into redundancy of the dog-ear

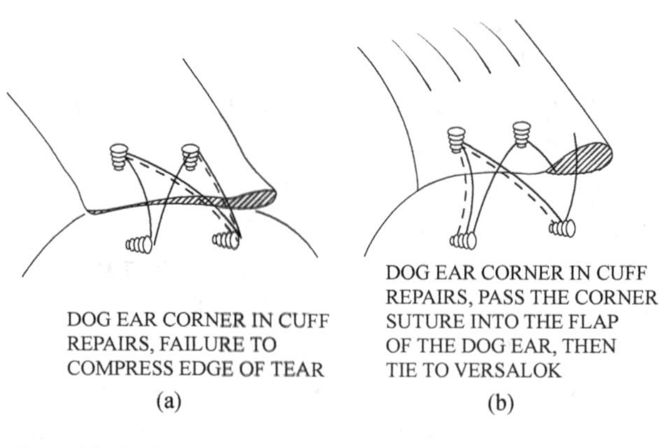

Fig. 11: Dealing with the Dog-ear corners. (a) The dog-ear corner, a loose corner due to suture tension not evenly spread out. (b) A technique to even out the tensions. Before the sutures are tied to the lateral row, the nearest suture is passed into the dog-ear. This evens out and distributes the suture tensions.

corners (Fig. 11(b)). Even a small bite is adequate to flatten the protruding corner and spread out the sutures more evenly over the repair.

(g) **Suture configurations: Standard and variations**

(i) **Standard box-like configuration (2–3 cm wide tears), 2 medial suture points**

- Symmetrical tears 2–3 cm wide (in AP length).
- Dual-loaded medial row anchor.
- Mentally, visualise the tear divided into two halves of equal length.
- Pair of sutures are passed antegrade by the lead-suture technique, to the middle of the anterior half, as deep as the suture passer permits. The other pair can be passed to the posterior half antegrade or retrograde. No tying is needed as each pair of sutures are passed out together. *This is the author's preferred technique.*
- Alternatively, pass each suture individually, equally spaced to the anterior and posterior halves of the tear. Then tie the anterior and posterior pairs of sutures.
- One suture limb from each pair is retrieved and tied to lateral row anchors (Versalok PEEK anchor), one anterior and another posteriorly (Fig. 12).
- This technique, knotted or knotless, provides a simple box-like suture configuration with adequate suture crossing in the middle.

(ii) **Standard box-like configuration (3–4 cm wide tears), 3 medial suture points**

- Symmetrical tears 3–4 cm wide (AP length).
- For these larger tears, a triple-loaded medial row anchor is used.
- Pass a pair of sutures by the lead-suture technique to the anterior third of the tear. The second pair of sutures are passed *individually* to the middle third of the tendon, which is usually the apex of the tear. The third pair of sutures can be retrieved retrogradely, either together or individually depending on how much posterior cuff needs to be recruited in the repair.
- Tie the second pair of sutures in the middle of the tear.

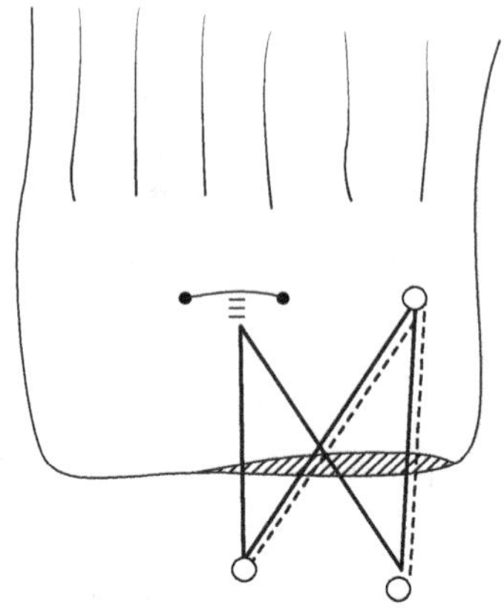

Fig. 12: Box-like configuration, two medial suture points.

- Then retrieve one suture limb from each of the three pairs of sutures from the lateral portal through an 8 mm cannula. Apply a firm tension on the sutures and use the cannula to hold down the sutures on the tendon, as a trial reduction, to visualise the spread of the sutures if the lateral row is fixed on that spot.
- If the sutures are bunched up and NOT spread out evenly, pass the sutures again, taking small bites but consciously spreading the sutures evenly apart.
- Then fix three suture limbs to the anterior lateral row anchor (Versalok PEEK anchor) and the other three limbs to the posterior lateral row (Fig. 13).

(iii) **V-shaped divergent (about 1 cm wide tear)**

- Tear is wide on the articular surface, narrows to a small opening on the bursal surface (Fig. 14(a)).
- Medial row anchor inserted either through the small tear on the bursal side (*preferred choice*) or use TransTend anchors (see Chapter 14). Dual-loaded medial row anchor is sufficient.
- Pass the anterior pair of sutures individually, as far anterior as possible to the anterior limits of the articular-sided tear.

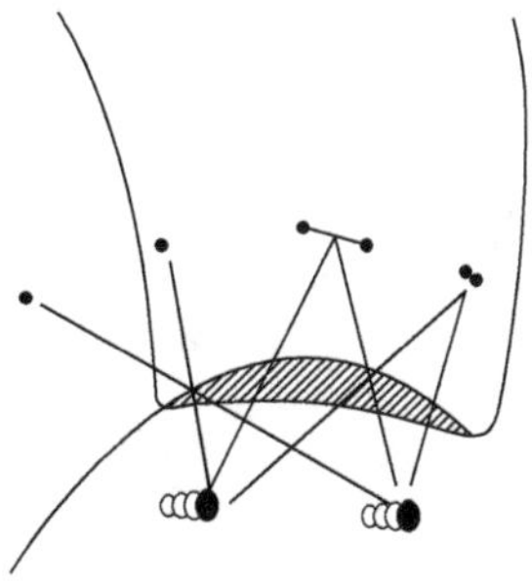

BOX CONFIGURATION, 3 MEDIAL PTS
Apex of tear is tied
Divergent suture, different depth
Near and far suture
Only middle suture, is tied, rest not tied

Fig. 13: Box-like configuration, three medial suture points.

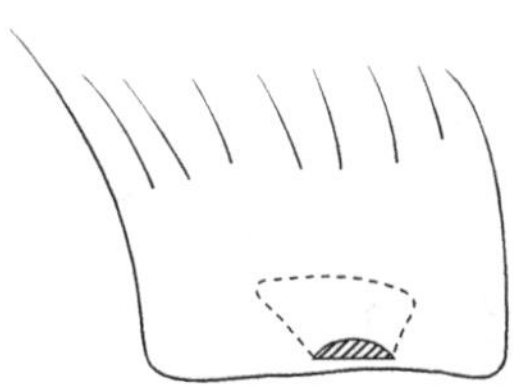

V-SHAPED DIVERGENT TEAR
(a)

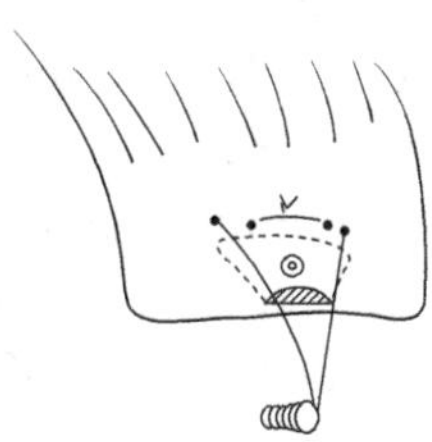

CONVERGENT REPAIR
1 X MEDIAL ROW
1 X LATERAL ROW
SINGLE PULLEY TIE
(b)

Fig. 14: V-shaped divergent tear. (a) Shows the tear. A medial row anchor (b) acts as a single pulley from which a horizontal tie is created. The loose ends are tied to the lateral row anchor.

- The posterior pair of sutures can be retrieved together in retrograde manner.
- One suture from each pair can be tied to each other, this will seal the articular side of the tear (transverse tie).
- The remaining suture limb from each pair can be tied to a single lateral row to mirror the tear configuration (Fig. 14(b)).

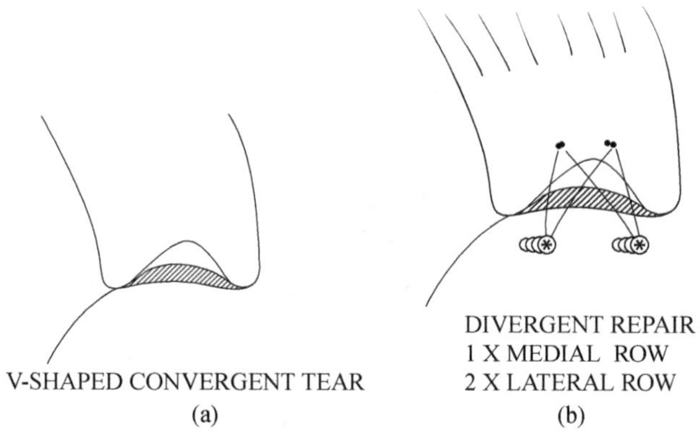

Fig. 15: Inverted V-shaped convergent tear. (a) Shows the tear. The suture configuration is similar to a box-like but spreads out to cover the wide bursal sided tear.

The tighter these suture limbs are pulled to the lateral anchor, the more compressed the repair will be (single-pulley technique).

(iv) **Inverted V-shape convergent**
- Tear is narrow on the articular surface and widens to a broad opening on the bursal surface (Fig. 15(a)).
- Single dual-loaded medial row anchor.
- Pass anterior pair of sutures antegrade by lead suture technique, then retrograde retrieval of posterior pair of sutures. Anterior and posterior bites need not be too wide, just enough cover the narrow articular side of the tear.
- Then one suture limb from each pair is retrieved to be secured to two lateral row anchors (Versalok PEEK). Position these lateral row anchors as wide as possible, about 5 mm from the intact tendon. The suture bridge thus compresses the tear, mirroring the tear morphology (Fig. 15(b)).

(v) **Margin convergence box**
- Small to mid-sized tears with medial-lateral extension (Fig. 16(a)).
- Single dual-loaded medial row anchor.
- Key to repair is to converge and bring the anterior and posterior halves of the tear together. Strength of repair is thus dependent on the number of sutures crossing the tear.

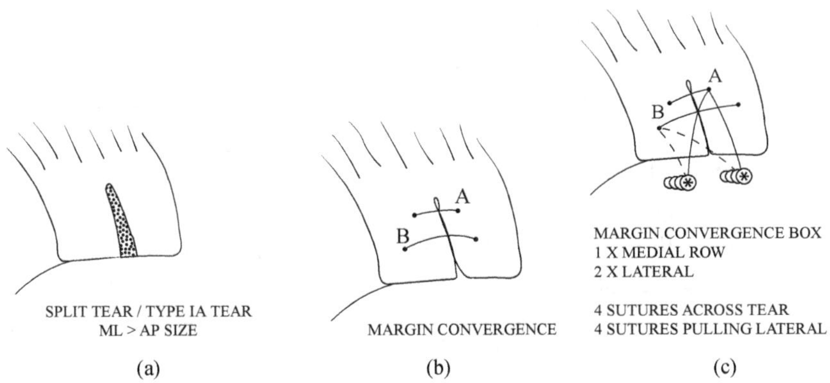

Fig. 16: Margin convergence Box configuration. (a) Shows the tear. From a medial row anchor, both sutures are passed to effect margin convergence as shown in (b). One suture limb from each is then tied to lateral row anchors. The effect is four sutures enforce the convergence and four pull the tendons laterally, as in (c).

- Pass one limb from suture (A) to the anterior half of the tear, as medial as the medial extension of the tear. Then pass the other limb from suture (A) to the posterior half. These sutures would thus converge the medial most portion of the tear (Fig. 16(b)).
- Similar procedure is repeated for suture (B), one limb passed anteriorly to a point more lateral than suture (A), closer to the insertion; another limb passed posteriorly.
- Tie sutures (A) first, converging the medial portions of the tear. Ensure that the anterior suture is the post, thus keeping the knot on the anterior half of the tear. Then tie sutures (B), keeping the knot on the posterior half by making the posterior suture the post (Fig. 16(b)).
- One suture limb from each suture is then taken and secured to a lateral row anchor (Versalok PEEK), one anterior and the other posterior. The lateral row anchors are positioned in line with the anterior- and posterior-most suture passes (Fig. 16(c)).
- The result would have four sutures traversing the tear (two margin convergence cross ties, and two diagonally crossing into the lateral row anchors. And all four sutures are tied to the lateral row anchors thus lateralising the tendon.

(vi) **Rip-stop technique**

- Concept is a technique whereby sutures tied to a lateral row cross perpendicularly over previously tied suture. This prevents the sutures from cutting out of the tendon. Useful in large tears where tension of repair may be high.
- Use a dual-loaded medial row anchor.
- Pass limbs from suture (A) to create a horizontal mattress tie. Pass the sutures far anteriorly and far posteriorly but take only small/shallow bites. This will create a wide but lateralised horizontal mattress tie (Fig. 17(a)).
- Pass limbs from suture (B) deep/more medial to sutures (A) but not as widely spread out as sutures (A). After sutures (A) are tied, pass sutures (B) perpendicularly over and secure them to a lateral row (Versalok PEEK) anchor (Fig. 17(b)).

(h) **Fixation to the lateral row of anchors**

- **How many lateral row anchors?**
  We recommend one lateral row anchor (Versalok PEEK) for every 8–10 mm of tear on the bursa side.
- **Where do we place them?**
  For small tears, they are placed in the middle of the tear (Figs. 5(b) and 5(c)). For larger tears, they should be in the

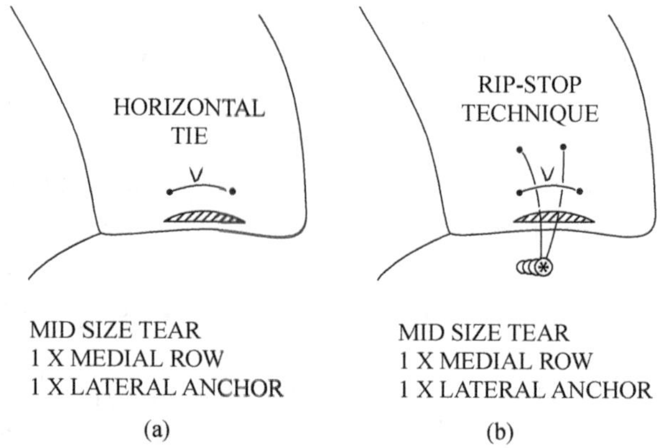

Fig. 17: The Rip-Stop technique. (a) Shows a typical tear, for which a horizontal tie was secured from a medial row anchor. The other pair of sutures are passed medial to the horizontal tie, and as they are secured to the lateral row anchor, they cross the horizontal sutures, shown in (b).

middle of equal halves of the tear. As a guide, they should be not more than 5 mm from the edge of the tear. Any closer the sutures would be compressing near the edge of the tear or even normal intact tendon, rendering the anchor unnecessary. More than 5 mm from the edge of the tear may cause fluid leakage and compromise the healing of the tear. In very large tears, more than two lateral row anchors may be needed, though this is not common. Space the lateral row anchors at least 10 mm from each other.

In the coronal plane, lateral row anchors should be placed below the prominence of the greater tuberosity, where the cortical bone is slightly thicker. This is achieved by abducting the arm when the anchors are secured and using cannulas in the lateral portal to aid visualisation.

- **Suture spread for better pull and compression**
  This point needs reiteration. Spread the sutures out so that when secured to the lateral row, the sutures evenly distribute the compression exerted and the tension applied to the tendon (Figs. 18(a) and 18(b)). Do a trial reduction before anchoring the sutures. Firmly pull on the selected sutures and use the cannula to hold them onto a proposed anchor position. Assess if the sutures are well and evenly spread out before accepting the position. If the sutures are bunched up, pass the sutures again to the edge of the tendon, taking small shallow bites but spread out.

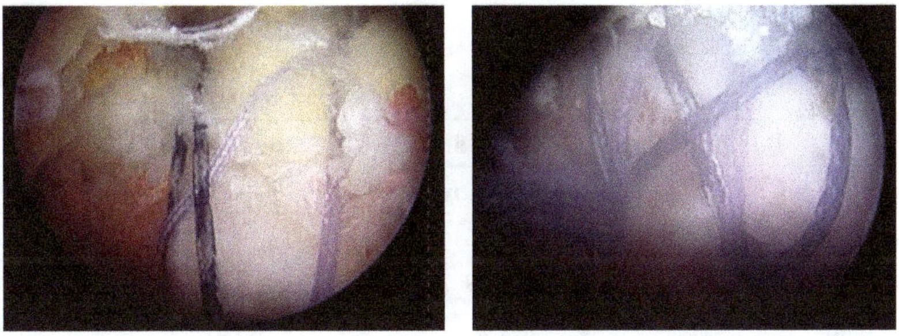

(a) (b)

Fig. 18: Suture spread. (a) Shows the suture bridge from two medial suture points and (b) shows from three medial suture points. Both show the sutures fairly spaced out, to evenly distribute the compression forces and uniformly pull the tendons laterally.

6. Post-op Management and Rehabilitation

Patients are typically admitted for overnight observation. However, should patients wish to be discharged on the same day as the procedure, they will be reviewed by a physiotherapist for prescription of an arm sling as well as education regarding post-operative activities. Patients are allowed passive ROM exercises from post-operation day 1, but only start strengthening exercises at 4–6 weeks post-operatively. They will be reviewed regularly by both the surgeon as well as a physiotherapist in the outpatient setting.

7. Outcomes

In our study, we followed up 210 patients with diagnosed, full-thickness rotator cuff tears confirmed on either ultrasonography or shoulder MRI treated surgically between May 2010 and June 2016. These 210 patients underwent arthroscopic double-row rotator cuff repair as described above. At 2 years post-operatively, there were significant improvements in post-operative ROM (both forward flexion and abduction), and the Visual Analogue Scale (VAS) for pain. There were also significant improvements in Constant Shoulder Score (CSS), University of California at Los Angeles (UCLA) Shoulder Rating Scale, and Oxford Shoulder Score (OSS) at 2 years post-operatively, as shown in Table 1. When patient satisfaction was collected at 2 years post-operatively as a binary outcome (satisfied versus dissatisfied surgery), the overall satisfaction rates were high at 95.8% [6].

Table 1. Outcomes after dual-row cuff repair [6].

Comparison between Pre- and Post-operative Variables			
Variable	**Pre-operative**	**2 Years Post-operatively**	***P*-Value**
Forward flexion	95 ± 36	130 ± 20	<0.05
Abduction	82 ± 39	122 ± 24	<0.05
VAS (pain)	6 ± 2	1 ± 2	<0.05
CSS	40 ± 19	71 ± 13	<0.05
UCLA shoulder rating scale	15 ± 5	30 ± 5	<0.05
OSS	32 ± 11	16 ± 7	<0.05

References

1. Neer CS 2nd. Impingement lesions. *Clin Orthop Relat Res* 1983;(173):70–77.
2. Lehman C, Cuomo F, Kummer FJ, Zuckerman JD. The incidence of full thickness rotator cuff tears in a large cadaveric population. *Bull Hosp Jt Dis* 1995;54(1):30–31.
3. Yamamoto A, Takagishi K, Osawa T, *et al*. Prevalence and risk factors of a rotator cuff tear in the general population. *J Shoulder Elbow Surg* 2010;19(1):116–120. doi:10.1016/j.jse.2009.04.006.
4. Yamaguchi K, Ditsios K, Middleton WD, Hildebolt CF, Galatz LM, Teefey SA. The demographic and morphological features of rotator cuff disease. A comparison of asymptomatic and symptomatic shoulders. *J Bone Joint Surg Am* 2006;88(8):1699–1704. doi:10.2106/JBJS.E.00835.
5. Tashjian RZ. Epidemiology, natural history, and indications for treatment of rotator cuff tears. *Clin Sports Med* 2012;31(4):589–604. doi:10.1016/j.csm.2012.07.001.
6. Lee M, Chen JY, Liow MHL, Chong HC, Chang P, Lie D. Critical shoulder angle and acromial index do not influence 24-month functional outcome after arthroscopic rotator cuff repair. *Am J Sports Med* 2017;45(13):2989–2994. doi:10.1177/0363546517717947.
7. Balke M, Liem D, Greshake O, Hoeher J, Bouillon B, Banerjee M. Differences in acromial morphology of shoulders in patients with degenerative and traumatic supraspinatus tendon tears. *Knee Surg Sports Traumatol Arthrosc* 2016;24(7):2200–2205. doi:10.1007/s00167-014-3499-y.
8. Kelvin G Tan, Denny TT Lie, Andy KS Yew, Siaw Meng Chou. Gap Formation after single lateral row vs dual-row suture bridge cuff repair: An ovine biomechanical model. *J Orthop Sci* 2019;Mar 23. https://doi.org/10.1016/j.jos.2019.03.005.

https://doi.org/10.1142/9789811249846_0016

Chapter 16

Large Rotator Cuff Tears: Classification and Approach Arthroscopic Margin Convergence (the Boot-Lace Technique) and Cuff Repair

Denny T.T. Lie and Gerald Zeng

Summary of Chapter

1. Introduction and epidemiology of large complete thickness tears
2. Clinical presentation and examination
3. Pathogenesis of tears
4. Imaging and approach
5. Surgical technique of arthroscopic margin convergence (boot-lace technique) and dual-row cuff repairs
6. Surgical technique of arthroscopic cuff repairs for type 1B and type 2 tears
7. Rehabilitation
8. Clinical outcomes

1. Introduction and Epidemiology of Large Cuff Tears

DeOrio and Cofield [1] classified rotator cuff tears on the basis of greatest dimension as either small (<1 cm), medium (1–3 cm), large (3–5 cm), or massive (>5 cm). The type and size of rotator cuff tears directly affect selection of treatment and surgical approach, post-operative prognosis, and tear recurrence. Large cuff tears are more commonly seen in the elderly population and may be challenging to address. Large and massive rotator cuff tear repairs are often associated with a high anatomical failure rate [2,3] ranging from 25% to in excess of 70% in older age group [4].

2. Clinical Presentation

2.1 *Symptoms*

The main symptom is pain, which is often insidious, and worse with overhead activities. Pain is often localised to the deltoid region. Patients with an acute traumatic tear may present with acute pain and weakness.

2.2 *Physical Examination*

The most common sign elicited is pain on resisted elevation (Jobe's test) and weakness of internal and external rotation. Specific considerations that may help characterise a tear include:

(a) Posterosuperior cuff tear (supraspinatus and infraspinatus).
- Loss of forward flexion, abduction and external rotation.
- Positive external rotation lag sign (unable to hold arm externally rotated at the side).

(b) Anterosuperior cuff tear (supraspinatus and subscapularis).
- Loss of forward flexion and abduction.
- Subscapularis involvement is suspected if patient demonstrated a positive Gerber's lift-off test.

(c) Larger tears involving teres minor.
- Positive Hornblower's test (patient unable to perform external rotation with shoulder in 90° of abduction and external rotation).

3. Pathogenesis of Large Tears

The pathogenesis of rotator cuff pathologies is multi-factorial. They are broadly divided into extrinsic (from structures surrounding the cuff) and intrinsic factors (degeneration within the cuff itself).

Extrinsic causes for development of rotator cuff disease include structural factors such as compression of tendons by bony impingement, or direct pressure from soft tissues [5]. Intrinsic factors include hypovascularity, local inflammation [6], and mechanical overuse. Demographic and anthropometric factors such as age, smoking, family history, obesity and corticosteroid [7] are known to play a role as well. Atraumatic rotator cuff tears, can at times, also be due to a normal aging process [8]. On the other hand, the mechanism of injury in younger patients is often acute avulsion.

In small tears, a large population of fibroblasts and other inflammatory cells facilitate an active reparative process. However, the recruitment of these inflammatory cells is markedly reduced as size of the tear in the rotator cuff increases [9], and reparative potential is limited.

4. Imaging, Diagnosis and Classification

1. **Imaging modalities**
   - **(a) Radiographs:** (see Chapter 13)
     - (i) **Anterior-posterior (AP)** view for assessing glenohumeral joint, osteophytes and sclerosis of the greater tuberosity (Fig. 1).
       - Critical shoulder angle (CSA) of more than 35° increases the risk of developing rotator cuff lesion.
       - Acromio-humeral index (AI) quantifies the lateral extension of the acromion. A high AI indicates increased lateral extension and significantly associated with rotator cuff tears.
       - Acromio-humeral distance (AHD) typical measures 7–14 mm in men and 7–12 mm in women. Abnormally low AHD suggests a defect of more than one rotator cuff tendon.

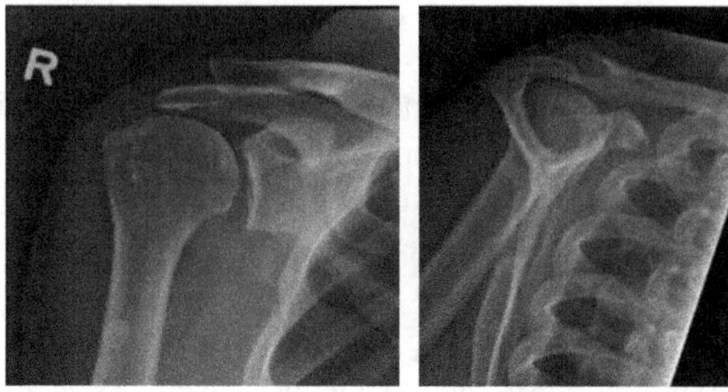

Fig. 1: X-rays of a patient with large cuff tear. This shows an AP and lateral X-ray views of the right shoulder of an elderly patient who sustained a large tear of the supraspinatus after a fall at home. Features include reduced AHI and broken Maloney's line, with no visible fractures.

(ii) **Scapular Y view** for assessing subacromial space and classifying the acromion type (Bigliani and Morrison classification).

(iii) **Axillary view** for evidence of os acromiale, a potential cause of secondary impingement.

(b) **Magnetic resonance imaging (MRI):** is used for assessing soft tissues, degree of muscle atrophy, and fatty infiltration with a sensitivity of 92% and specificity of 93% in detecting rotator cuff tears (Fig. 3). MRI is particularly useful to assess retraction of the tendon, based on the Patte classification (Fig. 2) and atrophy of the muscles (Fig. 5), based on the Goutallier staging (Fig. 4).

(c) **Ultrasound:** The ultrasound sensitivity and specificity is equivalent to those of MRI for diagnosis of complete rotator cuff injuries, and the size of the tear can be accurately measured (Fig. 6). However, it is largely dependent on the operator and the anatomy of the lesion cannot be fully appreciated, nor can atrophy be assessed.

2. **Classification** (Figs. 7 and 8).

   (a) **Type 1 tears:** These tears are morphologically symmetrical and hence mechanically well-balanced. The symptoms of pain and weakness tend to be well-tolerated till late, by which time the tears are large to massive by size and criteria. These are further sub-divided into:

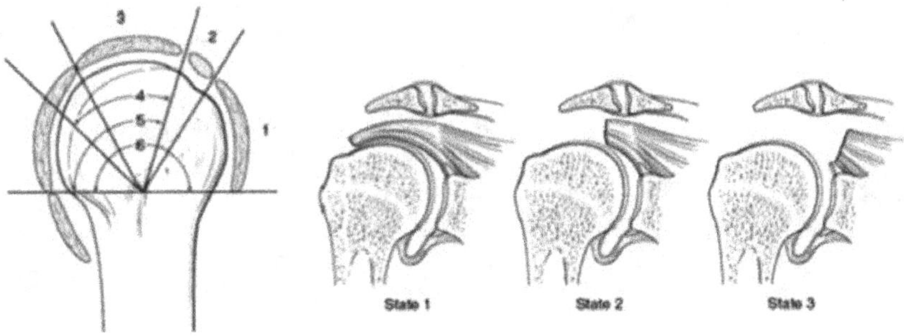

(a) (b)

Fig. 2: Patte classification. (a) shows the topography of tear in sagittal plane: segment 1 — subscapularis tear, segment 2 — coracohumeral tear, segment 3 — isolated supraspinatus tear, segment 4 — entire supraspinatus and half of infraspinatus tear, segment 5 — entire supraspinatus and infraspinatus tear, segment 6 — subscapularis, supraspinatus and infraspinatus tear. (b) shows the topography in coronal plane: stage 1 — proximal stump close to bony insertion, stage 2 — proximal stump at level of humeral head, stage 3 — proximal stump at level of glenoid [5].

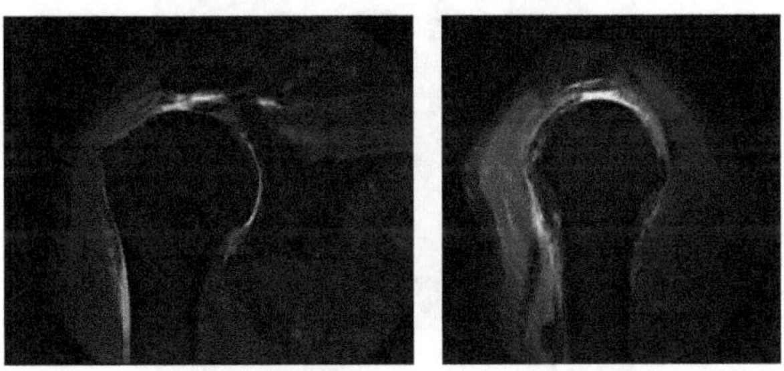

(a) (b)

Fig. 3: MRI of patient with large tear. (a) The coronal view of the right shoulder of the patient above, classified as Patte stage 2. (b) The sagittal view, tear is in segment 3 involving the entire supraspinatus.

- **Type 1A tears:** These tears are best described as **tendon split tears** ***along*** the tendon fibres, hence the medial-lateral (ML) dimension or retraction of the tear is more than the antero-posterior (AP) length. **Margin convergence** is recommended in such tears to reduce the large ML extension of the tear, after which dual-row repair is performed.

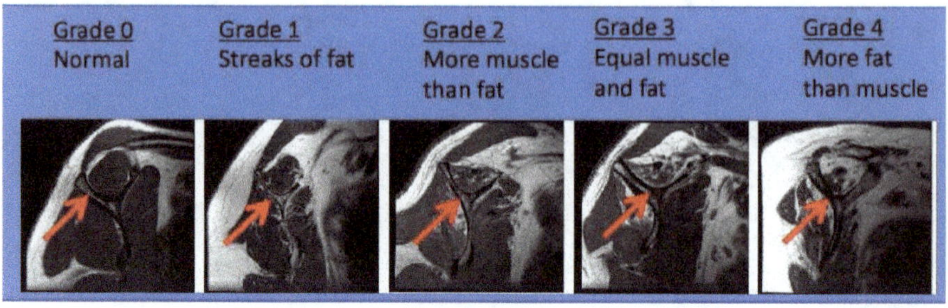

Fig. 4: Goutallier staging. Grade 1 shows only streaks of fat, grade 2 has more muscle than fats, grade 3 shows equal muscle and fat, and grade 4 shows more fat than muscle [6].

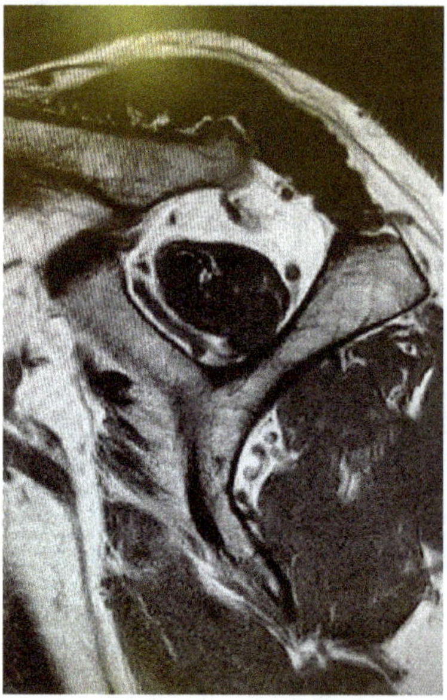

Fig. 5: Muscle atrophy. This sagittal view of an MRI of a patient with a large tear shows supraspinatus atrophy grade 2–3. It also shows infraspinatus atrophy.

- **Type 1B Tears:** these are the **true *detachments and avulsions*** of the tendons from the insertions at the footprint. Hence the AP length of the tear is wider than the ML split or retraction. These tears need extensive mobilisation then repaired with dual-row suture bridges using both near and far suture bites.

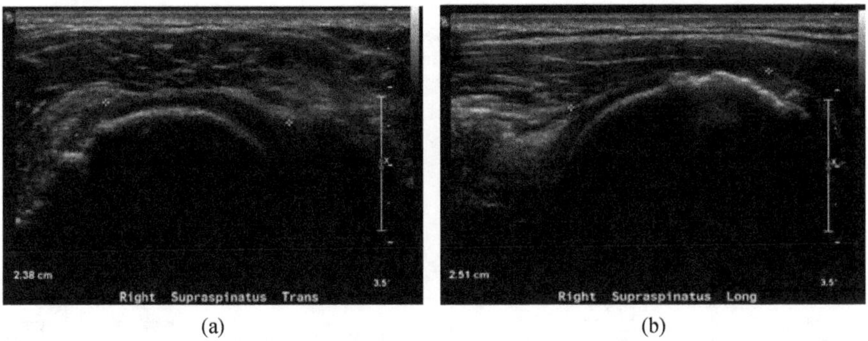

Fig. 6: Ultrasound scans. (a) A large tear od the right supraspinatus tendon measuring 2.38 cm in AP length and 2.51 cm in ML length or retraction, shown in (b).

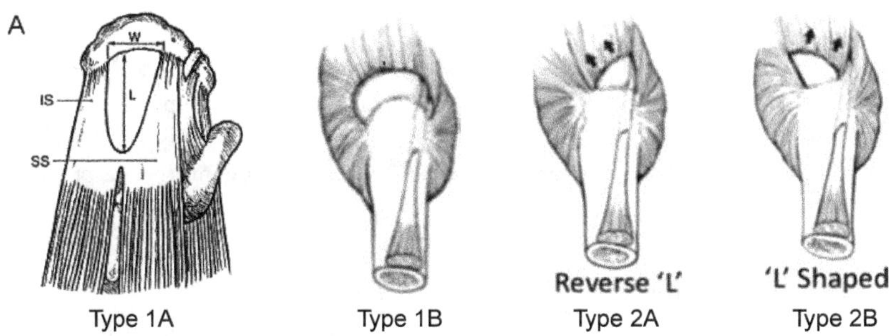

Fig. 7: Morphology of tears. Type 1 tears are balanced. Tear type 1A is longer in ML length than AP length. Type 1B is longer in AP dimension than ML dimension (minimal retraction). Type 2 tears are not balanced. Type 2A is an anterior type, described as reverse "L" and type 2B is posterior type, called the "L" shaped.

(b) **Type 2 tears:** These tears are **morphologically asymmetrical** and mechanically unbalanced; the symptoms of pain and weakness tend to be poorly tolerated and hence patients tend to appear early for surgery. The principles of surgery, employing dual-row repair, are similar; with the need to recognise the axis of the tear and focussing the suture lines of pull around this axis.

5. Arthroscopic Surgery

1. **Indications for surgery**
   - Any large tear that is symptomatic.
   - Asymptomatic tears are relative indications.

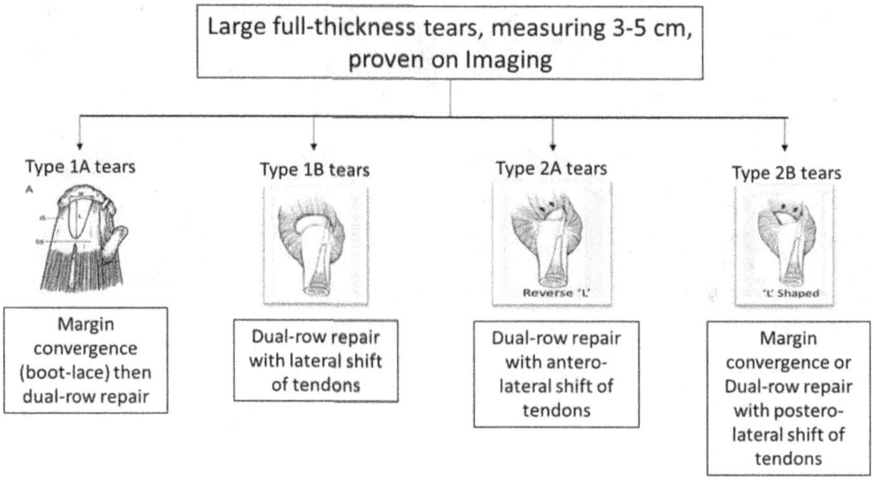

Fig. 8: Algorithm of surgical management based on morphology of tears. Type 1A tears need margin convergence before dual-row cuff repair can be done. Type 1B tears can be repaired with dual-row repair with a lateral shift of the repaired tendon; type 2A is repaired with antero-lateral shift of the tendon, and type 2B by margin convergence or postero-lateral shift of the tendon.

2. **Special instruments**
   - Mitek rotator cuff set, keep dermapatch graft on standby.
3. **Positioning and portals**
   - Posterior, anterior, antero-lateral and postero-lateral portals.

6. Arthroscopic Margin Convergence (The Boot-Lace Technique) and Dual-Row Cuff Repair for Type 1A Tears

6.1 *Mobilisation of the Tendons*

- The rotator interval must be cleared thoroughly, until the conjoint tendon is visualised. This will aid in the tendon mobilisation.
- The interval between the tendon and the superior labrum must similarly be debrided, adhesions here tend to limit the mobilisation and reduction of the tendon.

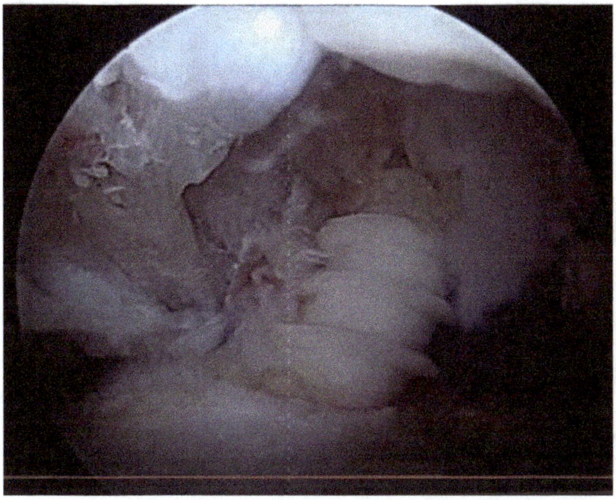

Fig. 9: Medial row anchor. Viewed from the glenohumeral joint, a Healix anchor is placed in the medial row.

- Perform a biceps tenotomy or tenodesis as indicated. A medial row anchor can be inserted (Fig. 9) at this stage, or it can be inserted after the margin convergence.
- The subacromial space needs to be meticulously cleaned (Fig. 10). Beware of the medial fat pad which hides a rich blood supply; this can bleed easily. There is a prominent vessel at the posteromedial corner of the subacromial space near the spine of the scapula. Be careful when cauterising the vessel, the supraspinatus nerve is perilously close. Adhesions also tend to form over the infraspinatus at the far posterior aspect of the subacromial space. View from the lateral portal and shave the posterior adhesions and bursa away.

6.2 *Margin Convergence Using Boot-Lace Technique*

- Keep the camera in the postero-lateral portal, and the working portal is the antero-lateral portal.
- A loose Orthocord suture is used in the margin convergence. Begin by passing the suture as medial as possible, at the medial limit of the tear (Fig. 11(a)). The sutures are always passed from below upwards

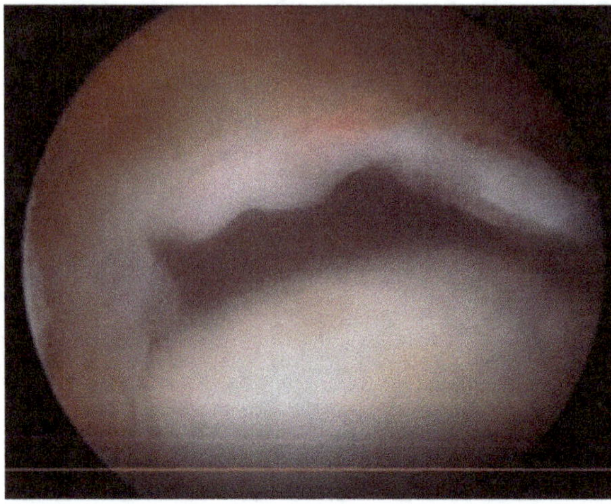

Fig. 10: Subacromial view. View of a large tear, camera from the posterolateral portal.

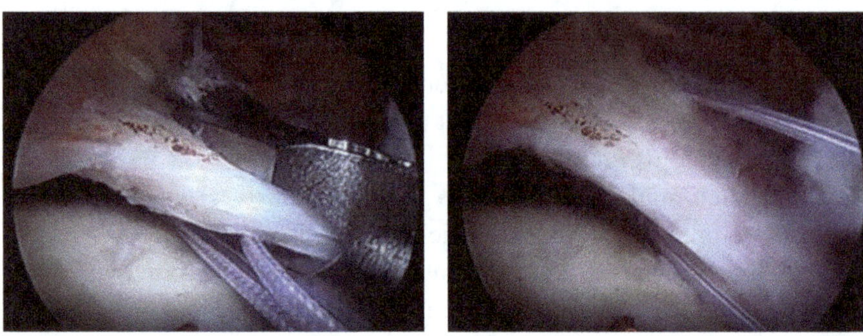

(a) (b)

Fig. 11: Anterior fold of margin convergence. (a) Shows a loose Orthocord suture being passed through the anterior fold of the tear and retrieved in (b) (limb A).

taking about 10 mm bites from the edge of the tear (Fig. 11(b)). The other end of the suture, limb B, is then passed to the posterior fold of the tendon (Figs. 12(a) and 12(b)). Suture limb (A) after being passed to the anterior fold of the tear, is then retrieved and used to bite the posterior fold of the tear about 5–7 mm lateral to the first pass of suture limb (B) (Figs. 13(a)–13(c)). Suture limb B, from the posterior fold is then passed to the anterior fold (Figs. 14(a)–14(c)). In this manner, instead of a single suture margin convergence, the same

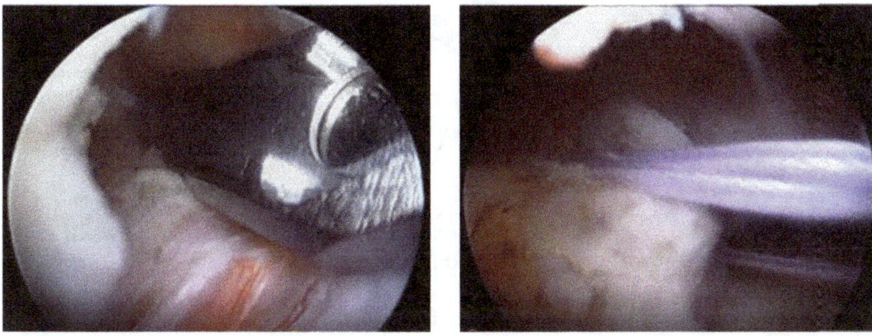

(a) (b)

Fig. 12: Posterior fold of margin convergence. The other end of the Orthocord suture (limb B) is then passed through the posterior fold of the tear, shown in (a) then retrieved in (b).

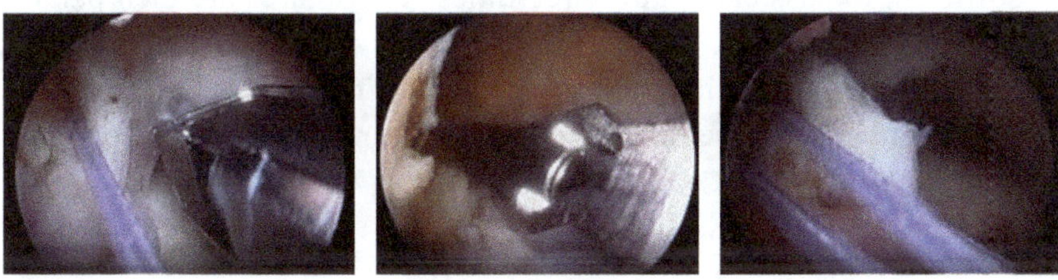

(a) (b) (c)

Fig. 13: Criss-crossing the sutures. Suture limb A from the anterior fold is then loaded (a) and passed to the posterior fold of the tear (b) with a deeper more posterior bite, and then retrieved (c).

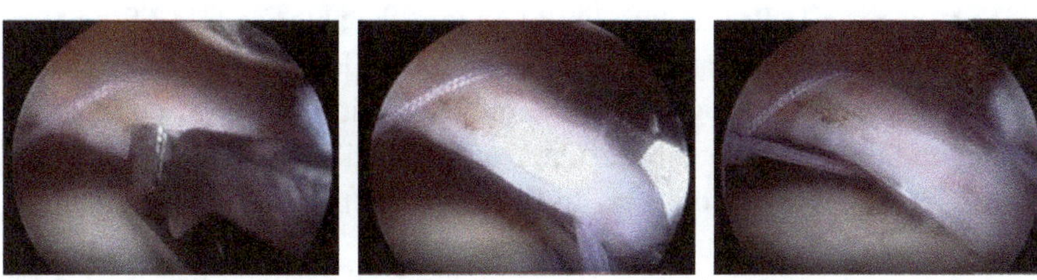

(a) (b) (c)

Fig. 14: The Boot-lace convergence. Suture limb B from the posterior fold is then loaded (a) and passed to the anterior fold of the tear (b) taking a deeper more anterior bite, then retrieved. The criss-crossing of sutures is clearly seen in (c).

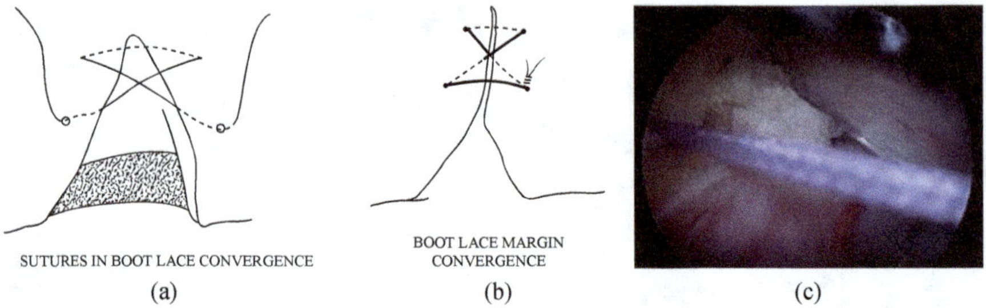

Fig. 15: Closing a large gap with the Boot-lace convergence. (a) Shows a schematic diagram of sutures passed interlacing with each other, like laces of a boot. When tied, the large gap can be minimised, as shown in (b) and (c).

suture is used to create interlacing and inter-locking margin convergence sutures, much like the laces of a boot (Fig. 15(a)). It is usually sufficient to pass each limb three times. The sutures are then parked at the anterior portal.

- Pull the sutures together to converge the tear together (Figs. 15(b) and 15(c)) and observe the residual gap of the tear, the area of the footprint thus exposed.

6.3 *Medial row anchor and sutures*

- A dual- or triple-loaded anchor is then placed in the middle of the footprint not covered by the tendon after margin convergence, medialised as much as possible (Fig. 16(a)).
- **Suture pair 1:** Pass suture limb (A) into the anterior fold of the tear, to the medial and anterior limit of the tear (Fig. 16(b)). Suture limb (B) is retrieved retrograde, at the medial limit of the tear, posteriorly, beyond the posterior limit of the tear. This will recruit the infraspinatus into the repair complex, to reduce the tension across the margin convergence. Park sutures in anterior portal.
- **Suture pair 2:** These sutures are placed at about the mid-point of the medial-lateral length of the tear, in contrast to suture pair 1, which are placed at medial limit of the tear, hence deeper from the working portal (Fig. 16(a)). Suture limb (A) is passed anteriorly, at the anterior limit of the tear. Limb (B) is retrieved posteriorly, as far posteriorly as

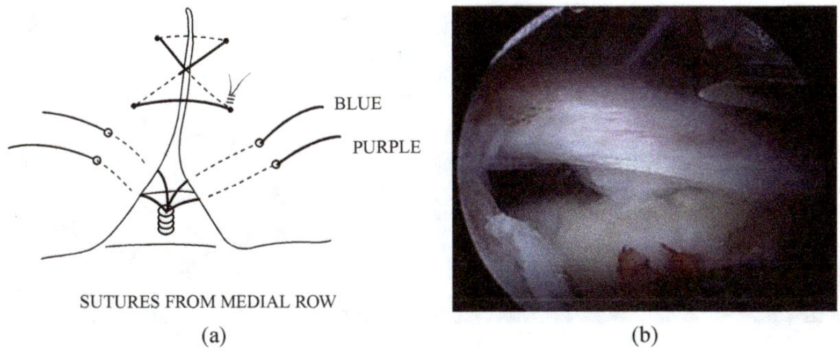

Fig. 16: Sutures from medial row anchor. (a) A schematic diagram showing sutures from the medial row anchor passed to the tendons. Each pair of the suture is passed to the anterior and posterior folds of the tear. (b) An ExpressSew passing the blue suture to the anterior tendon fold.

possible, beyond the posterior limit of the tear and more posterior than suture 1(B). Park sutures in posterior portal.

6.4 *Managing and Preparing the Sutures*

- Retrieve the margin convergence sutures in the antero-lateral portal (Fig. 17(a)) and tie with 6 half-hitches (Fig. 17(b)). Ensure the convergence is firm and snug. Corresponding pairs of sutures (blue and purple) from the medial row are then tied (Figs. 18(a) and 18(b)).

6.5 *Lateral Row Anchors*

- **Anterior anchor:** Retrieve one suture from the margin convergence, and one blue and one purple suture from the medial row (Fig. 19(a)). Suture (A) from the convergence provides a direct lateral pull while the blue and purple sutures from the medial row anchor provide an antero-lateral pull on the posterior fold. A trial reduction of the sutures is performed to ensure the sutures are well spaced out. This anchor is placed at the anterior limit of the tear, over the greater tuberosity. The arm is held in abduction and external rotation at this point.

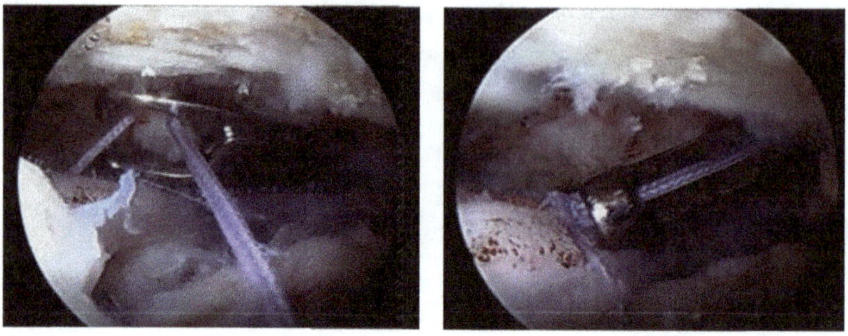

(a) (b)

Fig. 17: Tying the convergence sutures. (a) The convergence sutures being retrieved, then tied with 6 half-hitch knots, as shown in (b).

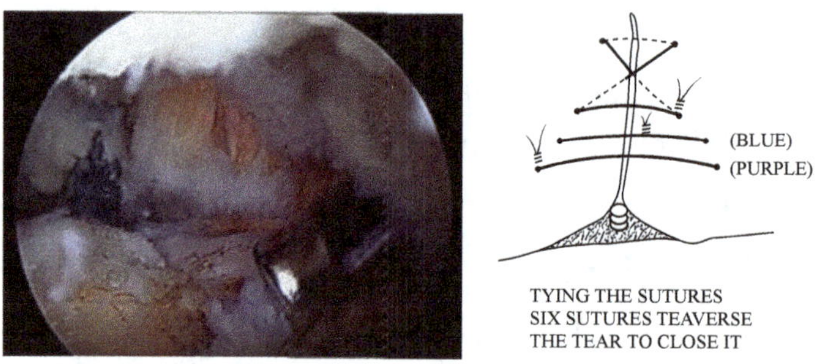

(a) (b)

Fig. 18: Tying the sutures from the anchor. (a) A knot pusher tying the purple suture from the medial anchor; the blue suture having been tied. (b) A schematic showing the tied convergence suture, and sutures from the medial row anchor. Sutures traversed the gap of the tear 6 times to ensure good closure.

- **Posterior anchor:** Retrieve the remaining suture from the convergence suture which pulls the posterior fold directly lateral, and the remaining blue and purple sutures, both of which pull the anterior fold postero-laterally. All three sutures, are then secured to the Versalok PEEK anchor positioned over the GT of the humeral head, at the posterior limit of the tear or slightly posterior to it (Fig. 19(b)). The suture construct is shown in Fig. 19(c).

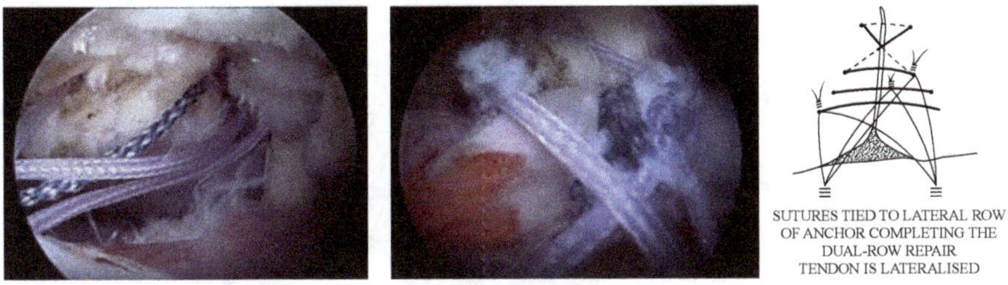

(a) (b) (c)

Fig. 19: Securing to the lateral row anchors. (a) Three sutures being secured to a Versalok anchor in the lateral row. This is repeated to secure all six sutures, to complete the dual-row repair, as shown in (b). (c) A schematic diagram to illustrate the completed dual-row repair. The large tear is thus approximated by sutures traversing the gap 6 times, then lateralised by six sutures.

7. Arthroscopic Dual-Row Cuff Repair Using Near and Far Sutures for Type 1B Tears

This technique has been described in Chapter 15. Here some tips and pointers are highlighted that might be useful for repair of type 1B tears, which are large tears with minimal retraction (AP length more than ML distance).

- Medialise the footprint, decorticate and prepare footprint.
- Use two medial row anchors (triple-loaded 5 mm Healix BR anchor).
- Pass one limb from suture 1 from anterior medial row, to the anterior limit of the large tear. The other limb remains attached to the anchor. When tied, suture 1 limits propagation of the tear and prevents formation of dog-ear at the corners (Fig. 20(a)).
- Suture pair 2 are passed together (lead suture technique) about 45° anterior to axis of tear, as deep as permitted by the bite of the suture passer (about 16 mm).
- Suture pair 3 are passed together directly in the axis of the tear in the medial direction, or in the middle of the wide tear (Fig. 20(a)).
- Suture pair 4 from the posterior medial row, is passed antegrade or retrieved retrograde, about 45° posterior to the axis of the tear.

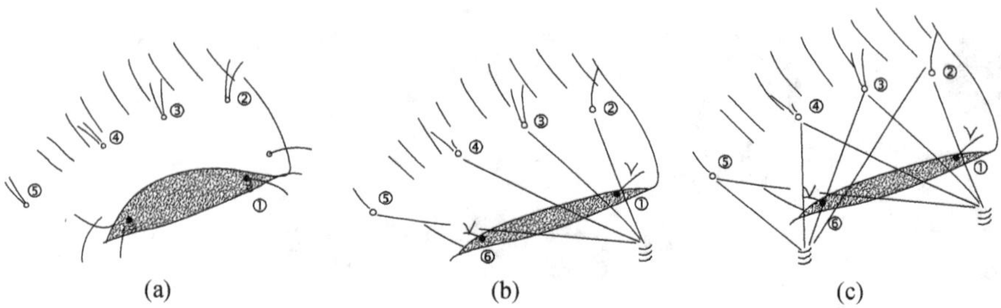

Fig. 20: Dual-row repair for type 1B tear. (a) shows a wide and large type 1B tear with two medial row anchors in place. Sutures 1 and 6 are placed at the anterior and posterior ends of the tear respectively. Sutures 2, 3, 4 and 5 are spaced out evenly over the torn tendon. (b) shows both sutures 1 and 6 are tied, thus limiting the tear from propagating. One limb from sutures 2–5 are retrieved and secured to the anterior Healix BR knotless anchor in the lateral row. (c) shows the remaining suture limbs tied to the posterior lateral row anchor.

- Suture pair 5 is retrieved retrograde, as far posterior as possible. This suture is the far suture that will recruit the infraspinatus into the repair complex, to ensure a wide suture spread and hence diffuse the high tension at the tear (Fig. 20(a)).
- Similar to suture 1, one limb from suture 6 is passed to the posterior limit of the tear and tied with a sliding knot of choice. Sutures are then cut (Fig. 20(b)).
- Suture 1 is then tied with a sliding knot and sutures cut.
- Retrieve one limb each from sutures 2, 3, 4 and 5; then these are secured to an anterior lateral row (5.5 mm Healix BR knotless anchor), positioned over the GT, close to or just posterior to the anterior limit of the tear (Fig. 20(b)).
- Another 5.5 mm Healix BR knotless anchor is used as a posterior lateral row, positioned at the posterior limit of the tear, or just anterior to it. The remaining suture limbs are retrieved and tied to this anchor (Fig. 20(c)).

8. Arthroscopic Dual-Row Cuff Repair for Type 2 Tears

These are asymmetric tears and tend to be mid-sized, occurring at the corners of the tendon. The anterior type 2 tears are far more common.

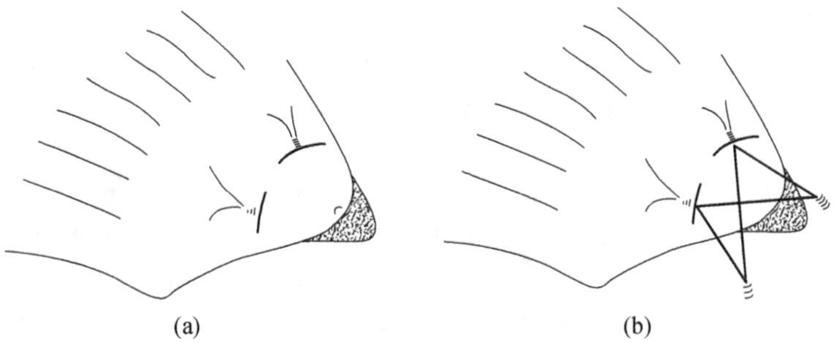

Fig. 21: Dual-row repair for type 2 tears. (a) The tear with a medial row anchor placed at mid-section and both pairs of sutures are passed individually. These are then tied. (b) One suture limb from each pair being tied to the Versalok anchor in the lateral row. Two such lateral row anchors are required.

Some tips are summarised below when dealing with anterior type 2 tears.

- After a thorough debridement, mobilise the tendon from the antero-lateral portal and reduce the tendon as anatomically as possible.
- Recognise the apex of the tear and hence the axis of pull required to reduce and repair the tear.
- Place a dual-loaded medial row anchor (5.5 mm Healix BR anchor).
- Pass both limbs of suture 1 individually, to the antero-medial part of the tendon (for anterior type 2 tears). Ensure the sutures are equally spaced apart. Similarly pass both limbs of suture 2 to the postero-lateral part of the tendon, equally spaced apart (Fig. 21(a)).
- Tie both sutures 1 and 2 with sliding knots (Fig. 21(a)).
- Retrieve one suture from each pair and secure to the lateral row of Versalok anchor. Two such lateral row of anchors may be needed (Fig. 21(b)).

9. Post-op Management and Rehabilitation

Rate of escalation of therapy for post-surgical rehabilitation should vary based on the size and extent of the tear. Tendon retraction should be assessed pre-operatively. If present, a slower rehabilitation course should be adopted in view of higher post-operative failure rate. During the first 6–8 weeks, it is recommended that the affected upper extremity placed in a sling with only passive mobilisation allowed in the pain-free range.

At 2 months post-operatively, active assisted range of motion can be allowed in the pain-free range and full passive range of motion can be allowed with light isometric exercises. From 3 months post-operatively onwards, resistance and strengthening exercises can be prescribed. Focus should be placed on advanced strengthening and dynamic stability from 6 months onwards.

10. Outcomes

Patient reported outcome measures (PROMs) are assessed post-operatively at 3, 6, 12 and 24 months. These include the visual analog scale (VAS), Constant shoulder score (CSS), Oxford shoulder score (OSS) and University of California, Los Angeles shoulder score (UCLASS). Significant milestones that can be assessed in specialist outpatient clinics include:

1. Clearance by physiotherapist.
2. Asymptomatic at rest, and with exercises or activities.
3. Sufficient range of movement to meet demands of occupation.
4. Good strength and endurance for patient's desired activities.

Our institution utilised the Boot Lace Margin Convergence Technique for arthroscopic repair of large to massive rotator cuff tears exceeding 3 cm. 80 consecutive patients of a single surgeon were identified through retrospective review of prospectively collected data from 2010 to 2015. Patients who underwent arthroscopic repair with boot lace margin convergence technique demonstrated significant improvement in range of motion, strength, pain scores and function scores (CSS, OSS, and UCLASS) post-operatively at 1 year and more than 80% were subjectively satisfied with this procedure.

References

1. DeOrio JK, Cofield RH. Results of a second attempt at surgical repair of a failed initial rotator-cuff repair. *J Bone Joint Surg Am* 1984;66(4):563–567.
2. Miller BS, Downie BK, Kohen RB, *et al.* When do rotator cuff repairs fail? Serial ultrasound examination after arthroscopic repair of large and massive rotator cuff tears. *Am J Sports Med* 2011;39(10):2064–2070. doi: 10.1177/0363546511413372.
3. Le BTN, Wu XL, Lam PH, Murrell GAC. Factors predicting rotator cuff retears: an analysis of 1000 consecutive rotator cuff repairs. *Am J Sports Med* 2014;42(5):1134–1142. doi:10.1177/0363546514525336.
4. Consigliere P, Polyzois I, Sarkhel T, Gupta R, Levy O, Narvani AA. preliminary results of a consecutive series of large & massive rotator cuff tears treated with arthroscopic rotator cuff repairs augmented with extracellular matrix. *Arch Bone Jt Surg* 2017;5(1):14–21.
5. Patte D. Classification of rotator cuff lesions. *Clin Orthop Relat Res* 1990;254:81–86.
6. Mellado JM, Calmet J, Olona M, Esteve C, Camins A, Pérez Del Palomar L, *et al.* Surgically repaired massive rotator cuff tears: MRI of tendon integrity, muscle fatty degeneration, and muscle atrophy correlated with intraoperative and clinical findings. *AJR Am J Roentgenol* 2005;184:1456–1463.

https://doi.org/10.1142/9789811249846_0017

Chapter 17

Massive Cuff Tears — Options and Approach

Arthroscopic Partial Repair with Superior Capsular Reconstruction Arthroscopic-Assisted Latissimus Dorsi Transfer

Denny T.T. Lie, Desmond Ong and Gerald Zeng

Summary of Chapter

1. Introduction and epidemiology of massive cuff tears
2. Clinical presentation and examination
3. Classification and approach
4. Imaging and diagnosis
5. Surgical technique of arthroscopic partial repair and superior capsular reconstruction (SCR)
6. Surgical technique of arthroscopic-assisted latissimus dorsi transfer
7. Rehabilitation
8. Clinical outcomes

1. Introduction and Epidemiology of Problem

Cofield *et al.* defined rotator cuff tears as massive when the anterior-posterior or medial-lateral dimension exceeds 5 cm [1] while Gerber *et al.* states that massive cuff tears should have at least involvement of 2 tendons [2]. Massive rotator cuff tears constitute approximately 20% of all rotator cuff tears [3]. Massive cuff tears can be challenging to treat, and variable re-tear rates of at least 20% and as high as 90% have been cited in preceding studies [3]. As discussed in the previous chapter, factors that should be taken into account when considering surgery include patient's symptoms and expectations, functional requirements, assessments based on objective scoring systems and chronicity of injury. While a fraction of patients remain asymptomatic, many suffer from pain, reduced function and quality of life, and may thus be good candidates for surgery with the ultimate goal of restoring function and relieving pain.

2. Clinical Presentation: ILEA, ILER, CLEER

The main symptom is weakness and difficulty in performing ADL (activities of daily living). Specific to massive irreparable cuff tears, three main deficits of active range of motion have been reported. These include isolated loss of active elevation (ILEA), isolated loss of active external rotation (ILER), and combined loss of elevation and external rotation (CLEER) [4]. Combination of two of three patterns may cause pseudo-paralysis of the shoulder.

3. Classification, Algorithm

The Hamada classification [5] (Fig. 1) divides patients with massive rotator cuff tears based on the acromiohumeral interval (AHI) and can provides a mechanistic explanation to the findings seen on the radiograph (Fig. 2).

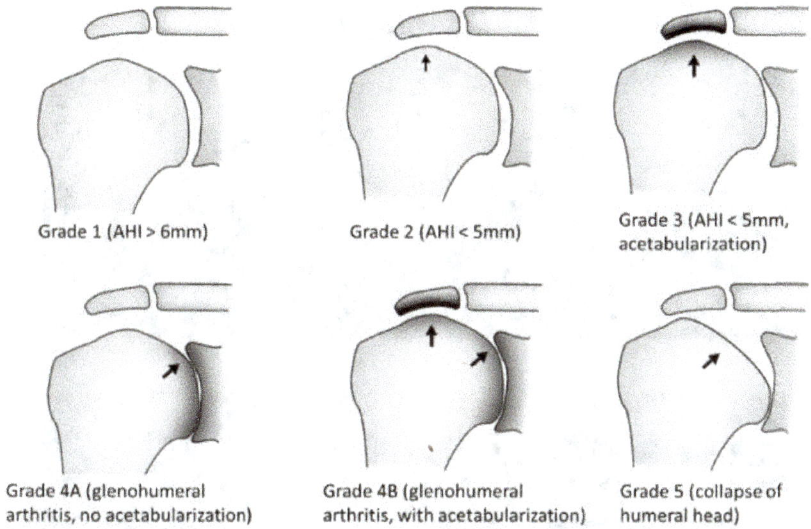

Fig. 1: Hamada classification of massive cuff tear and cuff arthropathy.

Grade 1: Preserved AHI or greater than 6 mm. Grade 2: AHI of 5 mm or less. Grade 3: AHI < 5 mm with acetabularisation of the acromion. Grade 4A: Glenohumeral arthritis without acetabularisation, AHI <7 mm. Grade 4B: Glenohumeral arthritis with acetabularisation, AHI ≤5 mm. Grade 5: humeral head collapse and cuff tear arthropathy (CTA).

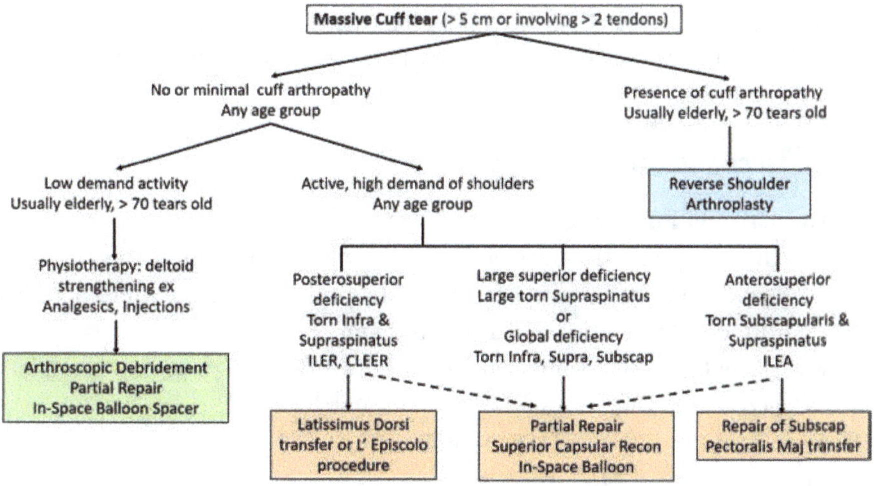

Fig. 2: Algorithm of treatment options in massive cuff tears. Treatment choices are dependent on presence of arthritis, age, activity and anatomical deficiencies.

4. Case Example and Imaging (Fig. 3)

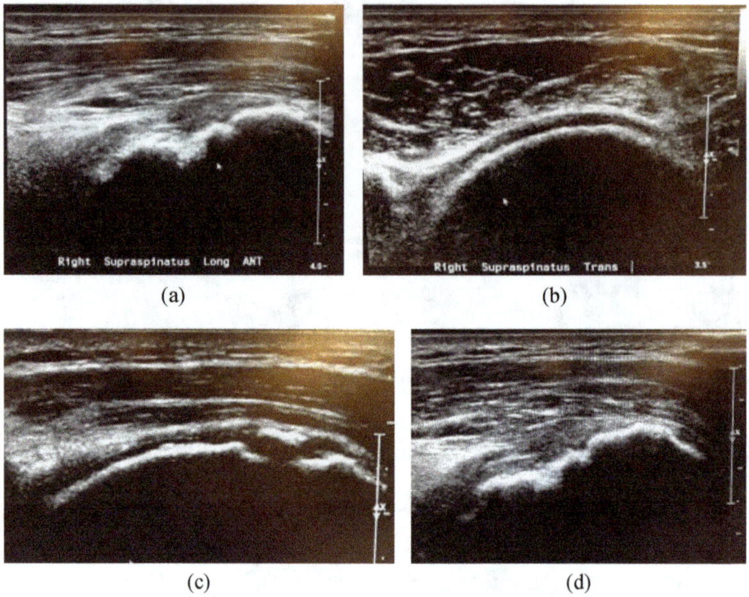

Fig. 3: Ultrasound images of case example. A 71-year-old active man presented with pain after a fall. His active forward flexion was limited to 90°, and active abduction to 80°. Power of Supra 3+/5, Infra 4/5, Subscap 5/5. US showed a complete tear of the supraspinatus tendon (a) and (b) extending into the anterior fibres of the infraspinatus tendon, (c) with diffuse fatty atrophy noted in the supraspinatus muscle. Fatty infiltration of the infraspinatus muscle is noted. Intact subscapularis (Fig. d).

5. Arthroscopic Surgery

1. **Indications for surgery**
   - Any symptomatic massive tear warrants consideration for surgery.
   - Pseudo-paralysis with loss of abduction and weak external rotation: consider latissimus dorsi transfer.
   - If weakness is mainly in abduction: consider superior capsular reconstruction.
2. **Special instruments:** Dermapatch graft.
3. **Positioning and portals**
   - Standard posterior for initial viewing, and anterior portal.
   - Postero-lateral for viewing throughout surgery.
   - Antero-lateral and lateral are the main working portals.

6. Arthroscopic Partial Repair with Superior Capsular Reconstruction

6.1 *The Partial Repair and Preparation*

(a) **Tendon mobilisation**

- The remnant tendons in massive cuff tears tend to be retracted postero-medially and are stuck down with inflammed adhesions.
- Slowly debride these adhesions, releasing the tendons and mobilising them. Be careful of the bleeding, which can be controlled with the RF cautery wand. Further haemostasis can be controlled by adding epinephrine into the fluid (1 mL per 3L saline) and by hypotensive anaesthesia.
- Keep the camera in the posterolateral portal, use the lateral and anterolateral portals to debride, preferably with the RF wand. Develop the plane between the tendons and the labrum beneath, and between the tendon and the bursa and acromion above. Debride deep medially and posteriorly, reaching over the posterior remnant of the tendon (infraspinatus).
- Mobilise and attempt to reduce the remnant tendons to the footprint, as much as it anatomically possible. Avoid excessive tension.

(b) **Measuring the defect and graft size**

- Measure the residual defect, the area left uncovered after the tendons are mobilised if they are tied down.
- From the anterior portal, insert a probe with alternating dark and light markings (each marking being 5 mm) and measure the AP length of the defect (AP 1) at the glenoid plane and the AP length of the defect over the footprint (AP 2) (Fig. 4(b)).
- From the lateral portal, measure the ML length of the defect, that is, the distance from the glenoid to the lateral most aspect of the anatomical footprint (Fig. 4(a)).
- The graft required is usually trapezoidal in shape, looking from the lateral portal. The top of the trapezoid is AP 1, add 0.5 cm at the anterior and posterior ends. The bottom is AP 2, and the height of the trapezoid in the ML distance. Hence the graft required measures at the top, AP 1 + 1 cm, at the base is AP 2 + 1 cm, and the height is ML + 1 cm (Fig. 4(c)).

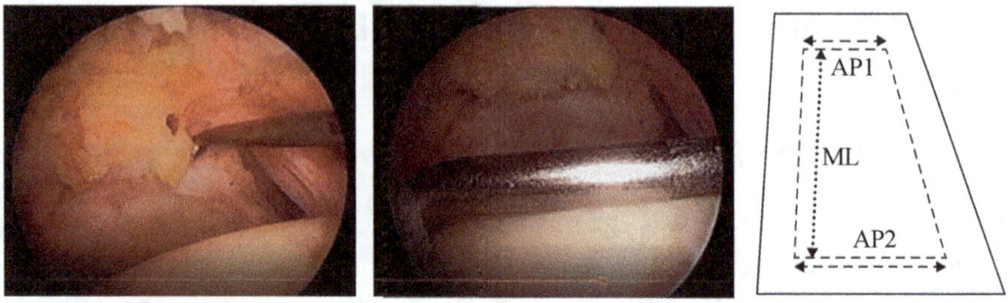

(a) (b) (c)

Fig. 4: Measuring the tendon defect. A calibrated probe is inserted to measure the medial-lateral (a) and antero-posterior (b) dimensions of the tear after debridement. (c) The sizing of the graft. The trapezoid-shaped graft measures AP 1 (+1) cm at the glenoid side, AP 2 (+1) cm at the humeral side and ML (+1) cm in height. The bursal (upper) side is then marked.

(c) **Medial row anchor and sutures**
- Medialise the footprint by decorticating the humeral head more medial than the anatomical footprint. Be careful not to decorticate too much and expose the cancellous bone, this will weaken the hold of the anchor in the bone.
- Insert a triple-loaded medial row anchor (5 mm Healix BR anchor) (Fig. 5(b)) at the area exposed and not potentially covered by the mobilised anterior tendon.

6.2 *Glenoid Anchors*

(a) **Nevaisier portal**
- This portal is created at the junction of the **inner** border of the spine of the scapula as it curves anteriorly to become the lateral process of the acromion. From the entry point, the needle is pointed laterally and will emerge at the superior aspect of the glenoid. The glenoid anchor can be inserted from the Nevaisier portal or from the antero-lateral portal (Fig. 5(a)), depending on the more appropriate trajectory.

(b) **Is one glenoid anchor sufficient?**
- In the author's opinion, **one** anchor is sufficient given the smaller size of the Asian glenoid. A 4 mm dual-loaded Gryphon anchor is

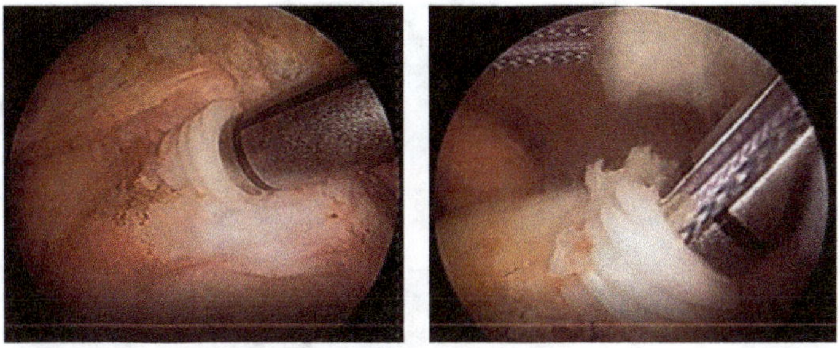

(a) (b)

Fig. 5: Anchor insertions: (a) Shows a Healix anchor inserted to the glenoid, and another fixed to the humeral head, as shown in (b).

adequate. The trajectory of the drill and hence anchor, should be pointing either directly from the top or from an angle of about 30° directed medially. The entry point is at least 7–10 mm from the superior edge of the glenoid.

6.3 *Graft Preparation*

(a) **Use of allograft instead of tensor fascia lata**
- The original description of SCR uses 7–8 mm thick tensor fascia lata. In the author's opinion the graft is too thick for the subacromial space, with inadequate space for manoeuvring, passing and tying of sutures.
- In this technique, with partial repair of the remnant tendon being performed, a dermal allograft (3–5 mm thick) is adequate to augment the repair, not to replace the tendon.

(b) **Cutting the graft to size**
- The graft is then cut to size according to measurement made above. It is usually trapezoidal in shape, the narrower top of the trapezoid will be attached to the glenoid and measures (AP 1 + 10 mm). The base of the trapezoid will be attached to the humeral head and measures (AP 2 + 10 mm) and the height of the trapezoid is (ML + 10 mm) (Fig. 4(c)).

(c) **Attachment of sutures to the graft**
- Retrieve one limb of suture from each of the two **suture pairs** from the glenoid anchor. Pass each limb at the top (glenoid end) of the

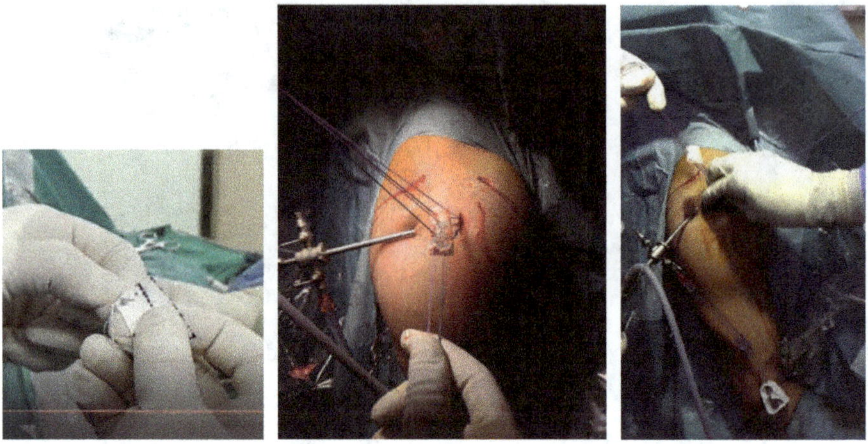

(a) (b) (c)

Fig. 6: Graft preparation. The graft is cut about 5–10 mm longer and wider than the size of the tear measured. The sutures from the glenoid anchor is retrieved and a horizontal tie is created at the apex of the graft, as shown in (a). This will be used to relay the graft in. Sutures from the humeral head anchors are then passed through the graft, as shown in (b). (c) Shows cleansing of the skin with iodine prior to insertion of the graft. This greatly reduces the risk of Cutibacterium Acne infection.

trapezoid graft (Fig. 6(a)). Then tie them together. The loose limbs of the sutures are kept in the Nevaisier or antero-lateral portal.

- Pass one pair of sutures from the medial row of anchor at the humeral head to the base of the trapezoid, near the corners, passing the suture from the under-surface upwards. The graft is then ready (Fig. 6(b)).

6.4 *Graft Insertion*

(a) **Iodine cleansing of the graft and portal**

- Generously douse the graft and the lateral portal with diluted iodine (Fig. 6(c)). The single biggest cause of infection in superior capsular reconstruction is from the graft, usually arising from *Cutibacterium acnes.* Hence it is the author's practice to routinely cleanse the graft and the portal to get rid of this skin pathogen.

(b) **Relaying the graft into the joint**

- The graft is rolled up side to side like a cigar, and the top end of the graft is gently held with a grasper, and delivered into the subacromial space. At the same time, the loose suture limbs from the glenoid anchor are gently pulled. These sutures thus relay the graft into place (Figs. 7(a) and 7(b)).
- It is common to see the graft bunching up over the glenoid, especially if only one anchor is used. Use a probe or an obturator to smoothen out the crumpled and bunched up edges (Fig. 7(c)).

(c) **Securing the glenoid sutures**

- One loose suture limb from the glenoid anchor is then retrieved and passed to the anterior fold of the tendon. Similarly, the other loose suture limb is passed to the fold of the tendon just posterior to the glenoid (Fig. 7(d)).

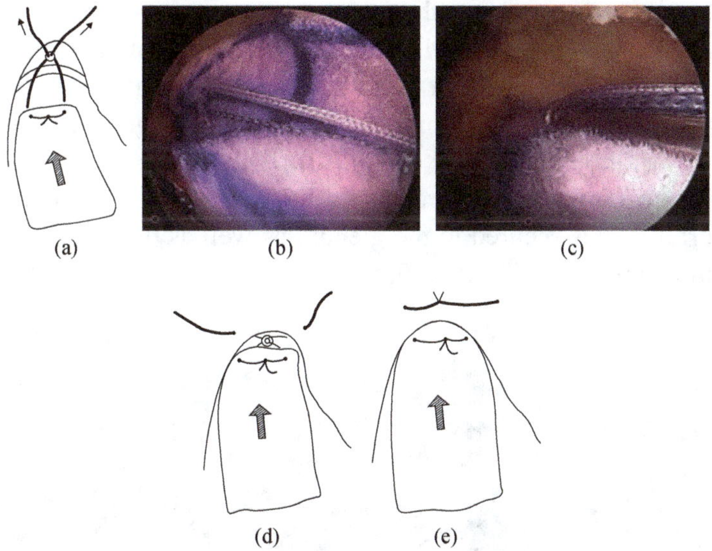

Fig. 7: Inserting the graft. The graft is relayed in, as shown in (a), by pulling on the loose glenoid sutures, with the anchor acting as a pulley. (b) Shows the graft neatly inserted. The edges of the graft are tucked in beneath the tendons (c). (d) Shows the loose sutures passed through the anterior and posterior tendon folds, after which they are tied (e) securing the graft to the glenoid.

- These two limbs of sutures are then tied using 6 half-hitch knots (Fig. 7(e)). This is effectively a convergence, bringing the medial most part of the massive tear together, usually covering the glenoid end of the graft (the top of the trapezoid), either partially or totally. The sutures can then be cut.

6.5 *Suture Management of the Graft*

(a) **Securing anterior and posterior edges of the graft**

- Retrieve a pair of sutures (purple sutures in Fig. 8) from the medial row anchor. Pass one limb of the suture to the anterior border of the graft, about 10 mm from the edge at about midway of the ML distance (Fig. 8(a)) and pass the other limb to the anterior fold of the tendon (Fig. 8(b)). Then tie both limbs of sutures but do not cut the sutures, park them in the anterior portal (Fig. 8(c)).
- Similarly retrieve the other pair of sutures from the medial anchor (striped blue suture in Fig. 9). Pass one suture limb to the posterior fold of tendon (Fig. 9(a)) and pass the other limb to the posterior part of the graft, 10 mm from the posterior edge and about midway of the ML distance (Fig. 9(b)). Then tie both limbs of sutures but do not cut the sutures, park them in the posterior portal. The graft is thus secured to the glenoid as well as the partial repair of the remnant tendon (Fig. 9(c)).

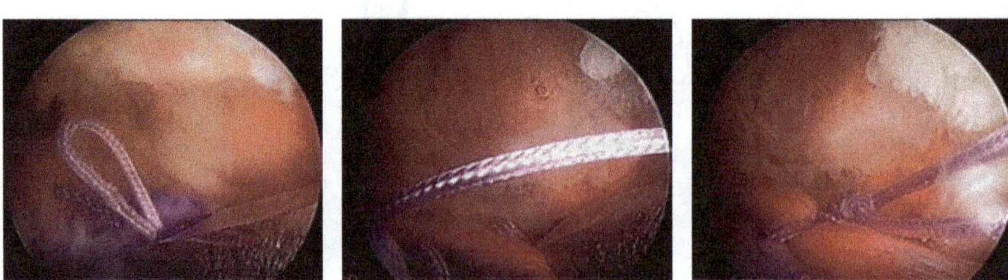

(a) (b) (c)

Fig. 8: Anterior tendon repair. (a) Shows the purple suture from the medial row anchor is passed to the graft, and to the anterior tendon fold, as shown in (b). This is then tied, as shown in (c), thus securing the graft to tendons and achieving a partial repair.

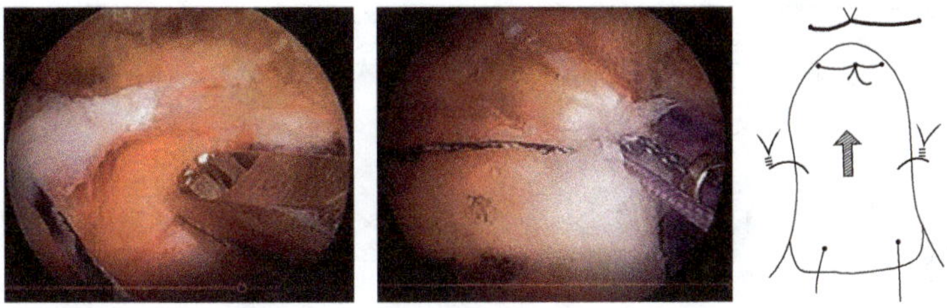

(a) (b) (c)

Fig. 9: Posterior tendon repair. Striped suture from the medial row anchor is passed to the posterior tendon fold, shown in (a) and to the graft, then tied, as shown in (b). (c) Shows the graft secured to both anterior and posterior tendon folds.

(b) **Suturing the lateral edge of the graft**

- Similar bunching up and crumbling of the edges can be seen at the lateral edge (the base of the trapezoid). Use an obturator to smoothen out the edges.
- The third pair of sutures from the medial row anchor attached earlier to the lateral edge of the graft is important here. Separate the sutures, and pull them from separate portals; the anterior limb from the antero-lateral portal and the posterior limb from the lateral portal. This divergent pull helps to reduce and prevent the bunching up often seen.

6.6 *Lateral Row Security*

(a) **Anterior lateral row**

Retrieve one limb of the blue suture(tied to the posterior tendon fold), one limb of the purple suture (tied to the anterior tendon fold) and one suture limb from the lateral edge of the graft, and secure these to the anterior lateral row anchor (Versalok PEEK anchor) (Figs. 10(a) and 10(b)).

(b) **Posterior lateral row**

Retrieve the remaining suture limbs (purple from the anterior tendon fold, striped blue from the posterior tendon and the suture from the lateral edge of the graft). Secure these sutures to the posterior lateral row anchor (Versalok PEEK anchor) (Fig. 10(c)).

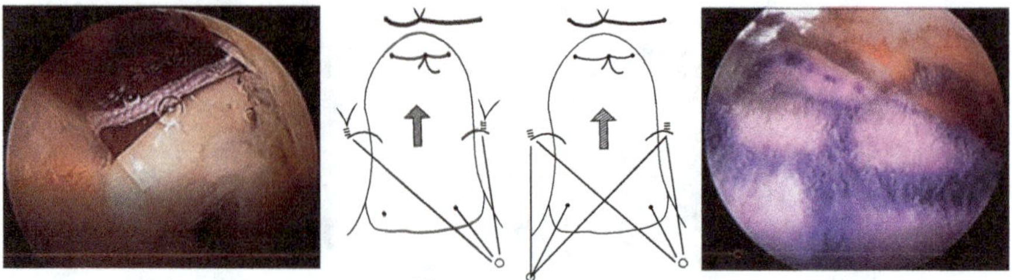

(a) (b) (c) (d)

Fig. 10: Final Check. Sutures from the medial row are then fixed to a Versalok anchor in the lateral row, as shown in (a), (b) and (c). (d) Shows the final check, with the graft well secured to the partial repair.

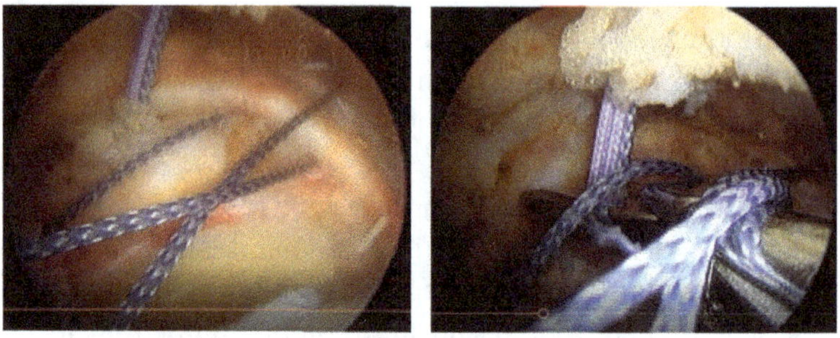

(a) (b)

Fig. 11: Partial repair augmented with SCR. (a) shows boot-lace margin convergence sutures prepared, and a glenoid anchor inserted. (b) shows the glenoid anchor sutures being retrieved beneath the convergence sutures, which will be used to relay the graft in.

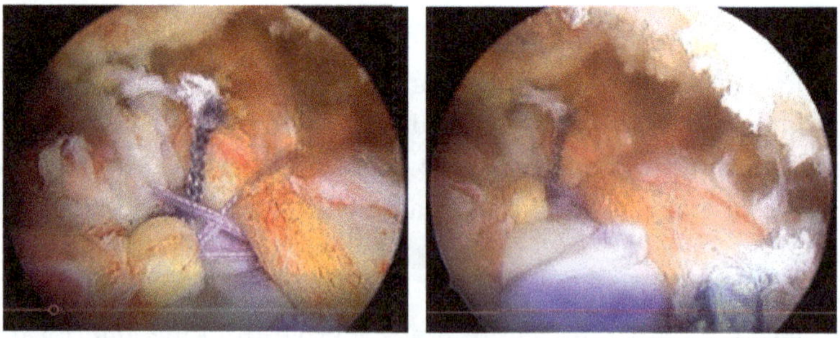

(a) (b)

Fig. 12: SCR tucked in. (a) and (b) show the tight partial repair of the tendons. The intervening gap is occupied by the SCR graft, tucked in and securely tied.

- The lateral row anchors thus provide a divergent pull on the graft, to avoid and reduce bunching up of the graft (Fig. 10(d)). Another example of SCR is shown in Figs. 11 and 12.

7. Arthroscopic-Assisted Latissimus Dorsi Transfer

7.1 *Anatomy of the Latissimus Dorsi Tendon*

(a) **Origin**
Spinous processes of lower six thoracic vertebra, thoracolumbar fascia, liiac crest, inferior three or four ribs and inferior angle of scapula.

(b) **Course**
Curves around the lower border of the teres major with which it may have adhesions and runs from the dorsum of the trunk to lie on the anterior aspect of the posterior axillary fold. Terminates as a quadrilateral tendon of about 7 cm.

(c) **Insertion**
Floor of the intertubercular grove and separated from the teres major insertion by a bursa.

(d) **Action**
By spanning the posterior trunk and crossing from the scapula to the humerus, its activation has an influence on scapular action. This synergistic line of action with other scapular stabilisers, e.g. lower and middle trapezius forms part of the basis of the transfer for massive rotator cuff tears. By shifting its insertion from the anterior humerus to the rotator cuff footprint, its action also changes from humeral internal rotation to external rotation. This corrects the external rotation deficit associated with massive rotator cuff tears.

7.2 *Positioning*

The patient is placed in the lateral decubitus position. A traction device is prepared as for a rotator cuff repair in the lateral position. The arm is however not attached to said device to allow free movement during tendon harvest.

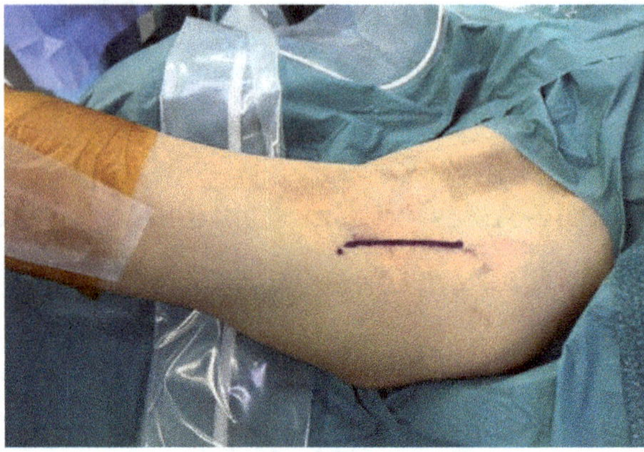

Fig. 13: Incision for tendon harvest. The tendon can be palpated at the posterior axillary fold. The patient is positioned in the lateral decubitus position. Figure 13 shows the incision for tendon harvest.

7.3 *Tendon Harvest*

- In a patient with average body habitus, the insertion of the latissimus dorsi can be palpated with the arm placed in the hand behind head position (Fig. 13).
- An incision of about 5–7 cm is made on the proximal anterior aspect of the posterior axillary fold. Following skin incision, blunt dissection is performed with the surgeon's finger to avoid neurovascular injury. To facilitate visualisation, retractors may be used to retract the skin but retraction of deep structures should be avoided to minimise the potential for neurovascular injury (Fig. 14).
- At the insertion on the humerus, the tendon can be easily isolated. The tendon is then freed from adjacent structures in a proximal to distal direction.
- The tendon is detached from humerus with a blade. The use of diathermy is avoided to prevent electrical/thermal injury to neurovascular structures. It is also not necessary as the tendon is relatively avascular (Fig. 15).

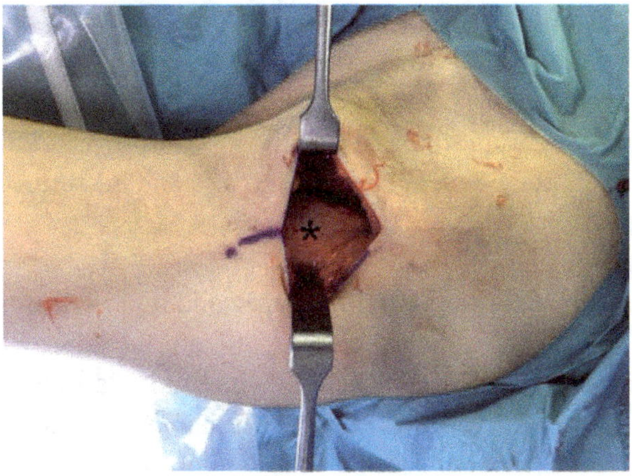

Fig. 14: Exposing the latissimus dorsi tendon. Blunt dissection is performed. Figure 14 shows the incision widely exposed by retractors, showing the latissimus dorsi tendon.

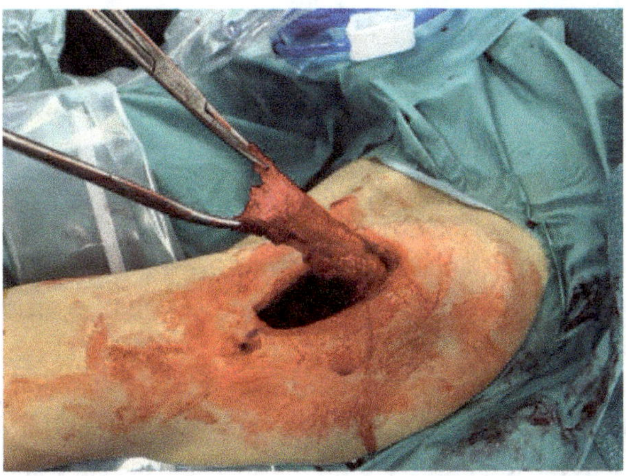

Fig. 15: Harvested tendon. The latissimus dorsi tendon is sharply detached from its attachment, avoiding the use of diathermy.

7.4 *Graft Preparation*

(a) **Suture placement**

The tendon is whip-stitched with a Fibrewire or equivalent suture. Placement of a single whip-stitch will tubularise the tendon which in the author's opinion will improve the suture pull-out strength of the construct compared to laying the tendon flat and spread out onto the rotator cuff footprint. No failure at the tendon-bone interface has been observed in the author's series with this suture configuration using Fibrewire or equivalent sutures. Usage of standard sutures however is not advised.

(b) **Mobilisation**

Using the suture for traction, the tendon and muscle is mobilised. It is freed of adhesions by finger dissection from the adjacent subcutaneous tissues and on its deep aspect off the trunk. Particular attention is paid to the inferior border of the scapular and teres major muscle which would affect the reach of the tendon. In a small patient, it is possible to reach the iliac crest and spinous processes of the vertebra.

7.5 *Arthroscopy*

(a) **Portals**

The arm is attached to the traction device in preparation for arthroscopy. A standard posterior viewing portal is made 2 cm inferior and medial to the posterior corner of the acromion. The working portal will be through an anterolateral portal made 1–2 cm lateral to the acromion at the junction of the anterior 1/3 and posterior 2/3 of the acromion (Fig. 16).

(b) **Arthroscopic fixation of the tendon**

- Subacromial decompression is performed although in the author's experience with massive rotator cuff tear the space and footprint is usually quite well visualised due to the extent of rotator cuff involved as well as the retraction (Fig. 17).
- The footprint is then roughened and prepared for graft attachment making sure not to decorticate excessively and exposing cancellous bone.
- Associated procedures such as biceps tenotomy can often be performed through these portals as well due to the size of the tear. However further glenohumeral procedures may have to be performed separately through more suitable and dedicated portals.

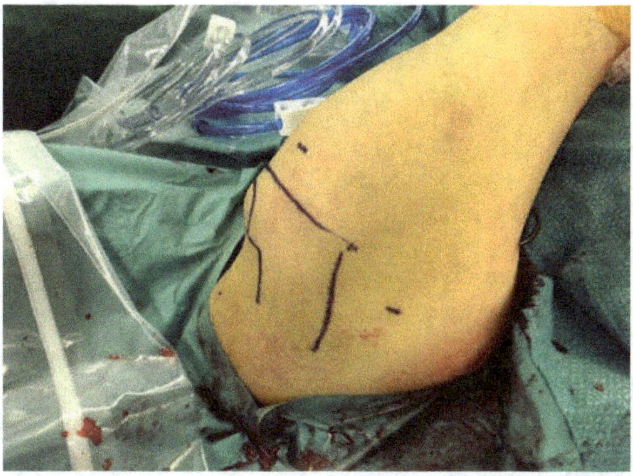

Fig. 16: Portals used. The main portals used in the arthroscopic tendon transfer are the posterior and antero-lateral portals.

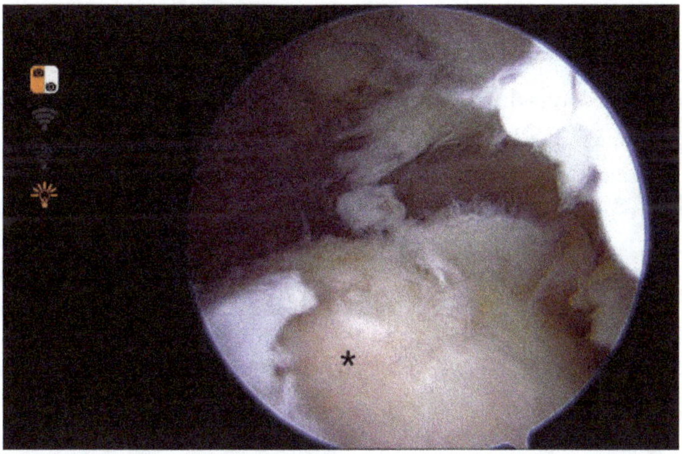

Fig. 17: Subacromial space. In massive and retracted tears, the subacromial space is wide and remnant tendons easily visualised.

- Attention is then turned to the posterior subdeltoid bursa. Arthroscopic dissection is carried out to reach the axilla incision. The tendon is then retrieved and brought into the subacromial space with an arthroscopic grasper coming through the anterolateral working portal.

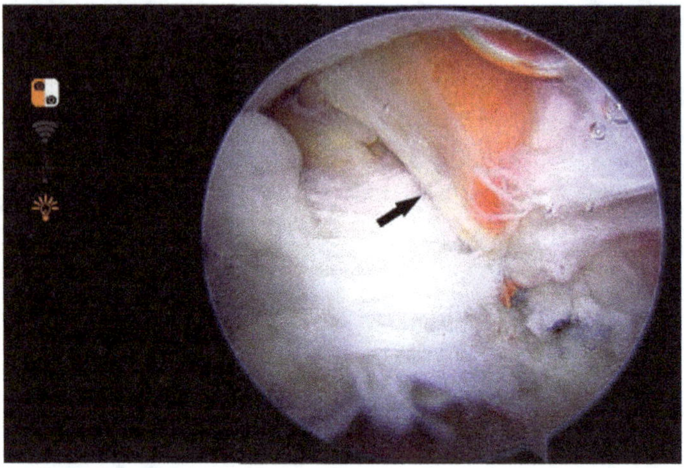

Fig. 18: The latissimus dorsi tendon transferred. The tabularised tendon is seen (black arrow) secured to the footprint.

- Tendon passage through the subdeltoid space superficial to the teres major and minor muscles would avoid the neurovascular structures passing through both the triangular and quadrilateral spaces.
- The tendon is then fixed to the footprint using the whip-stitch suture and a knotless rotator cuff anchor (Fig. 18).

8. Post-op Management and Rehabilitation

8.1 *Arthroscopic Partial Repair with Superior Capsular Reconstruction*

Rate of escalation of therapy for post-surgical rehabilitation should vary based on the size and extent of the tear. Tendon retraction should be assessed pre-operatively. If present, a slower rehabilitation course should be adopted in view of higher post-operative failure rate. During the first 6–8 weeks, it is recommended that the affected upper extremity placed in a sling with only passive mobilisation allowed in the pain-free range.

At 2 months post-operatively, active assisted range of motion can be allowed in the pain-free range and full passive range of motion can be allowed with light isometric exercises. From 3 months post-operatively onwards, resistance and strengthening exercises can be prescribed. Focus should be placed on advanced strengthening and dynamic stability from 6 months onwards.

8.2 *Latissimus Dorsi Transfer*

There is a wide variation in post-operative rehabilitative protocols for patients who had undergone this procedure. Most include 4–6 weeks of sling immobilisation fixed in slight abduction and close to full external rotation. Gentle external rotation and passive abduction may be considered immediately post-operatively to reduce risk of stiffness but patients should limit internal rotation and adduction for at least 6 weeks and remain on a sling. Progression to active range of motion exercises may be commenced thereafter.

9. Outcomes

Arthroscopic SCR has emerged as a feasible surgical option for addressing massive irreparable rotator cuff tears. A large case series involving 88 patients by Pennington *et al.* showed significant improvement in American Shoulder and Elbow Surgeons (ASES) score, visual analog scale pain scores, strength and range of motion post-operatively at 1 year, following SCR with dermal allograft.

Pooled analysis from a systematic review in 2019 by Sochacki *et al.*, including six articles involving 286 subjects showed clinically and statistically significant improvement in the American Shoulder and Elbow Surgeons (ASES) score, Visual analog scale (VAS) scores. A low rate of graft failure, complications and reoperations were observed.

References

1. Cofield RH. Subscapular muscle transposition for repair of chronic rotator cuff tears. *Surg Gynecol Obstet* 1982;154(5):667–672.
2. Gerber C, Fuchs B, Hodler J. The results of repair of massive tears of the rotator cuff. *J Bone Joint Surg Am* 2000;82(4):505–515. doi: 10.2106/00004623-200004000-00006.

3. Ok HS, Kim BG, Choi WC, Hong CG, Kim JW, Kim JH. Clinical relevance of classifying massive rotator cuff tears: results based on functional and radiological findings after arthroscopic repair. *Am J Sports Med* 2017;45(1):157–166. doi:10.1177/0363546516667498.
4. Kany J, Anis H, Werthel JD. Massive irreparable rotator cuff tears: treatment options, indications, and role of fully arthroscopic latissimus dorsi transfer. *Obere Extremität* 2018;13(4):246–254. doi:10.1007/s11678-018-0478-9.
5. Hamada K, Fukuda H, Mikasa M, Kobayashi Y. Roentgenographic findings in massive rotator cuff tears. A long-term observation. *Clin Orthop Relat Res* 1990;(254):92–96.
6. Seitz AL, McClure PW, Finucane S, Boardman ND, Michener LA. Mechanisms of rotator cuff tendinopathy: intrinsic, extrinsic, or both? *Clin Biomech (Bristol, Avon)* 2011;26(1):1–12. doi:10.1016/j.clinbiomech.2010.08.001.
7. Nho SJ, Yadav H, Shindle MK, Macgillivray JD. Rotator cuff degeneration: etiology and pathogenesis. *Am J Sports Med* 2008;36(5):987–993. doi:10.1177/0363546508317344
8. Gumina S, Candela V, Passaretti D, *et al.* The association between body fat and rotator cuff tear: the influence on rotator cuff tear sizes. *J Shoulder Elbow Surg* 2014;23(11):1669–1674. doi:10.1016/j.jse.2014.03.016.
9. Milgrom C, Schaffler M, Gilbert S, van Holsbeeck M. Rotator-cuff changes in asymptomatic adults. The effect of age, hand dominance and gender. *J Bone Joint Surg Br* 1995;77(2):296–298.
10. Longo UG, Berton A, Khan WS, Maffulli N, Denaro V. Histopathology of rotator cuff tears. *Sports Med Arthrosc Rev* 2011;19(3):227–236. doi:10.1097/JSA.0b013e318213bccb.
11. Pennington WT, Bartz BA, Pauli JM, Walker CE, Schmidt W. Arthroscopic superior capsular reconstruction with acellular dermal allograft for the treatment of massive irreparable rotator cuff tears: short-term clinical outcomes and the radiographic parameter of superior capsular distance. *Arthroscopy* 2018;34(6):1764–1773. doi:10.1016/j.arthro.2018.01.009.
12. Sochacki KR, McCulloch PC, Lintner DM, Harris JD. Superior capsular reconstruction for massive rotator cuff tear leads to significant improvement in range of motion and clinical outcomes: a systematic review. *Arthroscopy* 2019;35(4):1269–1277. doi:10.1016/j.arthro.2018.10.129.

https://doi.org/10.1142/9789811249846_0018

Chapter 18

Arthroscopic Reconstruction of the Acromio-Clavicular Joint

Denny T.T. Lie and Hamid Rahmatullah Bin Abd Razak

Summary of Chapter

1. Introduction and epidemiology of ACJ injuries
2. Clinical presentation and examination
3. Diagnosis and imaging
4. Surgical technique of arthroscopic ACJ reconstruction using dog-bone sutures
5. Rehabilitation
6. Clinical outcomes

1. Introduction, Epidemiology and Pathophysiology

Acromioclavicular joint (ACJ) dislocation is a relatively common injury that accounts for 50% of all sports-related shoulder injuries [1, 2]. ACJ dislocation is associated with acromioclavicular (AC) and coracoclavicular (CC) ligament injuries [3]. ACJ dislocations can be caused by both direct and indirect trauma. Direct trauma is caused by a vertically oriented superior impact ono the lateral aspect of the shoulder, forcing the ACJ in an inferior direction [4]. Indirect trauma usually results from falling on an adducted and outstretched arm causing the humeral head to be driven into the inferior aspect of the acromion and the ACJ itself [5]. The severity of ACJ injuries is related to the force of the impact. ACJ injuries can range from a simple sprain of the AC and CC ligaments, which are responsible for holding the joint in its anatomic and physiologic position without displacement, to frank dislocation of the distal third of the clavicle inferiorly or posteriorly.

2. Clinical Presentation

Patients usually present with localised pain over the ACJ with varying degrees of difficulty in moving the shoulder joint following a history of trauma. The pain can also be referred to the trapezius. On examination, there is almost always lateral clavicle or ACJ tenderness. A prominent swelling or palpable deformity can be seen and felt on the injured side in more severe injury. Shoulder range is typically reduced by pain. The presence of associated injuries should always be examined for. Provocative tests for ACJ pathology like the cross-body test, can be helpful to distinguish other causes of shoulder pain. These tests may be particularly useful in milder injury in which there might not be any visible swelling or palpable deformity.

3. Diagnosis, Imaging and Treatment Algorithm

Standard shoulder radiographs (anteroposterior [AP], lateral) (Fig. 1) should be undertaken to exclude other causes of traumatic shoulder pain. ACJ injuries may not always be obvious on standard radiographic views. Additional views include the Zanca view, and AP view performed by tilting the beam 10° to 15° cranial, as well as bilateral AP views to compare displacement to the normal shoulder. Stress views may also be undertaken with weights when the diagnosis is equivocal on standard AP views. If there still is uncertainty in diagnosis, ultrasound or magnetic resonance imaging (MRI) may also be considered.

ACJ injuries are classified by the Rockwood classification system into types I–VI on the basis of radiographic criteria [6]. The Rockwood classification system is based on the magnitude and direction of dislocation.

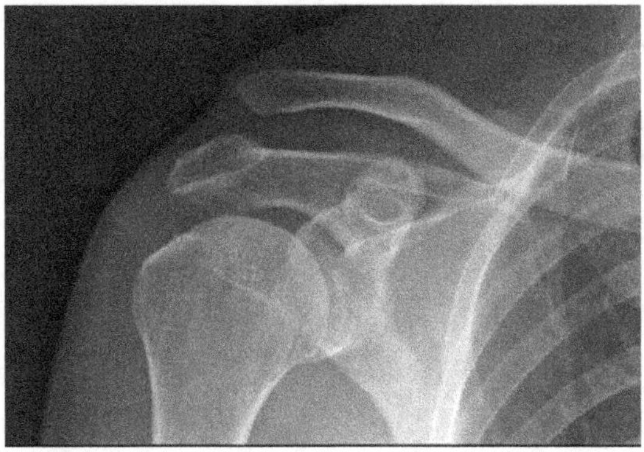

Fig. 1: X-ray AP view of right ACJ injury. The history is a 30-year old male who fell during a cycling accident. X-rays show the lateral clavicle had dislocated superiorly, making it type III injury.

Types I and II respond to short-term conservative treatment. However, surgical treatment is usually recommended for types IV–VI (Fig. 2). Management of type III injuries is still controversial regarding conservative versus surgical management [7,8].

4. Arthroscopic Surgery

(a) **Indications for surgery:**
- Symptomatic (pain and weakness) ACJ types III, IV and V injuries
- ACJ injuries types I and II in overhead athletes and certain individuals with physically demanding occupations

(b) **Special instruments:**
- Athrex ACJ reconstruction with dog-bone

(c) **Positioning and portals:**
- **Posterior** portal for viewing initially, later moved to the **anterolateral or biceps** portal
- **Anterior** portal, just lateral to the coracoid tip
- Skin incision over the lateral third of the clavicle that is to be reduced, can be extended laterally over the ACJ

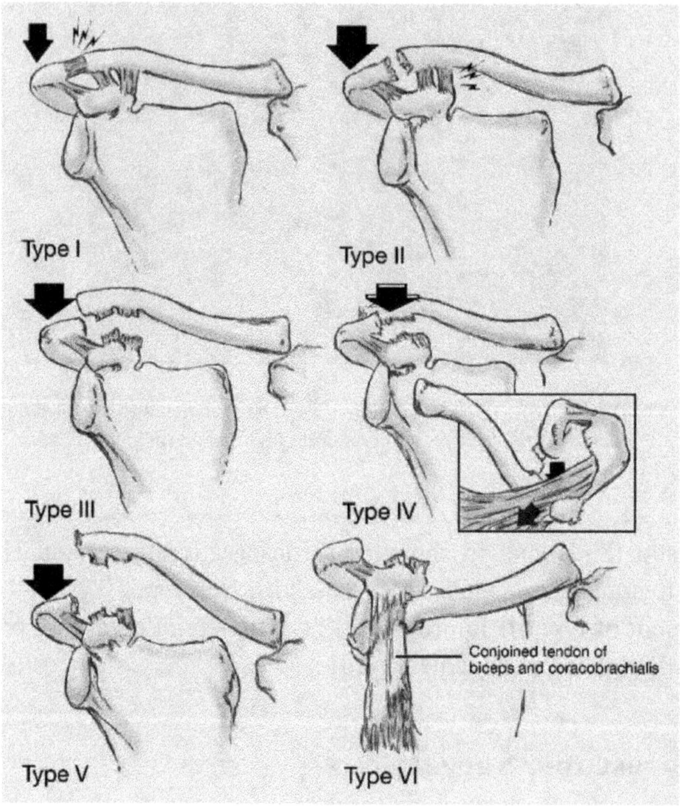

Fig. 2: Rockwood classification of ACJ injuries. Type I is a strain or stretching of the AC ligaments. Type II is a complete rupture of ACJ and strain of CC ligaments resulting in 50% subluxation. Type III is a rupture of both ACJ and CC ligaments, causing 100% subluxation. Type IV is a posterior subluxation over the acromion (rare). Type V is superior subluxation, and type VI is an inferior subluxation beneath the coracoid (very rare) [6].

4.1 *Arthroscopic Reconstruction of the Acromio-clavicular Joint — Acute Injuries*

This technique is best suited for acute ACJ injuries, that is, within 6 weeks. It is often recommended that chronic ACJ injuries require a biological graft.

(a) **Gleno-humeral inspection and debridement**

- The glenohumeral joint is routinely inspected for synovitis and associated injuries, and debridement done. Depending on the specific trauma cause, ACJ injuries in the elderly may be associated with rotator cuff tears and must be excluded. Look out for SLAP tears, the deep-seated pain of which can mimic ACJ injuries.

(b) **Rotator interval clearance, preparing the coracoid tip**

- The rotator interval must be thoroughly cleared, and haemostasis secured with RF cautery. Be careful to avoid injuring the biceps tendon and the biceps sling at the confluence of the biceps with the subscapularis.
- The fascia in the interval is often thickened in adhesive capsulitis, these need to be debrided till the muscle layer of the anterior deltoids is visible.
- The conjoint tendon is visible and can be probed. Be careful when debriding the tendon, avoid blindly thrusting the shaver anywhere medial to the conjoint.
- Follow the conjoint tendon upwards to the coracoid tip. Shave and cauterise the under-surface of the coracoid clean without decorticating the coracoid. Remove any soft tissue and fascia that may block visualisation (Fig. 3).

(c) **Drilling and reaming, passage of sutures**

- The Arthrex ACJ drill guide is now used, inserted from the anterior portal, while the camera is transferred to the antero-lateral portal (Fig. 4(a)). The author's preference is to use the older guide with a broader aiming device, as opposed to the newer narrow aiming device.
- The broad aiming guide straddles the under-surface of the coracoid, thus ensuring the drilling would be in the middle of the coracoid. If the drill hole is too medial or lateral, there is a danger it will weaken the coracoid, which can then fracture. Medial drilling has the additional danger of injuring the nearby neurovascular structures. Position the aiming device in the middle of the base of the coracoid (Fig. 4(b)).

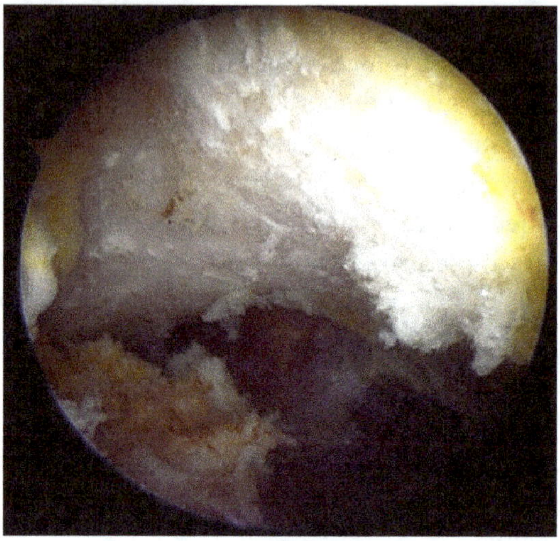

Fig. 3: Under surface of the coracoid. The coracoid tip is debrided clear of soft tissues and decorticated as shown above.

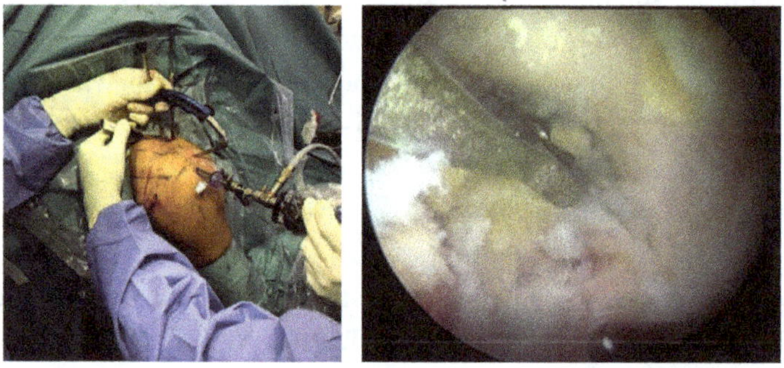

(a) (b)

Fig. 4: Inserting the drill guide. The drill guide is inserted via the anterolateral portal as shown in (a) with the drill sleeve positioned over the lateral clavicle. The guide itself is positioned on the under surface of the coracoid as shown in (b).

- The wire is to be drilled from the lateral third or quarter of the dislocated clavicle. Make a small stab incision over the clavicle and firmly press down the drill guide (Figs. 5(a) and 5(b)).
- After drilling the wire, check the position with image intensifier (Figs. 6(a) and 6(b)). Ensure it is satisfactorily in the middle of the coracoid (neither too medial nor lateral).

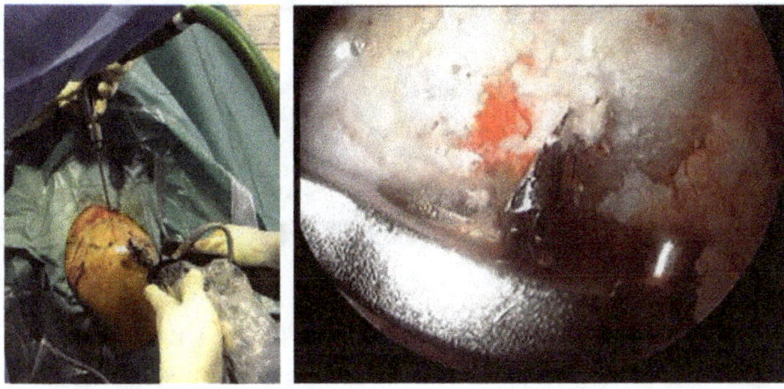

(a) (b)

Fig. 5: Drilling the wire. A wire is drilled from the lateral clavicle, through the coracoid tip shown in (a). The guide prevents over-drilling of the wire, seen in (b).

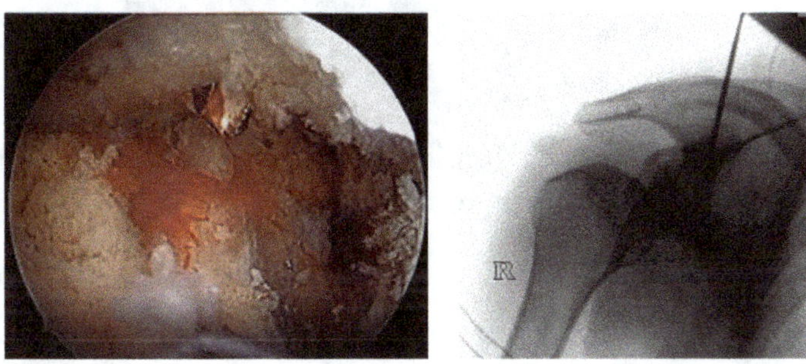

(a) (b)

Fig. 6: Position of the wire. The position of the wire at the coracoid is assessed after the drill guide is removed, shown in (a). An X-ray is done to ensure that the wire traverses across the coracoid, to exit in the middle of the coracoid, shown in (b).

- Ream with 4 mm reamer and leave the reamer, uncoupling the drill and removing the wire (Fig. 7(a)).
- Then insert a passing monofilament wire with the loop down (Fig. 7(b)), and retrieve from the anterior portal (Fig. 7(c)). Use the passing wire to pass an Ethibond suture upwards, keeping the loop of Ethibond below the coracoid and outside the joint.
- The dog-bone sutures (Fig. 8) are then passed into the Ethibond suture loop, and shuttled upwards (Figs. 9(a) and 9(b)), to exit above the clavicle (Fig. 10(a)).

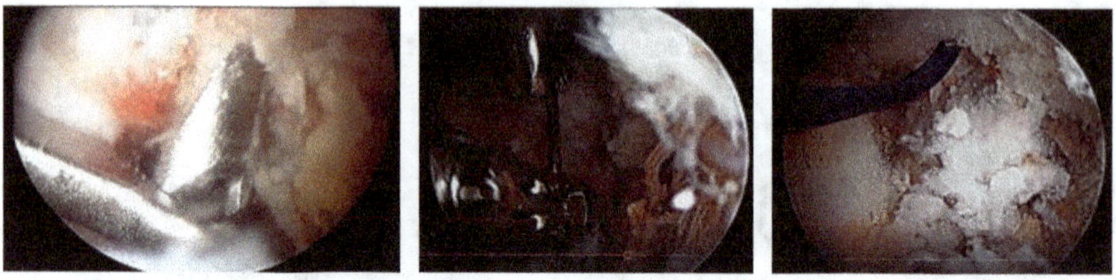

(a) (b) (c)

Fig. 7: Reaming: (a) Shows the reamer drilling over the wire, onto the drill guide. A monofilament is then passed into the reamer, as shown in (b). The reamer is then removed and the filament retrieved out of the portal, seen in (c).

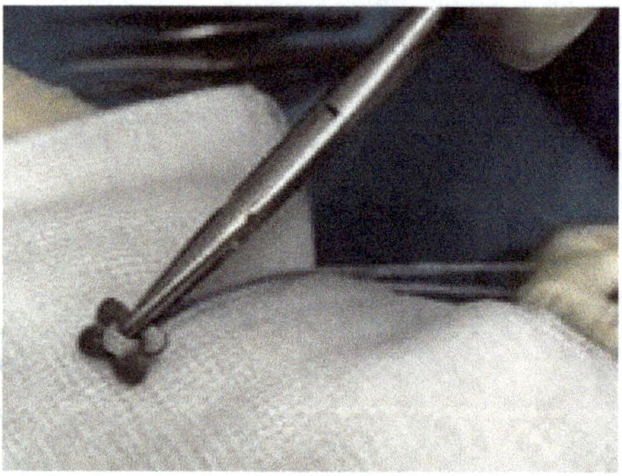

Fig. 8: The dog-bone plate. Sutures are prepared at the dog-bone plate as shown.

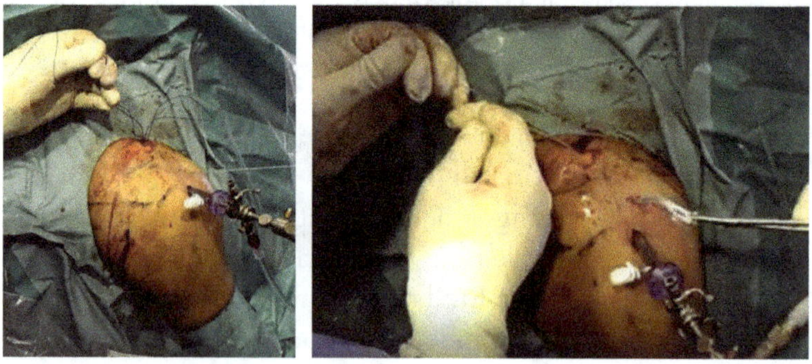

(a) (b)

Fig. 9: Shuttling the sutures. The mono-filament shuttles the sutures into the joint (a). (b) Shows the sutures and the dog-bone plate being pulled into position.

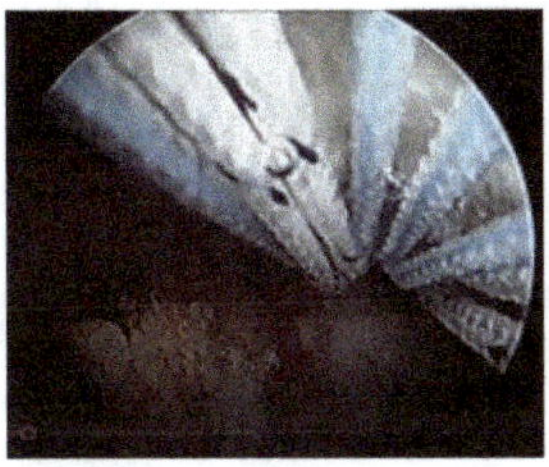

(a)

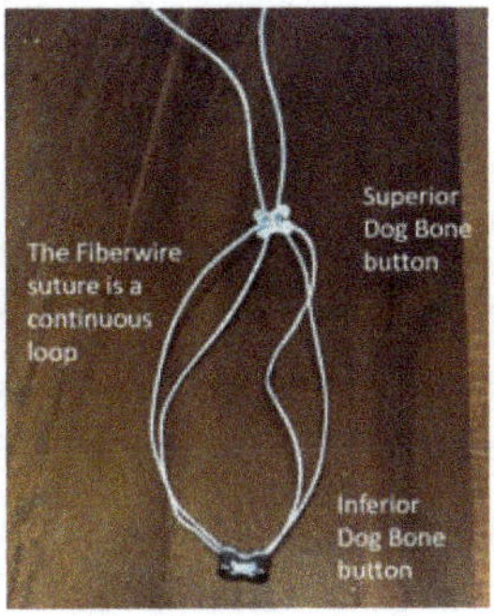

(b)

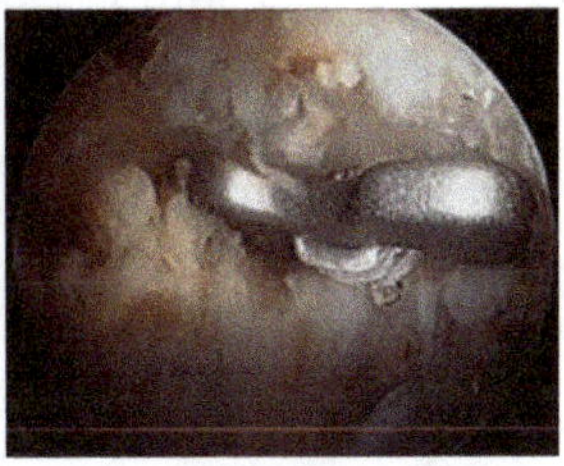

(c)

Fig. 10: The dog-bone plate in position. (a) Shows sutures being pulled into the joint. (b) Illustrates the modification, by using a continuous loop of suture over the dog-bone plates. (c) Shows the dog-bone plate in position, snug on the under surface of the coracoid.

(d) **A note on the sutures**

- The original tightrope device is similar to an endo-button, and was inserted antegrade, from the clavicle downwards to the coracoid. The suture is actually a continuous loop. From one end at the top, it goes down to loop at an endo-button beneath the coracoid. The suture goes up to loop again over an endo-button above the clavicle. The suture traverses down to make a third loop at the endo-button beneath the coracoid before going up.
- Being a continuous loop means that as both free limbs above the clavicle are pulled, the sutures are shortened, thus reducing the clavicular dislocation.
- The current dog-bone device is bigger than the endo-button of the tightrope. Thus, it spreads the high pressure over a wider area and reduces the risk of fracturing the coracoid. The dog-bone employs two separate sutures, tied directly over both the superior and inferior dog-bone devices.
- It is possible to create a continuous suture loop with the dog-bone device (Fig. 10(b)). From one end of the suture, loop the suture over a dog-bone device (intended to be the inferior device, beneath the coracoid). Then create another loop (meant to loop over the superior dog-bone device) and hold the loop up with another free

suture. The suture then goes down to make the third loop over the inferior dog-bone device before going up. Thus, at the inferior end are two suture loops over the dog-bone device and at the superior end are two free suture limbs and a loose suture holding up the free loop, which will go over the superior dog-bone device.

(e) **Reducing the dislocation, tying the sutures**

- As the two free suture limbs and the separate suture holding the free loop are shuttled up from the coracoid to exit above the clavicle, ensure the inferior dog-bone fits snugly to the under-surface of the coracoid (Fig. 10(c)).
- The ACJ dislocation/subluxation is reduced by pressing down at the lateral edge of the clavicle, while at the same time, lifting the ipsilateral arm and girdle upwards (Fig. 11(a)). The ACJ must be palpated to ensure it is flat and well reduced.
- The loose suture loop is then placed over the superior dog-bone device. Ensure it sits snugly over the clavicle, then tie the two free suture limbs over the dog-bone device (Fig. 11(b)).
- A repeat Image Intensifier may be done to ensure the reduction is adequate (Fig. 12).

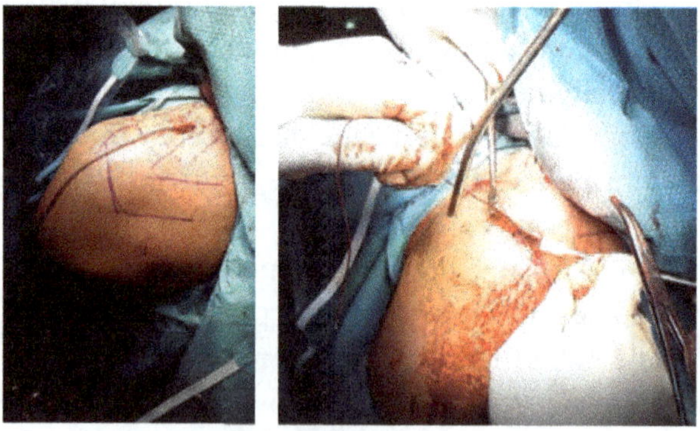

(a) (b)

Fig. 11: Tying the clavicle end. (a) shows sutures emerging from the clavicle and incision. A dog-bone plate is affixed to the sutures above the clavicle. The ACJ subluxation is then reduced and sutures tied over the dog-bone plate over the dog-bone plate, as shown in (b).

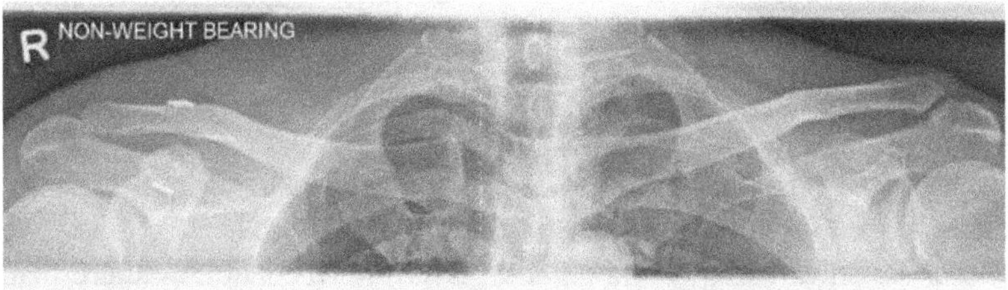

Fig. 12: Post-op X-rays. The non-weight bearing X-ray performed after the surgery, shows the ACJ reduced to its anatomical position, similar to the contralateral side.

5. Post-operative Management and Rehabilitation

The operated shoulder is immobilised for 3 weeks. Pendulum exercises should be started in the immediate post-operative period and gradually progressed to achieve passive and passive-assisted abduction and flexion up to the horizontal plane. Loading and full active range of motion should only be allowed after 6 weeks. Heavy lifting or any other activity that would cause significant downward displacement of the upper extremity should be avoided for 3–4 months post-operatively. The rehabilitation protocol should ideally be conducted under supervision of a physiotherapist.

6. Outcomes of Arthroscopic ACJ Reconstruction Following Acute Injuries

In a study of patients operated on by the senior author of this chapter [9], short-term outcomes were found to be good. In 17 patients who underwent arthroscopic TightRope® fixation, the mean flexion and abduction at 6 months were 78 ± 36° and 74 ± 35°, respectively. This improved to 132 ± 15° and 140 ± 22°, respectively, at 1 year following surgery. Other functional scores such as the Constant Score, University of California at Los Angeles (UCLA) Shoulder Score and the Oxford Shoulder Score also improved significantly up to 1 year post-operatively. The mean coracoclavicular distance improved from 29.3 ± 11.1 mm pre-operatively to 11.4 ± 1.6 mm at 6 months and 11.8 ± 1.7 mm at 1-year following surgery.

References

1. Oussedik S. Injuries to the clavicle and acromioclavicular joint. *Br J Hosp Med* 2007;68:M68–M70.
2. Willimon S, Gaskill T, Millett P. Acromioclavicular joint injuries: anatomy, diagnosis, and treatment. *Phys Sport* 2011;39:116–122.
3. Rieser G, Edwards K, Gould G, *et al.* Distal-third clavicle fracture fixation: a biomechanical evaluation of fixation. *J Shoulder Elbow Surg* 2013;22:848–855.
4. Greenspan A. *Orthopaedic Imaging*, 4th edn. Lippincott Williams and Wilkins, Philadelphia, 2004.
5. Johansen JA, Grutter PW, McFarland EG, Petersen SA. Acromioclavicular joint injuries: indications for treatment and treatment options. *J Shoulder Elbow Surg* 2011;20:S70–S82.
6. Rockwood C, Williams G, Young D. *Fractures in Adults*, vol. I, 4th edn. Lippincott-Raven, Philadelphia, 1996.
7. Philips A, Smart C, Groom A. Acromioclavicular dislocation: conservative or surgical therapy. *Clin Orthop Relat Res* 1998;353:10–17.
8. Spencer EJ. Treatment of grade III acromioclavicular joint injuries: a systematic review. *Clin Orthop Relat Res* 2007;455:38–44.
9. Bin Abd Razak HR, Yeo EN, Yeo W, Lie TD. Short-term outcomes of arthroscopic TightRope® fixation are better than hook plate fixation in acute unstable acromioclavicular joint dislocations. *Eur J Orthop Surg Traumatol* 2018;28:869–875.

https://doi.org/10.1142/9789811249846_0019

Chapter 19

Arthroscopic Bursoscopy and Debridement of the Scapula

Denny T.T. Lie and Gerald Zeng

Summary of Chapter

1. Introduction and epidemiology of scapula bursitis
2. Clinical presentation and examination
3. Pathophysiology of the problem
4. Diagnosis and imaging
5. Surgical technique of Arthroscopic Scapula Bursoscopy and Debridement
6. Open Debridement and Partial Scapulectomy (Muscle Tuck technique)
7. Rehabilitation
8. Clinical outcomes

1. Epidemiology of Scapula Bursitis

Few epidemiologic and clinical studies have been performed to evaluate the prevalence and aetiology of scapulothoracic bursitis and its available treatment options. While the true incidence of scapulothoracic bursitis is not well established, it is known to usually affect patients aged between 40 and 60 years old [1]. However, it is known that shoulder pain has an estimated annual incidence of 14.7 per 1,000 patients, and lifetime prevalence of up to 70% [2]. Out of these cases, 10% arise from abnormalities in periscapular soft tissue [3], of which about 40% are due to anatomic abnormalities such as a prominent tubercle of Luschka [4].

2. Clinical Presentation and Examination

Scapulothoracic bursitis is a significant clinical condition that can limit day-to-day function of patients. Symptoms of scapulothoracic bursitis typically include pain and difficulty with overhead activity, worse with repetitive motion. The pain patients experience is often described as deep and severe, often penetrating to the chest. In left scapula bursitis, it may be mistaken for cardiac pain. There is also an aching dull pain around the scapula which affects ADL. This is often associated with a clicking, crunching, grating, or snapping sensation. Patients may occasionally present with referred pain to the neck or radiculopathy precipitated by activity. Examination specific to the scapula includes palpation for periscapular tenderness, feeling for scapular crepitus as the shoulder is passively moved, winging of the scapula and the scapula retraction test (see Chapter 1).

3. Pathophysiology of the Problem

Various causes of scapulothoracic bursitis and crepitus have been proposed. A prominent superomedial border, known as the tubercle of Luschka [2], is often the cause of patients' symptoms. Other proposed mechanisms for bursitis include overuse, abnormal scapula morphology, glenohumeral dysfunction, post-surgical or post-traumatic changes (from malunion or surrounding callus formation due to fracture), osseous and soft tissue masses and scapular dyskinesis [2–4]. Early recognition is crucial to reduce unnecessary disability [5].

4. Diagnosis and Imaging

Scapular bursitis is ultimately a clinical diagnosis. A suspicion is raised during the history-taking, and often confirmed on examination. X-rays done are to exclude other causes of scapula pain and crepitus like fractures or obvious bony exostosis and protuberances like enlarged tubercle of Lushka. Magnetic resonance imaging (MRI) is deemed most useful amongst in detecting and characterising soft lesions and avoiding misdiagnoses [4]. MRI is useful for differentiating malignant soft tissue lesions from benign soft tissue, and also aiding preoperative planning, such as identification of fibrous bands (which would need to be sectioned or excised) and guiding the extent of resection for the superomedial border [6] (Figs. 1–3).

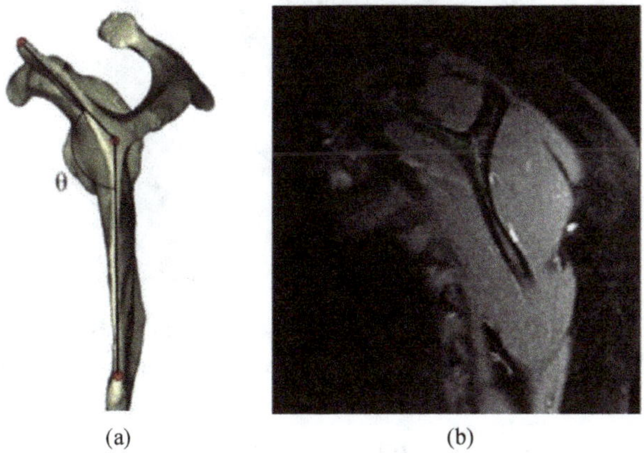

Fig. 1: The costomedial angle. (a) shows a schematic diagram of the costomedial angle, between the superior and inferior wings of the scapula. In the MRI example of (b), it measures about 130°.

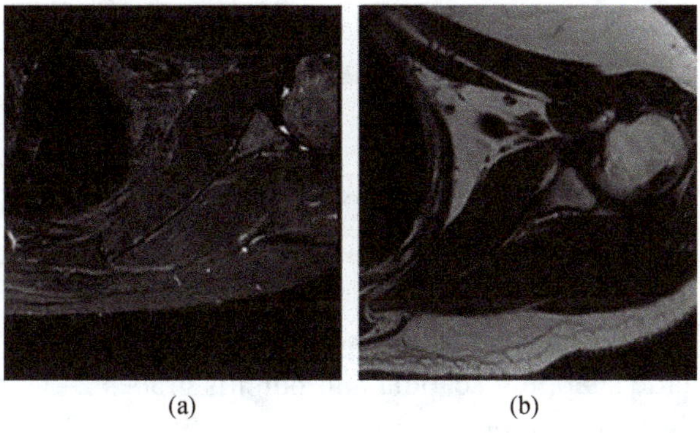

Fig. 2: Scapular morphology. Of the three types of scapula shapes (straight, concave, S-shaped), two are shown in the figure above. (a) Shows straight-shaped scapula, and (b) shows concave-shaped scapula.

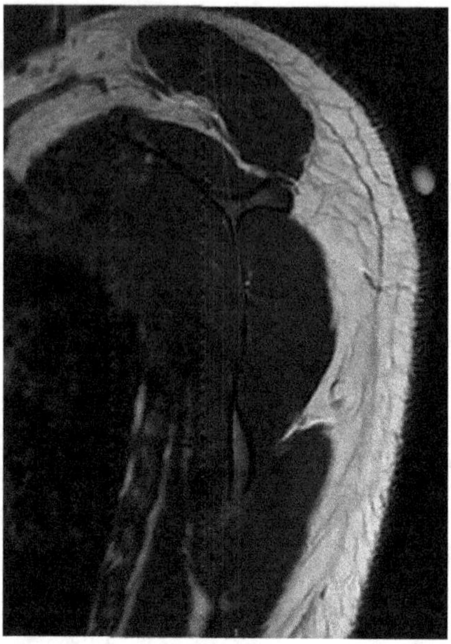

Fig. 3: Anterior offset. This is the horizontal distance from an estimated scapular body plane to the superomedial point of the scapula, drawing a value of 27.12 mm.

5. Treatment Approach

Non-operative treatment such as physiotherapy, which involves periscapular strengthening, combined with oral or intramuscular analgesia [4,7] is effective for symptoms due to scapular dyskinesias or benign, non-osseous lesions [8,9]. On the other hand, surgical management is considered if there are osseous lesions or if patients have failed a prolonged trial of conservative therapy [10]. Surgical management can be classified into arthroscopic or open surgery, with open surgery increasingly falling out of favour with improvement in arthroscopic techniques.

5.1 *Surgical Indication*

- Symptomatic snapping scapula and bursitis grades 2–3
- Scapula dyskinesia types 1 and 2 may benefit
- Failed physiotherapy and injections for at least 6 months
- Activities of daily living (ADL) and occupation affected

5.2 *Arthroscopic Bursoscopy and Debridement of the Scapula*

(a) **Positioning and Portals**

- The patient is placed in prone position, with both the ipsilateral arm and posterior thorax prepared and draped in a sterile fashion. The arm is secured with tape to ensure a stable position. The patient's arm is internally rotated in extension (the chicken wing position) as demonstrated in Fig. 4.
- This creates artificial winging of the scapula, thereby increasing the amount of space between the scapula and the thorax, to facilitate easier portal placement. Three arthroscopic portals are created, guided by skin demarcations as illustrated in Fig. 5.
- The **medial portal** is first created at the level of scapula spine, 3 cm medial to medial border of scapula (Fig. 5(a)). This is medial to the dorsal thoracic nerves and vessels which run just beside the edge of the scapula.

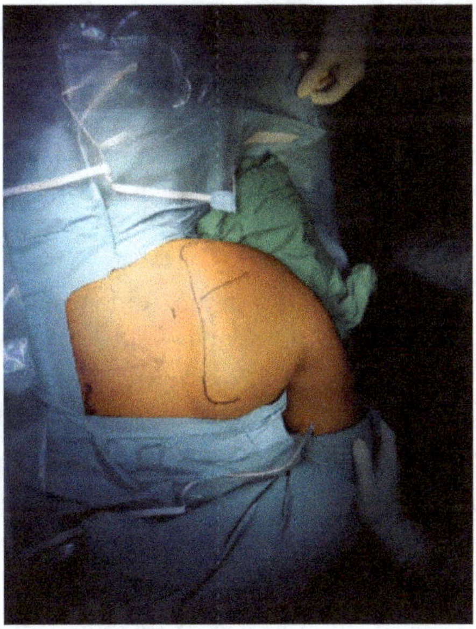

Fig. 4: The chicken-wing position. The arm is placed in internal rotation (chicken wing position) and draped as shown.

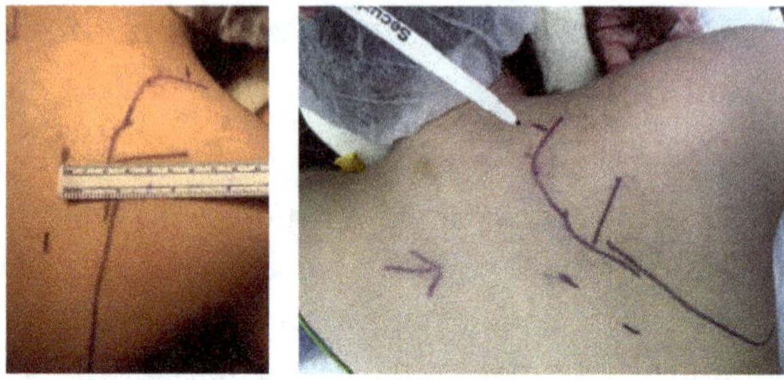

(a) (b)

Fig. 5: Surface markings of portals used. (a) is the medial portal at the level of scapula spine, 3 cm medial to medial border of scapula. (b) shows the superior portal which is at the junction of the medial and middle third of scapula, 1–2 cm superior to the scapula's superior border.

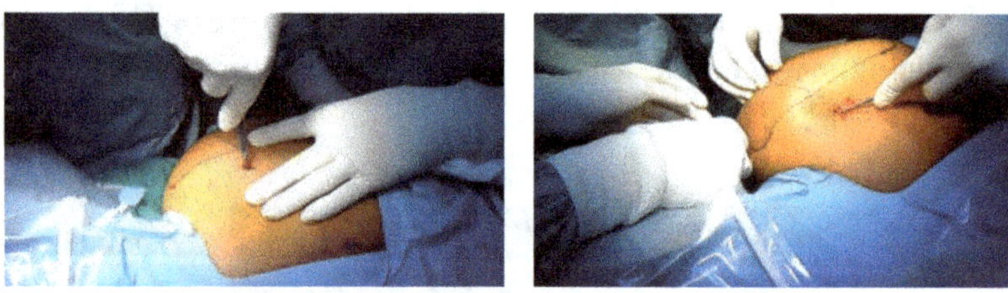

(a) (b)

Fig. 6: Portal preparation. After skin incision, the medial portal is widened bluntly with forceps, as shown in (a). A trocar is inserted to develop the scapulo-thoracic plane, shown in (b).

- The **superior portal (Bell's portal),** identified by the junction of the medial and middle third of scapula, 1–2 cm superior to the scapula's superior border (Fig. 5(b)). A 30° 3.5 mm diameter arthroscope is used.
- The last **inferior portal** is placed 4 cm inferior to the medial portal, and is optional.

(b) **Arthroscopic Bursoscopy and Debridement of the Scapula**

- After the creation of the portals (Figs. 6(a) and 6(b)), diagnostic bursoscopy is performed to assess the supero-medial border. The camera is inserted from the medial portal (Fig. 7(a)) and the bursal layer is identified. It is analogous to the subacromial space.

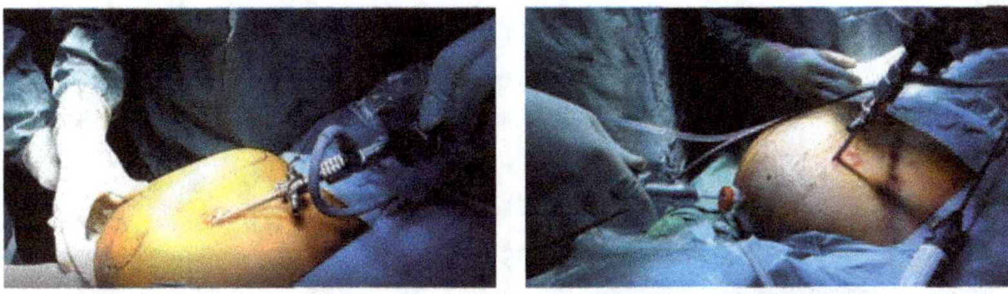

(a) (b)

Fig. 7: Scapula bursoscopy and debridement (a) shows the camera being inserted in the medial viewing portal. A shaver is used to debride the bursa and bony medial edge of the scapula, shown in (b).

The roof of the space is the scapula and the floor is occupied by the posterior intercostal muscles lining the posterior thoracic wall.

- In contrast to the subacromial space, there are no recognisable limits to the sub-scapular space, neither superior, inferior, lateral nor medial. *The greatest worry are the dorsal thoracic nerves which run just beside the medial border of the scapula. By entering the space medial to the vessels, they are kept above the instruments. Another precaution is not to debride or dig deep into the floor of the space, which are the posterior intercostal muscles.*

  Hence it is critical to have the viewing and working portals orthogonal to each other, to help visualisation of the working instruments.
- Debridement is performed using a 4.5-mm arthroscopic shaver blade, inserted from the superior portal, to clear the scapula borders and improve visualisation (Fig. 7(b)). A radiofrequency device is employed to ensure haemostasis and also to clear bony edges of the scapula (Fig. 8(b)).
- The prominent superior border of the scapula, the tubercle of Luschka is identified, burred, shaved and co-planed till flat (Fig. 8(a)).
- A switching stick may be employed to rotate the working and viewing portals, which can provide better visualisation for more optimal resection.

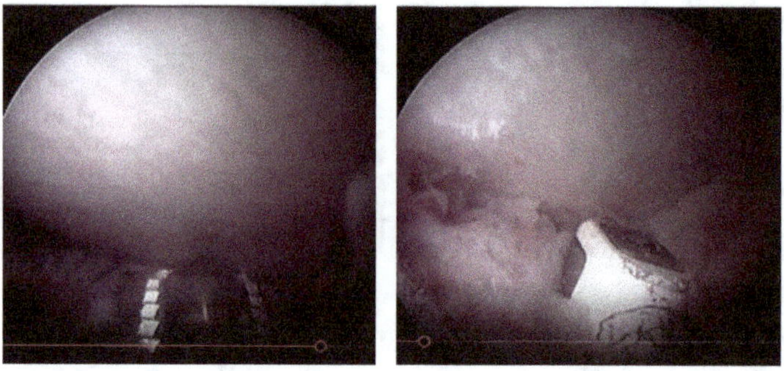

(a) (b)

Fig. 8: Intra-arthroscopic views of the supero-medial corner of the scapula. (a) Shows a shaver from the superior portal burring the tubercle flat. The RF clears the prominent tubercle of Lushka of the bursa, shown in (b).

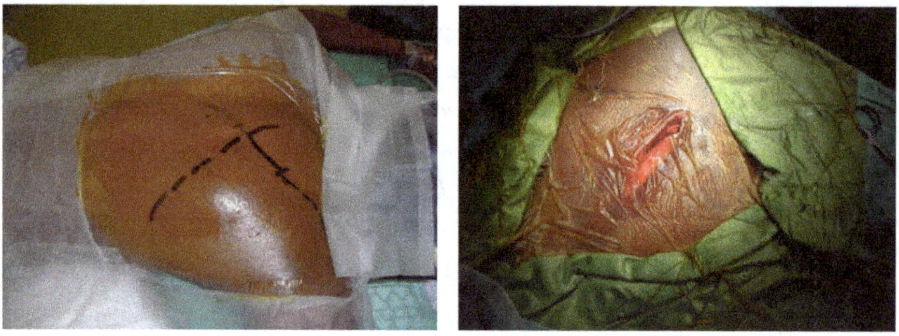

(a) (b)

Fig. 9: Skin markings and incision in open scapula debridement. (a) Shows the skin markings on medial border and spine of scapula. The skin incision is made and fascia developed, as shown in (b).

5.3 *Open Bursoscopy and Debridement of the Scapula, the 'muscle-tuck' Technique*

(a) **Incision**

- Make a paramedial incision about 4 cm long, along the upper part of the medial border of the scapula (Fig. 9(a)). This can be extended and curved superiorly along the supero-medial corner of the scapula.

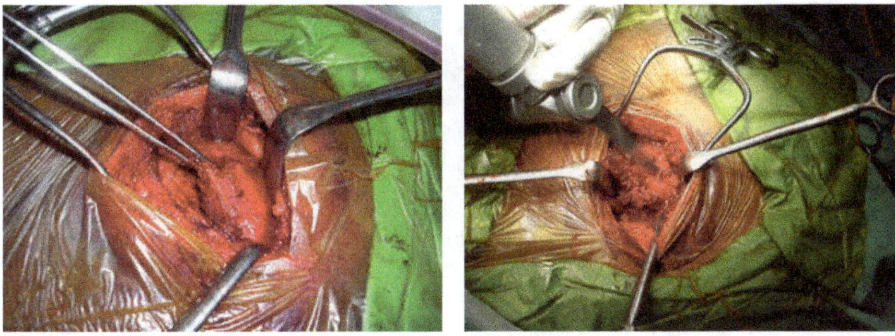

(a) (b)

Fig. 10: Open partial scapulectomy. (a) Shows the superomedial corner of the scapula stripped of its muscle attachments. Then an oscillating saw is used to remove superomedial corner of scapula, shown in (b).

- Deepen the incision and separate the fascia (Fig. 9(b)), developing the plane and separating the attachment of the rhomboids to the medial and superomedial corner of the scapula (Fig. 10(a)).
- Cauterise to stop the bleeding of the muscles.

(b) **Partial scapulectomy**

- Having isolated the upper medial border and supero-medial corner, perform a partial scapulectomy using a narrow osteotome or oscillating saw (Fig. 10(b)), and nibbler to remove the supero-medial corner and the prominent bulbous medial border. It is sufficient to remove a bone fragment about 3 cm long by about 2 cm.

(c) **Muscle re-attachment**

- Pass Ethibond sutures in a mattress fashion, to the detached rhomboids and parts of the lower trapezius, about 1 cm from the edge of the muscle. Place a mattress suture for every 2 cm of detached muscle, evenly spaced out (Fig. 11(a)).
- To the proposed site of re-attachment, make a small hole on the scapula edge. It is tougher than it looks and requires drilling with 1.6 mm drill bits (Fig. 11(b)).
- Pass one suture limb of the mattress suture through the hole on scapula from BELOW the scapula upwards. Then tie the sutures together. This brings the muscles to be re-attached below

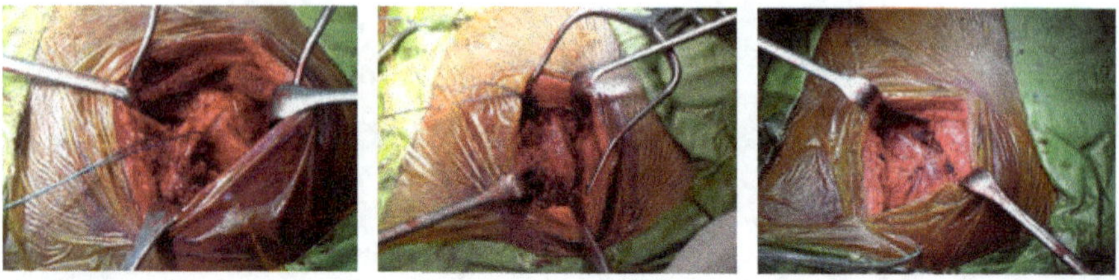

(a) (b) (c)

Fig. 11: Re-attachment of muscle by tucking in. (a) Shows sutures placed at the edge of the muscles. In Fig. 11(b) the scapula after the partial scapulectomy, holes are drilled for re-attachment of the muscles. The surrounding muscles are attached below the scapula, tucked beneath, as shown in (c).

the scapula, tucking the muscle beneath the scapula. This will prevent the scapula from grating on the posterior rib cage below (Fig. 11(c)).

- Repeat the mattress suturing and re-attaching below the edge of the scapula as necessary.
- Close the fascia and skin in layers.

6. Post-operative Management

Post-operatively, all patients were placed on an arm sling, and engaged in passive ROM exercises with senior physiotherapists prior to discharge. Passive exercises are then escalated to active range of motion exercises at around 1 week, followed by strengthening exercises by the end of the first month. Post-operative rehabilitation focuses on restoring scapular kinematics and strengthening relevant muscles such as the levator scapulae and rhomboids with the ultimate aim of allowing return to sports or overhead activity.

7. Outcomes

There are no validated outcome measures specifically targeting scapular disorders. Commonly utilised PROMs for shoulder surgery, which include Constant Shoulder Score (CSS), Oxford Shoulder Score (OXF), University of California at Los Angeles (UCLASS) Shoulder Rating Scale) and visual analog scale (VAS), can be used to gauge progress. In a case series by our institution involving eight patients, arthroscopic scapula debridement and resection provided satisfactory mid-term clinical outcomes post-operatively at 2 years. VAS scores decreased significantly from 8 (pre-op) to 1.3 (post-op). Statistically significant improvement was observed in all outcome measures. UCLA scores averaged 13.8 (pre-op) improved to 32.1 (post-op), as did Constant scores (from 50.2 pre-op to 91.4 post-op) [11].

References

1. Boneti C, Arentz C, Klimberg VS. Scapulothoracic bursitis as a significant cause of breast and chest wall pain: underrecognized and undertreated. *Ann Surg Oncol* 2010;17(S3):321–324. doi:10.1245/s10434-010-1232-8.
2. Cadogan A, Laslett M, Hing WA, McNair PJ, Coates MH. A prospective study of shoulder pain in primary care: prevalence of imaged pathology and response to guided diagnostic blocks. *BMC Musculoskelet Disord* 2011;12:119. doi:10.1186/1471-2474-12-119.
3. Vecchio P, Kavanagh R, Hazleman BL, King RH. Shoulder pain in a community-based rheumatology clinic. *Rheumatology* 1995;34(5):440–442. doi:10.1093/rheumatology/34.5.440.
4. Conduah AH, Baker CL, Baker CL. Clinical management of scapulothoracic bursitis and the snapping scapula. *Sports Health* 2010;2(2):147–155. doi: 10.1177/1941738109338359.
5. Parsons TA. The snapping scapula and subscapular exostoses. *J Bone Joint Surg Br* 1973;55(2):345–349.
6. Osias W, Matcuk GR, Skalski MR, *et al.* Scapulothoracic pathology: review of anatomy, pathophysiology, imaging findings, and an approach to management. *Skeletal Radiol* 2018;47(2):161–171. doi:10.1007/s00256-017-2791-6.
7. Warth RJ, Spiegl UJ, Millett PJ. Scapulothoracic bursitis and snapping scapula syndrome: a critical review of current evidence. *Am J Sports Med* 2015;43(1):236–245. doi:10.1177/0363546514526373.
8. Gaskill T, Millett PJ. Snapping scapula syndrome: diagnosis and management. *J Am Acad Orthop Surg* 2013;21(4):214–224. doi:10.5435/JAAOS-21-04-214.
9. Groh G, Simoni M, Allen T, Dwyer T, Heckman M, Rockwood C. Treatment of snapping scapula with a periscapular muscle strengthening program. *J Shoulder Elbow Surg* 1996;5(2):S6. doi:10.1016/S1058-2746(96)80089-9.

10. Chang WH, Kim YW, Choi S, Lee SC. Comparison of the therapeutic effects of intramuscular subscapularis and scapulothoracic bursa injections in patients with scapular pain: a randomized controlled trial. *Rheumatol Int* 2014;34(9):1203–1209. doi:10.1007/s00296-014-2966-6.
11. Gerald Joseph Zeng, Ken Lee Puah, Ying Hao, Denny Lie. Arthroscopic management of scapulothoracic bursitis: Clinical outcomes and assessment of novel bony parameters on magnetic resonance imaging. *Orthop J Sports Med* 2021;9(4). doi:10.1177/2325967121998273.

https://doi.org/10.1142/9789811249846_0020

Chapter 20

Proximal Humeral Head Fracture Fixation — The Fibula Graft Strut Technique

Denny T.T. Lie, Wong Merng Koon and Edwin Tan

Summary of Chapter

1. Epidemiology of proximal humeral fractures
2. Case example
3. Pathophysiology of problem
4. Diagnosis and imaging, algorithm
5. Surgical technique of fracture fixation with fibula strut graft
6. Post-op management and rehabilitation
7. Clinical outcomes

1. Epidemiology of Proximal Humeral Fractures

Proximal humeral fractures account for approximately 4–5% of all fractures [1]. They are the second most common upper-extremity fracture and the third most common non-vertebral fracture, in patients who are older than 65 years of age [2]. Women suffer this injury at twice the incidence of men [3] and it is postulated that these fractures are related to osteoporosis [4]. Although the overwhelming majority of proximal humeral fractures are either non-displaced or minimally displaced and can be treated with sling immobilisation and physical therapy, approximately 20% of displaced proximal humeral fractures will require operative treatment [5].

2. Case Example and Presentation

We present the sentinel case that changed our technique. She was a housewife, 62 years of age then, with no significant past history of note. She suffered a right proximal humeral fracture after a fall on 10th February 2009 (Fig. 1). An open reduction and internal fixation surgery (Fig. 2) was then performed on 11th February 2009 and she was discharged well on the third post-op day. The patient started physiotherapy 2 weeks after the surgery and she even started swimming 6 weeks post-surgery. However serial X-rays by her surgeon did not show evidence of bony union and this was confirmed on CT scan 11 months post-op, in January 2010. She was given a single dose of Aclasta then. Several months of physiotherapy and non-surgical treatment continued, including electromagnetic stimulation.

She was subsequently referred to us in September 2010, about 18 months after the initial surgery and presented with persistent pain that affected her daily life, loss of function and inability to swim, which made

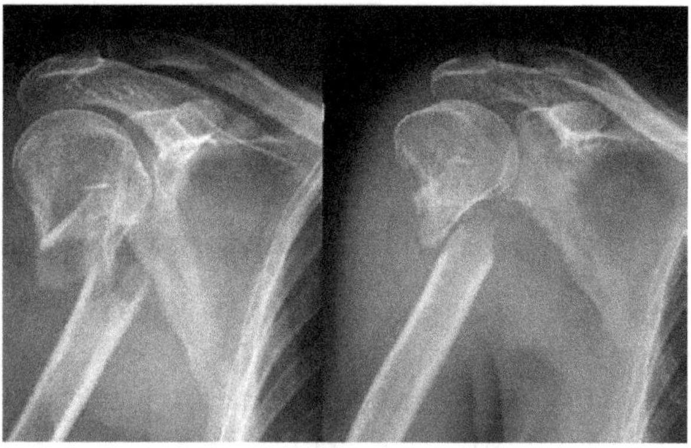

(a) (b)

Fig. 1: Pre-op X-rays of right shoulder. (a) and (b) show a displaced oblique fracture of the right proximal humerus.

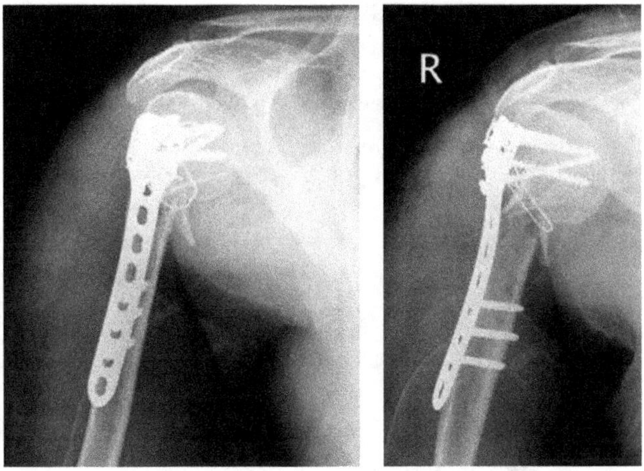

(a) (b)

Fig. 2: Post-op X-rays of right shoulder, soon after first surgery. (a) Oblique view and (b) AP view, show the initial fixation with locking plate and screws. There is insufficient bony support in the medial calcar. In fact, the loose fragment is held by the cerclage wire, which served to strangulate the blood supply to the humeral head.

her upset. CT scan done then reported absence of bony union. X-ray of her right shoulder (Fig. 3) showed non-union of the fracture with varus angulation, broken plate with a screw backing out. Our priorities then were to preserve as much as possible, the intact rotator cuff enveloping an otherwise intact glenohumeral joint, as the fracture was extra-articular. We recognised the high risk of avascular necrosis (AVN). Any intervention had to be strong and should enable the patient to resume her active lifestyle.

Our options then were:

(1) **Revision ORIF:** This preserves the joint but structurally, the humeral head is like an empty shell. A strong support is needed without compromising the blood supply. Thus, we chose the option of **revision ORIF with intramedullary strut graft**, which would preserve the joint and blood supply, yet provided a strong mechanical repair (Fig. 4).
(2) **Humeral hemiarthroplasty:** This would have been an option if the humeral head was fractured, dislocated, or showed signs of AVN or post-traumatic arthritis.

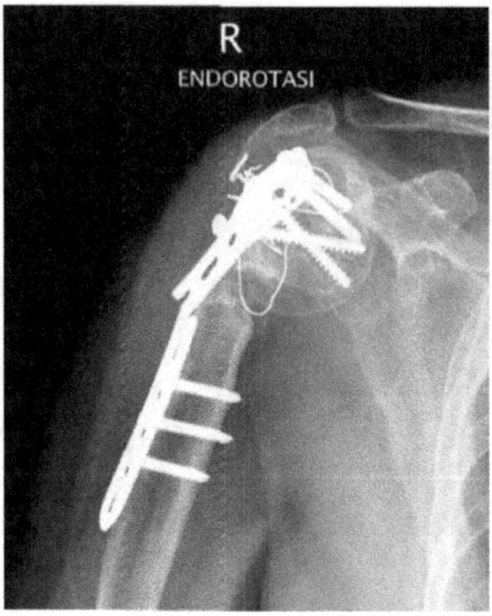

Fig. 3: X-rays of right shoulder, 18 months after first surgery. It shows the AP view X-ray of the right shoulder when she presented some 18 months after the initial surgery. The fracture had gone into avascular atrophic non-union, causing the proximal humerus to varus angulate. This exceeded the bending stress of the plate causing it to break. The patient was experiencing pain and limitation of motion.

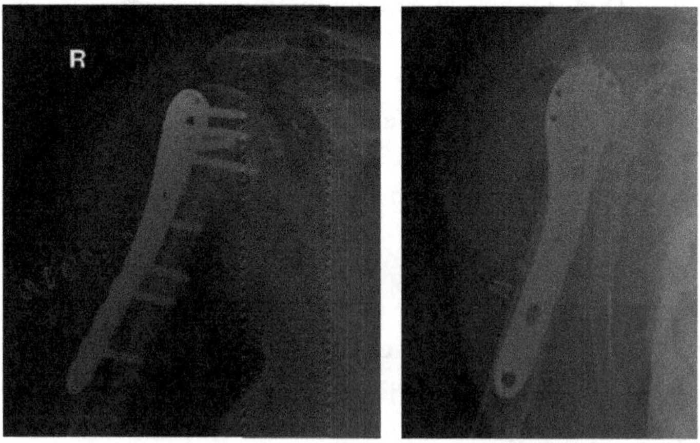

(a) (b)

Fig. 4: X-rays of right shoulder after revision surgery. (a) AP view and (b) lateral view, show the fibula strut graft in the intramedullary cavity of the right humeral head and shaft. The fracture was stable after revision fixation with locking plate and screws, and went on to heal.

(3) **Total shoulder arthroplasty or reverse shoulder arthroplasty:** These are viable options if AVN or post-traumatic arthritis was evident, but these were not options we entertained in this case.

3. Pathophysiology of Problem

The typical patient is an elderly lady presenting with shoulder pain and bruising after a relatively low-energy fall. In such demographic, the mechanism of injury is typically low energy, whereby the incident occurred at ground level. Younger individuals commonly present after a higher energy injury, and this can occur after a road traffic accident, fall from height or high impact sports. In such cases, it is essential to exclude concomitant soft tissue and neurovascular injuries, such as axillary nerve injury or more uncommonly, arterial injury.

HERTEL'S PREDICTORS OF ISCHAEMIA
<8 mm calcar length
Disrupted medial hinge
Comminuted fracture
>10 mm displacement
>45 deg angulation

The fracture may be observed across the surgical neck, anatomic neck, greater tuberosity, and lesser tuberosity. As such fractures can be complex, devascularisation of the fracture fragments may occur. The main arterial supply to the humeral head arises from the anterior and posterior humeral circumflex arteries, which form numerous anastomoses within the proximal humerus. Vessels from the rotator cuff contribute to the vascularity of the humeral head, and hence, complexity of the fracture pattern would determine risk of ischemia.

Hertel *et al.* [6] described several predictors of humeral head ischemia, namely, less than 8 mm of calcar length attached to the humeral head; disrupted medial hinge; increasing complexity of fracture configuration; displacement of more than 10 mm; and angulation of more than 45°. As such, it is essential to thoroughly evaluate the fracture configuration and complexity prior to determining the surgical technique to employ.

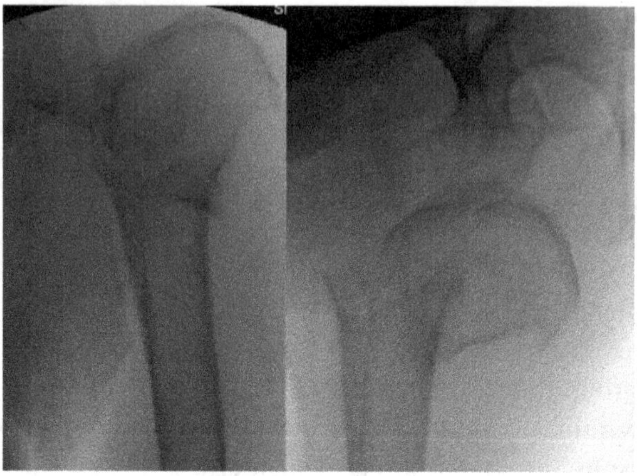

(a) (b)

Fig. 5: X-rays of Proximal Humeral fracture. (a) AP view and (b) axial view show a displaced proximal humeral fracture.

4. Diagnosis and Imaging, Algorithm

The patient may present with complaints of pain and swelling over the shoulder after an injury. The arm is commonly held close to the torso and movement aggravates the pain. Examination would reveal extensive ecchymosis of the chest and affected arm.

Imaging studies would aid in achieving a diagnosis as well as guide management. Initial studies should include radiographs of the affected shoulder. An anterior-posterior view of the shoulder (Fig. 5(a)) with scapular Y view would provide the surgeon with the necessary information. If possible, an axillary view (Fig. 5(b)) should be performed as it may be difficult to exclude a glenohumeral dislocation in certain situations. Additional views such as the apical oblique view, Velpeau views may be acquired if necessary. In preparation for surgical intervention, it is recommended that a CT scan be performed as it would allow for better visualisation of the fracture pattern and fragments, to aid in surgical planning (Fig. 6). Should the head fragment be involved, considerations can then be given to arthroplasty rather than fixation.

There are various classification systems employed and are constantly being refined. The Neer classification (Fig. 7) of proximal humerus fractures is most commonly used [7].

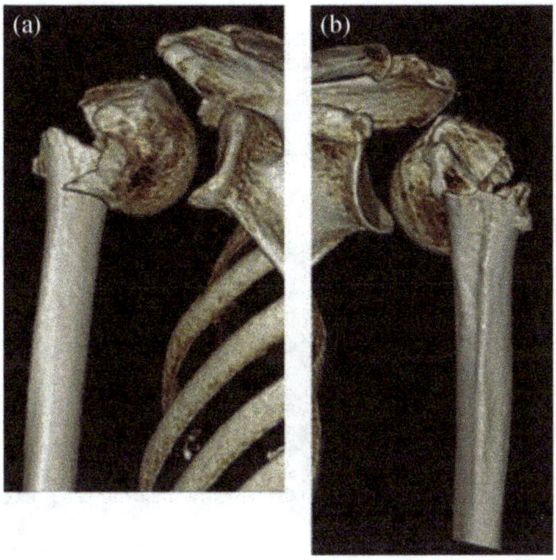

Fig. 6: 3D recon of Proximal Humeral fracture. (a) Anterior view and (b) posterior view of the displaced proximal humeral fracture.

5. Surgical Technique by Prof Wong MK

5.1 *Fracture Reduction*

- Surgery is performed with the patient in the beach-chair position on a radiolucent table. We prefer the delto-pectoral approach as this approach permits the extensile ability for extensive debridement, and reduction of the fracture.
- The fracture is reduced and provisionally stabilised with threaded Kirschner wires (Fig. 8(a)). This reduction is evaluated for adequacy with use of image intensification. *It is imperative to ensure the medial calcar has adequate bony contact and support, whilst maintaining the blood supply.*

5.2 *Preparation of the Strut Graft*

- A 10 cm fibula strut allograft was shaped to splint and span the fracture in the intramedullary site (Fig. 8(b)). This is pivotal to the success of the surgery as it provides several key benefits:
  - (i) Intramedullary reduction.
  - (ii) Prevention of humeral head varus.

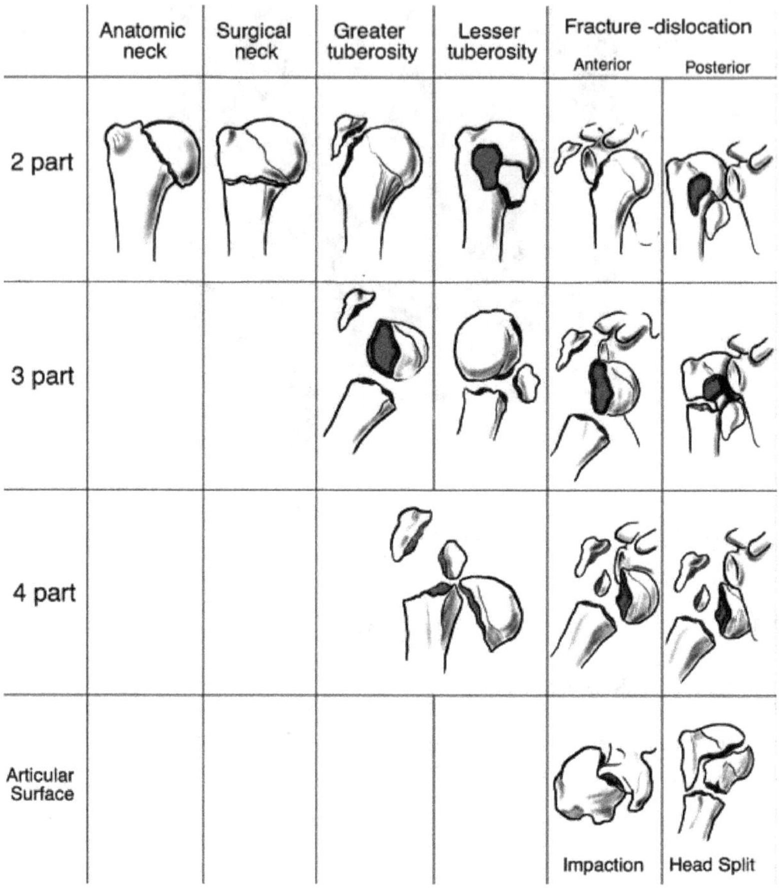

Fig. 7: Neer classification of Proximal Humeral fracture. Displaced 2-part, 3-part, 4-part and articular fractures are indications for surgery.

(iii) Purchase of proximal set of screws without need to gain screw tip purchase of subchondral humeral head bone. This reduces greatly the possibility of screw penetration if avascular necrosis occurs. This complication has a high likelihood due to the prolonged history of non-union.

(iv) Rotation stability of the reduction.

(v) Can provide a neocortex for the lateral wall of the neck of humerus.

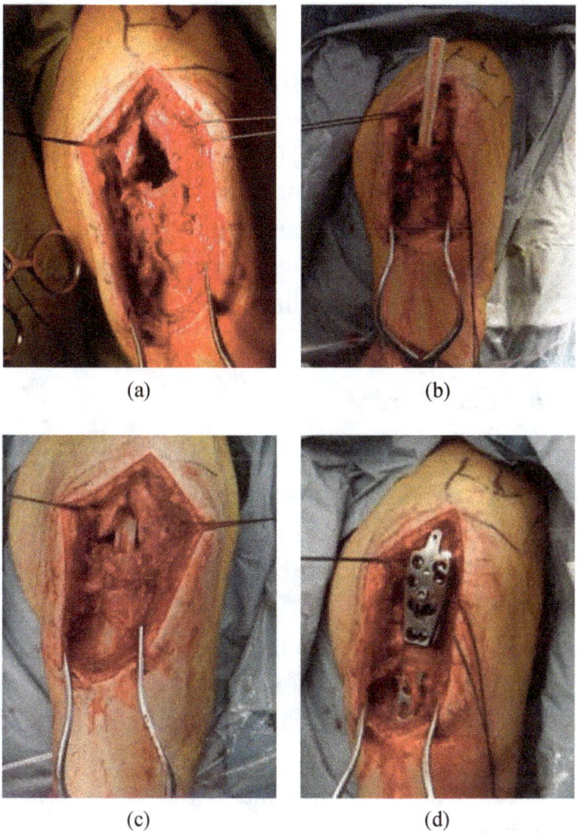

Fig. 8: Surgical fixation of proximal humeral fracture with strut graft and plate fixation. (a) Shows an extensile delto-pectoral approach with good exposure of the fracture, whose fragments are tagged. In (b), the strut graft has been inserted into the humeral shaft. The graft was then trimmed, and the humeral head skilfully manoeuvred over to cap the graft, as shown in (c). Temporary fixation is achieved by K-wires or sutures, before final fixation is done using a plate and screws, in (d).

- The strut graft preparation and burring needed great finesse as the medullary cavity is large proximally and narrows down the shaft. Further, the cavity is not a cylinder and neither is the fibular strut. There is a twist both in the fibular graft as well as the humeral intramedullary cavity. Hydrating the graft adequately is critical as otherwise cracks in unwanted directions can occur.

5.3 *Inserting the Strut Graft*

- The strut is introduced in the narrow distal humeral cavity. It is often necessary to distract the fracture site to enable the humeral head to cap over the strut graft (Fig. 8(c)).
- After successful introduction of the graft, bending and rotational stability at the fracture site is obvious. We further address the biological deficiency of the fracture healing with transplantation of cancellous bone grafts harvested from the iliac crest.

5.4 *Plating the Fracture*

- The plate is positioned, with the help of a mounted aiming device, at least 8 mm distal to the upper end of the greater tuberosity and 2 mm posterior to the bicipital groove, with care being taken to ensure that a sufficient gap was maintained between the plate and the tendon of the long head of the biceps.
- A Kirschner wire is inserted into the proximal guide hole of the insertion guide below the rotator cuff so that it aims at the proximal joint surface. Drill sleeves are inserted and Kirschner wires placed within (Fig. 8(d)).
- A position check with the image intensifier is performed, and screw length is determined (Fig. 9). The plate is fixed definitively with the insertion of angular stable screws into the humeral head.
- A final image intensifier check is performed to verify correct screw placement and length (Fig. 10).

6. Post-op Management and Rrehabilitation

Post-operatively, the arm was immobilised in an arm sling and passive range-of-motion exercises were started. Additionally, the patient may perform pendular exercises from post-op day 1. Controlled active mobilisation with abduction and flexion beyond 90° was started three weeks postoperatively, depending on the stability of the osteo-synthesis and the bone quality. In situations where the rotator cuff was repaired, rehabilitation may be tailored to the individual surgeon's preference and protocols.

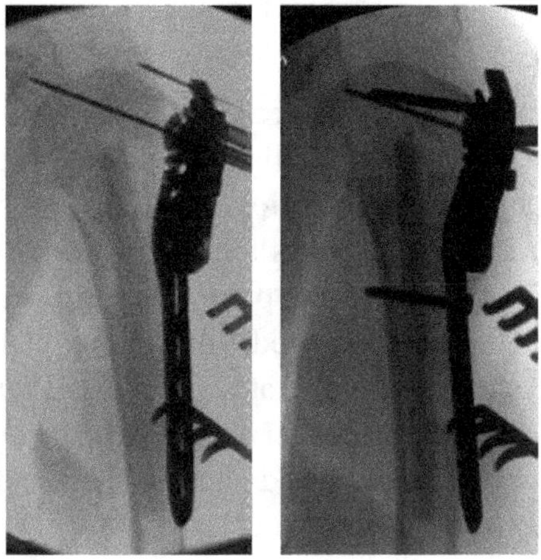

(a) (b)

Fig. 9: Intra-op X-rays. (a) Shows K-wires in the proximal humeral head, while (b) shows plate fixation in progress.

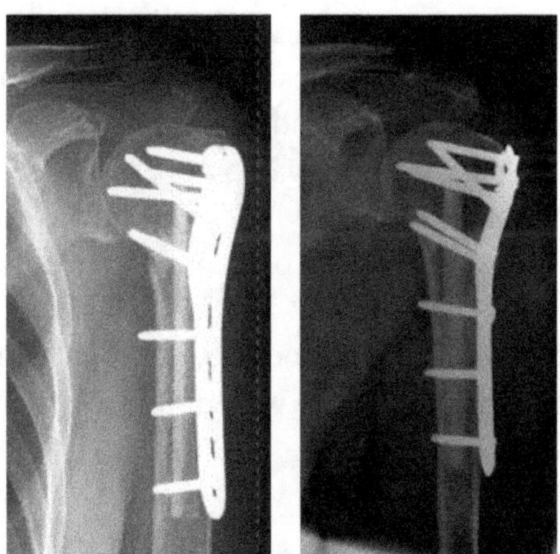

(a) (b)

Fig. 10: Post-op X-rays. (a) An oblique and (b) the AP view of the humerus after strut grafting and plate fixation.

7. Outcomes of Fixation of Proximal Humeral Fractures

For union in osteoporosis related fractures of the humerus, stable fixation is required. However, standard plating techniques have been associated with failure rates as high as 70% [8,9]. The addition of an autograft has been suggested to improve union.

In vivo studies with cadaveric specimens have concluded the improved strength of fixation with intramedullary strut graft augmentation. Craig Mathison *et al.* found that the addition of the graft increased the failure load of the constructs by 1.72 times and the initial stiffness of the construct 3.84 times. They studied six pairs of embalmed specimens, with each pair having one humerus repaired with locking plate fixation, and the other humerus repaired with plate fixation and intramedullary fibular allograft. The constructs were tested in bending to determine the relative movement between the humeral head and the shaft under bending loads, and the failure loads of both constructs [10].

Biomechanical testing has proven that the locking plate is superior in torsional rigidity and stiffness as compared with a blade plate for 2-part proximal humeral fractures. With the increased stiffness and reduced motion at the fracture site, an improved mechanical environment may enhance healing [11].

In our study of early outcomes after strut grafting and plating of proximal humeral fractures [12], head-shaft angles were maintained as the fractures went on to heal, with no varus collapse. The head-shaft angles were maintained between 130° and 145° with good restoration of ROM. By achieving a stiffer construct in osteoporotic bone, we postulate that fracture healing would be improved. The advantages of the allograft strut are that it provides added bone stock to improve fixation, and its use avoids the complications associated with donor site morbidity from autograft harvesting.

References

1. Helmy N, Hintermann B. New trends in the treatment of proximal humerus fractures. *Clin Orthop Relat Res* 2006;442:100–108.
2. Baron JA, Barrett JA, Karagas MR. The epidemiology of peripheral fractures. *Bone* 1996;18(3 suppl):209S–213S.
3. Kristiansen B, Barfod G, Bredesen J, *et al.* Epidemiology of proximal humeral fractures. *Acta Orthop Scand* 1987;58:75–77.

4. Jones G, Nguyen T, Sambrook P, Kelly PJ, Eisman JA. Progressive loss of bone in the femoral neck in elderly people: longitudinal findings from the Dubbo osteoporosis epidemiology study. *BMJ* 1994;309:691–695.
5. Nho SJ, Brophy RH, Barker JU, Cornell CN, MacGillivray JD. Management of proximal humeral fractures based on current literature. *J Bone Joint Surg Am* 2007;89(suppl 3):44–58.
6. Hertel R, Hempfing A, Stiehler M, Leunig M. Predictors of humeral head ischemia after intracapsular fracture of the proximal humerus. *J Shoulder Elbow Surg* 2004;13(4):427–433. doi: 10.1016/j.jse.2004.01.034.
7. Lasanianos N.G., Makridis K. Proximal Humeral Fractures. In: Lasanianos N., Kanakaris N., Giannoudis P. (eds) *Trauma and Orthopaedic Classifications*. Springer, London, 2015.
8. Walch G, Badet R, Nove-Josserand L, *et al*. Nonunions of the surgical neck of the humerus: surgical treatment with an intramedullary bone peg, internal fixation, and cancellous bone grafting. *J Shoulder Elbow Surg* 1996;5: 161–168.
9. Nayak NK, Schickendantz MS, Regan WD, *et al*. Operative treatment of nonunion of surgical neck fractures of the humerus. *Clin Orthop Relat Res* 1995;313:200–205.
10. Mathison C, Chaudhary R, Beaupre L, Reynolds M, Adeeb S, Bouliane M. Biomechanical analysis of proximal humeral fixation using locking plate fixation with an intramedullary fibular allograft. *Clin Biomech* 2010; 25:642–646.
11. Weinstein DM, Bratton DR, Ciccone WJ, *et al*. Locking plates improve torsional resistance in the stabilization of three-part proximal humeral fractures. *J Shoulder Elbow Surg* 2006;15:239–243.
12. Edwin Tan TS, Denny TT Lie, Wong MK. Early outcomes of proximal humerus fracture fixation with locking plate and intramedullary fibular strut graft. *Orthopedics* 2014;37(9):e822–e827.

https://doi.org/10.1142/9789811249846_0021

Chapter 21

Humeral Hemiarthroplasty for Humeral Head Fractures

Denny T.T. Lie and Puah Ken Lee

Summary of Chapter

1. Introduction
2. Case example
3. Diagnosis and imaging
4. Surgical technique of humeral hemiarthroplasty
5. Post-op management and rehabilitation
6. Clinical outcomes

1. Introduction

Proximal humerus fracture account for 6% of fractures and have a bimodal distribution between the young patient with high-energy trauma with good quality bone which is amenable to surgical fixation and the elderly patient with low energy trauma and osteoporotic bone whom apart from surgical fixation, may need to consider the use of arthroplasty [1].

Arthroplasty options for elderly patients with 3 or 4-part proximal humerus fractures include hemiarthroplasty and increasingly, reverse shoulder arthroplasty [2]. For arthroplasty in general, the loss of normal anatomical landmarks creates a challenge in implant positioning with regards to prosthesis height and retroversion. For proximal humerus hemiarthroplasty, there is a further challenge of rotator cuff tensioning and tuberosity healing.

2. Case Example and Presentation

The example presented is a 68-year-old lady with no significant co-morbidities, who had a fall during her holidays, sustaining a fracture of the right proximal humerus in May 2018 (Fig. 1(a)). She underwent open reduction and plate fixation in May 2018 (Fig. 1(b)). Post-op she underwent numerous sessions of physiotherapy but complained of gradually increasing right shoulder pain on active movement. This was associated with inability to actively flex and abduct. However, there was no rest pain and no numbness.

She presented with in our clinic with severe right shoulder pain about 1 year after the initial surgery. Examination showed active forward flexion 0°–80°, passive flexion 0°–120°; active abduction 0°–90°, passive abduction 0°–120°; intact rotator cuff power with no evidence of nerve injury. X-rays showed collapse of the right humeral head, either due to AVN or osteoporosis, with several screws having penetrated the head (Fig. 2). Ultrasound showed biceps tendinosis with no rotator cuff tear. The only reasonable option is **humeral hemiarthroplasty** while keeping the option of total shoulder arthroplasty in mind.

3. Diagnosis and Imaging

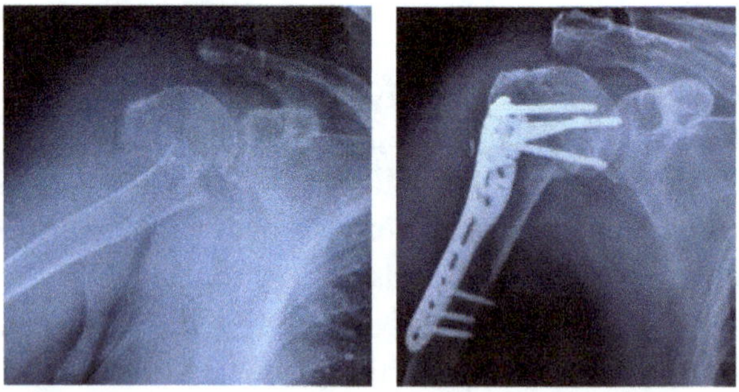

(a) (b)

Fig. 1: Initial X-rays. (a) Shows the initial X-ray of the displaced humeral head fracture after the fall. (b) Shows the initial post-op X-ray, the head was reduced and well fixed.

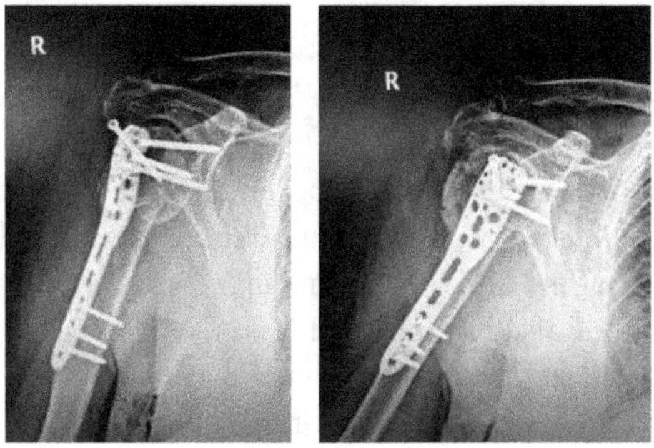

(a) (b)

Fig. 2: X-rays at time of presenting. (a) The AP X-ray of the right shoulder 1 year after fixation, the humeral head has undergone AVN and collapsed, and the screws have cut out. (b) The lateral view of the right shoulder.

4. Surgical Techniques

4.1 *Indications for Surgery*

- Comminuted fractures of the humeral head.
- Fracture-dislocation of the humeral head that carries a high risk of AVN.
- Failed ORIF of the humeral head with screws penetrating the head.
- AVN of the humeral head due to various causes.
- Arthritis of the head with no or minimal involvement of the glenoid.

4.2 *Special Instruments*

- Depuy Global Unite/Fx.

4.3 *Position*

- Easy beach-chair inclined at about 30°.

4.4 *Humeral Hemi-arthroplasty for Fractures*

A. The Delto-Pectoral approach including subscapularis take-down and biceps tenodecis

- The patient is positioned in a beach chair, inclined at about 30°. It is important that the affected humerus is allowed to hang vertically at the side of the table. The arm can be supported on a Mayo table or freely mobilised as the need arises.
- Surface marking is made, from the coracoid tip to the insertion of the deltoid, hence approximating the anterior contour of the deltoid.
- A skin incision is made along this marking; from the tip of the coracoid extend downwards for about 7–10 cm. The incision can be extended later. Deepen the incision into the fascia. Identify the cephalic vein.
- Develop the plane between the anterior deltoid and the pectoralis major, in which the cephalic vein sits. Mobilise the vein laterally with the deltoid, cauterising and tying the medial branches of the vein. Tip: a guide to this plane is that the vein is accompanied and surrounded by a fatty plane. Then lift the deltoid using a broad retractor.
- The upper third of the pectoralis insertion into the humeral shaft can be detached. This will help with manoeuvring during surgery.
- Identify the biceps tendon, if still present. Cut it as it emerges from the groove, and tag it with Ethibond 2/0 sutures.
- Medial to the biceps is the subscapularis tendon, detach it from the insertion at the lesser tuberosity, preserving as much tendon as possible. At the inferior border of the subscapularis are the circumflex humeral vessels, these can be cauterised and need not be preserved.
- Detach the capsule from the anterior to the inferior humeral head, detach completely using a diathermy probe. Tip: sometimes it is difficult to dislocate the humeral head, often it is due to adherent inferior capsule. Detaching this would free the head.
- The supraspinatus tendon, if still present, can be cut. Then dislocate the humeral head by bringing the arm to external rotation and levering the head out (Fig. 3).

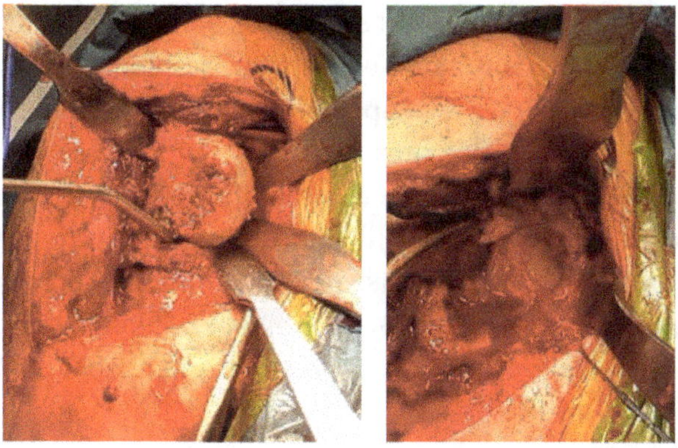

(a) (b)

Fig. 3: Intra-op findings of the case example. The humeral head is seen to have collapsed as shown in (a). The glenoid is relatively well preserved, as shown in (b), hence a hemiarthroplasty is correctly indicated in this example.

B. Stem and Proximal Body:

- Standard stem diameter ranges from 6 to 16 mm (most common is 10 mm).
- Proximal Body component ranges from 10 to 16 mm in height, with minor variations of –5, 0 or +5 mm in height. Most common is 10 (0) mm proximal body.

C. Head and Suture Collar:

- Humeral head diameter ranges from 40 to 56 mm, thickness of either 15, 18 or 21 mm. Both normal and eccentric heads are available. Most commonly used are the 44 and 48 mm diameter heads, 18 mm thick.
- Suture collar diameter mirrors size of the humeral head, ranging from 40 to 56 mm, most common are the 44 and 48 mm suture collars.

D. Concept of suture management

- The key to a successful hemi-arthroplasty is the position and integrity of the greater tuberosity, and hence the function of the rotator cuff tendons.
- There are many variations of suturing techniques described for securing the fragments of the tuberosities during a hemiarthroplasty.

- Conceptually **3 columns** of suture ties are planned: anterior to hold the lesser tuberosity and subscapularis, antero-lateral to hold the greater tuberosity and supraspinatus, and lateral to fasten the supraspinatus-infraspinatus tendons.
- Each column should fasten together the **shaft of the humerus, the humeral head implant and the tuberosity-tendon complex**.
- The construct thus consists of 3 columns of 3 suture bites, with 1 circumferential suture over the suture columns, to hold the fragments together. Hence this technique is often labelled the **"3/3/3+1 suture technique"**.

E. Surgical technique

- Drill **four of 2-mm diameter holes** into the upper part of the humeral shaft, about 3–5 cm below the fracture line (Fig. 4(a)). These holes should be equally spaced apart, 2 such holes anterior and another 2 holes in the lateral aspect of the shaft (labelled holes 1–4 from medial to lateral).
- Pass 3 Ethibond sutures from the outside in, in horizontal mattress fashion. Pass the first suture through holes 1 and 2 (Fig. 4(b)), then the second Ethibond through holes 2 and 3, and the third suture through holes 3 and 4 (Fig. 4(c)). These should be prepared before cementing and implantation.

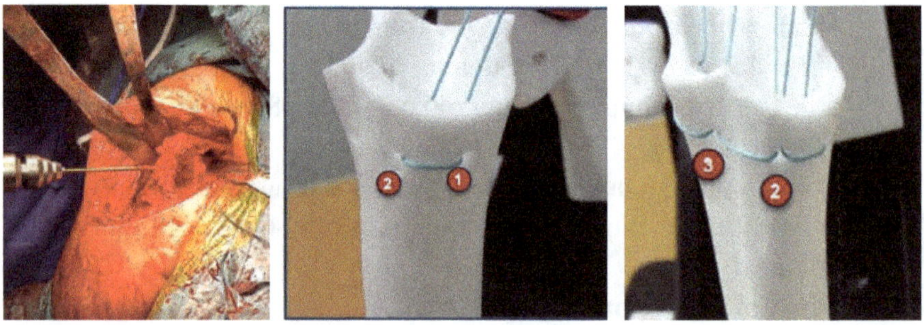

(a) (b) (c)

Fig. 4: Humeral shaft sutures, first layer of sutures. (a) Holes are drilled in the humeral shaft for the passage of sutures. (b) A mattress suture prepared in the sawbone model. Three such columns are prepared in the shaft, shown in (c).

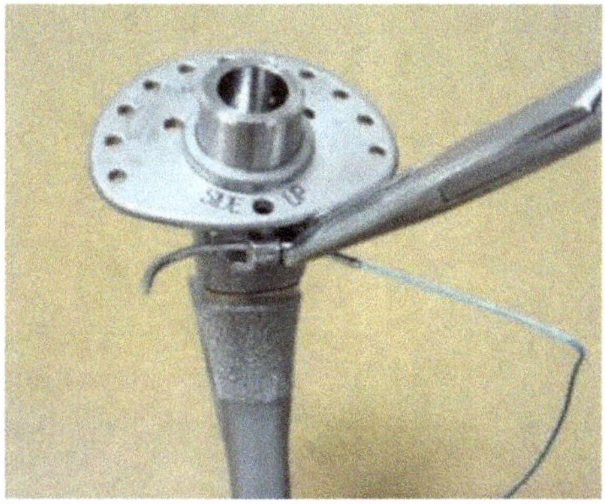

Fig. 5: The circumferential suture. Prior to insertion of the humeral stem, a suture is threaded through the stem, to be used as a circumferential suture tie.

- The bone cement, when doughy and ready, is hand packed into the humeral shaft. The implant is then slowly inserted in; it is important not to push in the implant too rapidly as it will cause the doughy cement to separate and thus interrupt the cement mantel.

  Pay attention to the **version** of the implant and orient the implant in the anatomical version if possible. Remember the planned **height** of the implant, it would be safer to leave it to leave the implant a little higher and proud. This will ensure the Deltoids are under tension and hence improve stability.
- Pass an Ethibond suture at the medial collar hole of the implant, this is the circumferential suture (Fig. 5).
- Pass the first pair of Ethibond sutures through two holes in the anterior part of the suture collar (Figs. 6(a) and 6(b)). Likewise, the second Ethibond suture through the two holes in the anterolateral part of the collar and finally the third suture through holes at the posterolateral part of the collar.
- The humeral head is then secured and locked in place by giving it a few gentle blows.
- **Lateral column:** Pass the third pair of sutures at the insertion of the infraspinatus to the greater tuberosity (Fig. 7(a)). Then reduce the greater tuberosity to its anatomical position below the suture

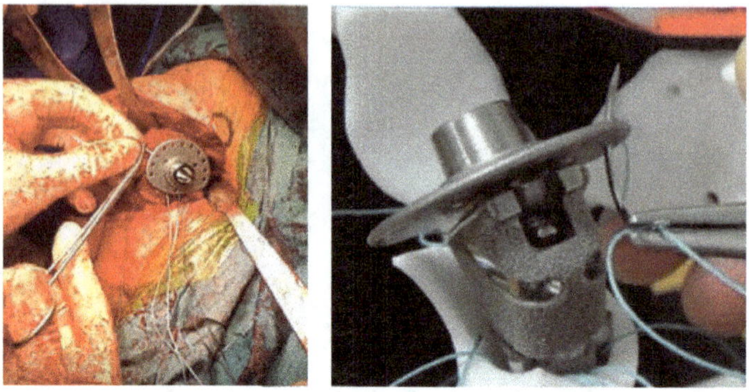

(a) (b)

Fig. 6: Implant sutures, second layer of sutures. After the humeral stem is inserted, sutures from the three columns of the sutures from the shaft are threaded through the suture collar as shown in (a) and in the model in (b).

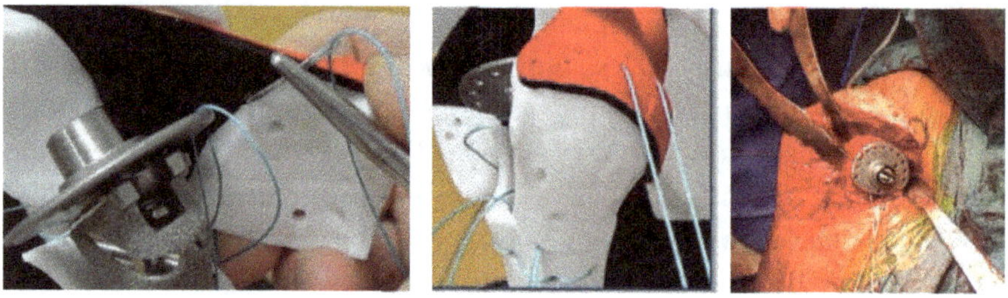

(a) (b) (c)

Fig. 7: Tendon-tuberosity sutures, third layer of sutures. (a) Shows sutures from the suture collar of the implant is passed through the tendon, which will reduce and hold the tuberosity down, as shown in (b). Reducing and fixing the tuberosity is shown in (c).

collar, bringing the entire rotator cuff tendons to cover the humeral head almost completely (Figs. 7(b) and 7(c)).

- Suture limb (A) of the third suture pair is passed under its own horizontal mattress suture from holes 3 and 4 (Fig. 8(a)). This creates the lateral column of suture bridge holding down the supraspinatus-infraspinatus and GT complex (Fig. 8(b)).
- **Antero-lateral column:** Pass the second pair of Ethibond sutures at the junction of the greater tuberosity and supraspinatus tendon, about 1 cm apart from each other (Fig. 9(a)).

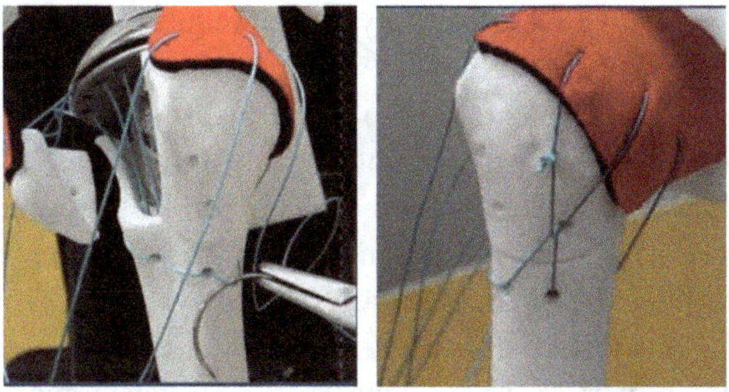

(a) (b)

Fig. 8: The suture-bridge column. One suture limb is then passed under the horizontal mattress suture, as shown in (a) and tied to the other limb, shown in (b). This creates a suture-bridge column. Three such suture columns are thus created to tie down the tuberosities.

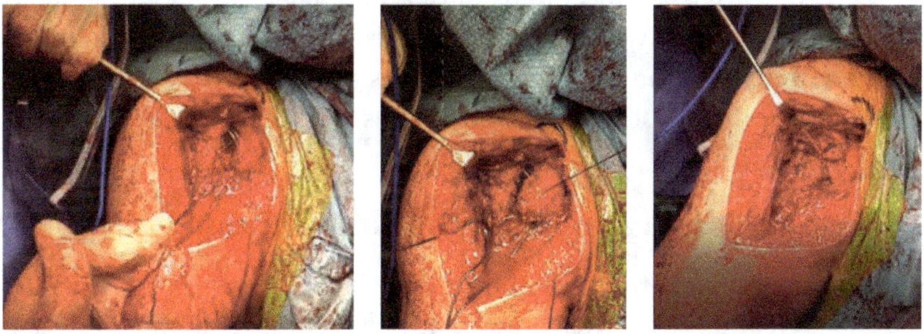

(a) (b) (c)

Fig. 9: Tying the tuberosities. The anterior column holds down the lesser tuberosity and subscapularis, while the lateral column holds down the greater tuberosity and supraspinatus. (a) The antero-lateral column, that will close the gap between the greater and lesser tuberosities. (b) The sutures of the antero-lateral column, which will tie the tuberosities together, as shown in (c).

- Pass suture limb (A) of the second suture under its own horizontal mattress base, threaded earlier through holes 2 and 3. Tying suture limbs (A) and (B) will secure the antero-lateral column of suture bridge holding down the supraspinatus and GT.
- **Anterior column:** Take large and deep bites, passing the first pair of sutures at the junction of the lesser tuberosity-subscapularis

insertion. The lesser tuberosity is then reduced anatomically, bringing it below the suture collar, and the subscapularis anterior to the humeral head implant. Then pass the suture limb (A), the one with the needle, below the horizontal mattress suture of its own suture, passed earlier through holes 1 and 2. Then tie suture limbs (A) and (B) together. This creates an anterior column of suture bridge, securing the lesser tuberosity and subscapularis (Figs. 9(b) and 9(c)).

- The **circumferential suture**, threaded earlier through the hole at the medial part of the implant, is then retrieved and tied over the suture columns, bringing the GT and LT fragments together.
- **In summary, the GT and LT fragments during a humeral hemiarthroplasty are secured by the 3 suture columns (anterior, antero-lateral and lateral), and the circumferential suture.**

F. **Closure**

- The deltoids and pectoralis muscles are tagged to close the interval, though a water tight closure is not critical. No drains are required as long as obvious bleeders are cauterised. The fascia is closed in layers and skin with sutures of choice.

5. Post-op Management and Rehabilitation

Patients are kept overnight with the arm immobilised in an armsling (Fig. 10). Gentle passive ROM especially internal-external rotations and pendular exercises are encouraged as tolerated in the first 2 weeks. Passive

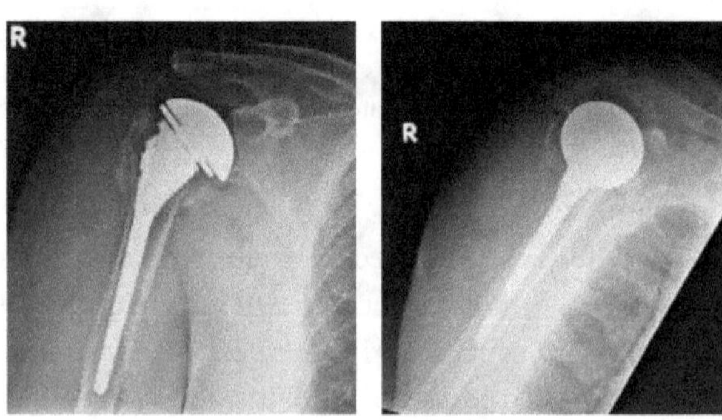

(a) (b)

Fig. 10: Post-op X-rays. (a) The AP view of the post-op X-ray after a hemiarthroplasty was performed. (b) The lateral view.

ROM is increased gradually from weeks 3 to 6. Active ROM and strengthening is started only after 6 weeks.

6. Outcomes

Hemiarthroplasty reduces pain compared to non-surgical management for proximal humerus fractures but does not improve range of motion or function as reported by Olerud *et al.* [3]. A systematic review by Kontakis *et al.* reported a similar finding of pain relief with marked or limited function at follow-up [4]. In our study of 30 patients [5], the mean age of our patients was 67.5 ± 12.6 years and they were followed up for 7.7 ± 4.6 years. At 2 years, the mean forward flexion was 93.7°. The mean UCLA score at 2 years was 24.8. Only 9 (31.3%) patients had a good or excellent UCLA score as defined by a score of more than 27. Twenty-four (82.7%) patients were satisfied with their surgery. We found that in our series of elderly patients with proximal humerus fractures, proximal humerus hemiarthroplasty provides overall good pain relief and satisfaction. This is consistent with existing literature on proximal humerus hemiarthroplasty for fractures which report good pain relief but uniformly poor range of motion and strength [3,6,7].

References

1. Bell J-E, Leung BC, Spratt KF, *et al.* Trends and variation in incidence, surgical treatment, and repeat surgery of proximal humeral fractures in the elderly. *J Bone Joint Surg Am* 2011;93:121–131. doi: 10.2106/JBJS.I.01505.
2. Bufquin T, Hersan A, Hubert L, Massin P. Reverse shoulder arthroplasty for the treatment of three- and four-part fractures of the proximal humerus in the elderly: a prospective review of 43 cases with a short-term follow-up. *J Bone Joint Surg Br* 2007;89:516–520. doi: 10.1302/0301-620X.89B4.18435.
3. Olerud P, Ahrengart L, Ponzer S, *et al.* Hemiarthroplasty versus nonoperative treatment of displaced 4-part proximal humeral fractures in elderly patients: a randomized controlled trial. *J Shoulder Elb Surg* 2011;20:1025–1033. doi: 10.1016/j.jse.2011.04.016.
4. Kontakis G, Koutras C, Tosounidis T, Giannoudis P. Early management of proximal humeral fractures with hemiarthroplasty: a systematic review. *J Bone Joint Surg Br* 2008;90:1407–1413. doi: 10.1302/0301-620X.90B11.21070.

5. Puah Ken Lee, Isaac Ng, Denny TT Lie. Radiographic parameters for proximal humerus hemiarthroplasty for fractures do not affect clinical outcome, submitted to Science Direct, 2020.
6. Simovitch R, Flurin PH, Wright T, *et al.* Quantifying success after total shoulder arthroplasty: the minimal clinically important difference. *J Shoulder Elb Surg* 2018;27:298–305. doi: 10.1016/j.jse.2017.09.013.
7. Andrés-Cano P, Galán A, Arenas J, *et al.* Results of uncemented hemiarthroplasty as primary treatment of severe proximal humerus fractures in the elderly. *Eur J Orthop Surg Traumatol* 2014;25:273–280. doi: 10.1007/s00590-014-1487-z.

https://doi.org/10.1142/9789811249846_0022

Chapter 22

Reverse Shoulder Arthroplasty: Tips and Pearls

Denny T.T. Lie, Mak Wai Keong and Ruben Manohara

Summary of Chapter

1. Introduction: How common is cuff arthropathy?
2. Pathophysiology of cuff arthropathy
3. Diagnosis and imaging, algorithm
4. Overview of biomechanics of RSA
5. Surgical technique of reverse shoulder arthroplasty
6. Post-op management and rehabilitation
7. Clinical outcomes

1. Introduction: How Common is Cuff Arthropathy?

Rotator cuff pathology places a growing burden on our aging society. It is estimated that cuff arthropathy affects about 2% of patients above 80 years of age [1]. Degeneration of the rotator cuff leads to arthropathy, first reported in the literature by Neer *et al.* in 1983 [2]. The authors described cuff tear arthropathy as a rare pathologic entity characterised by rotator cuff insufficiency, degenerative changes of the glenohumeral joint, a subcutaneous effusion, humeral head collapse, acetabularisation of the acromion, diminished acromiohumeral distance, and erosions of the skeletal architecture of the shoulder.

2. Pathophysiology of Cuff Arthropathy

The true etiology of rotator cuff tear arthropathy is unclear. In 1981, Halverson *et al.* proposed a crystal-mediated theory of rotator cuff tear arthropathy [3]. Deposition hydroxyapatite crystals induce phagocytic degeneration of the rotator cuff tendons and articular cartilage. The inflammatory process induced deposition of further crystals thereby propagating the cycle. This proposed mechanism implied that the rotator cuff underwent a physiologic process of severe degeneration due to a crystal-induced arthropathy.

Neer *et al.* hypothesised in 1983 [2] that a massive rotator cuff tear was the inciting event in the development of rotator cuff tear arthropathy, that both mechanical and nutritional factors contributed to the subsequent progression of the arthropathy. In the absence of a functioning rotator cuff, there is humeral head superior and anterior migration as a result of the unopposed contraction of the deltoid. The loss of joint stability and position is postulated to cause pseudoparalysis.

1. Additionally, leakage of synovial fluid into the surrounding soft tissue along with the decrease in the quality of the synovial fluid remaining within the compartment reduces nutrient delivery required for sustain healthy articular cartilage [4].
2. Decreased shoulder activity secondary to pain further reduces the delivery of synovial nutrients, hastening articular cartilage degeneration and disuse osteopenia
3. The progressive migration of humeral head and glenoid injury eventual results in femoralisation of the humeral head and acetabularisation of the acromion [5,6].
4. The Hamada classification of CTA depicts this process of progressive superior migration of the humeral head, beginning with a decrease in acromiohumeral distance (stage II), progressing to acetabularisation of the acromion (stage III), followed finally by glenohumeral arthritis (stages IV and V) (see Chapter 17).

3. Diagnosis and Imaging, Algorithm

Diagnosis of rotator cuff arthropathy can be done via clinical examination and standard radiographic views. Patients with rotator cuff tear arthropathy may present with anterosuperior escape of the humeral head from the glenoid and marked atrophy of the shoulder musculature. Some patients will demonstrate a tolerable range of active shoulder motion because of compensation by the deltoid muscle and a relatively stable fulcrum of motion, whereas others will present with pseudo-paralysis during attempted abduction and forward flexion [7].

Characteristic radiographic findings include femoralisation or erosion of the greater tuberosity, acetabulisation of the acromial arch and destruction of the superior glenoid (Fig. 1). Additionally, complications of arthropathy such as osteopenia of the humerus and glenoid, osteophyte formation and joint space narrowing may be observed [8,9].

Computed tomography (CT) of the glenohumeral joint can provide useful preoperative information regarding the glenoid bone stock and version. Magnetic resonance imaging (MRI) is useful for assessing the integrity of the rotator cuff (Fig. 2). An algorithm proposing a treatment approach to cuff arthropathy is shown in Fig. 3.

4. Overview of Biomechanics of RSA

The Reverse Shoulder Arthroplasty was designed as a solution to the shortcomings of the Neer total shoulder replacement. Initial designs had

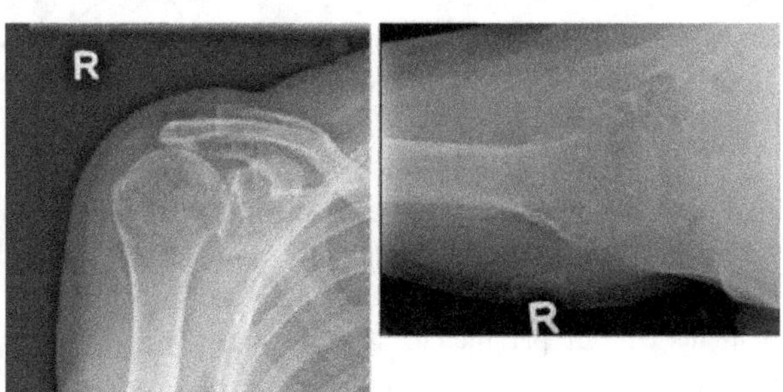

Fig. 1: X-rays of 70-year-old patient with cuff arthropathy. There is narrowing of the joint space, osteophytes, acetabularisation of the acromion and rounding of the humeral head (Hamada stage 4B).

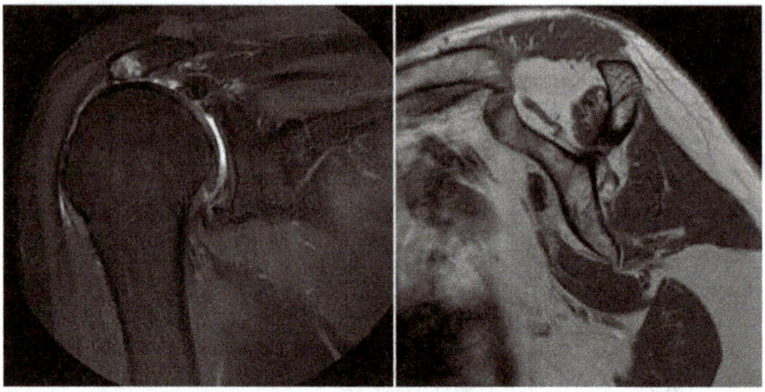

Fig. 2: MRI of patient with cuff arthropathy. There is massive tendon tear and retraction, and Goutallier stage 4 atrophy of the supraspinatus and infraspiantus muscles. This is irreparable cuff tear.

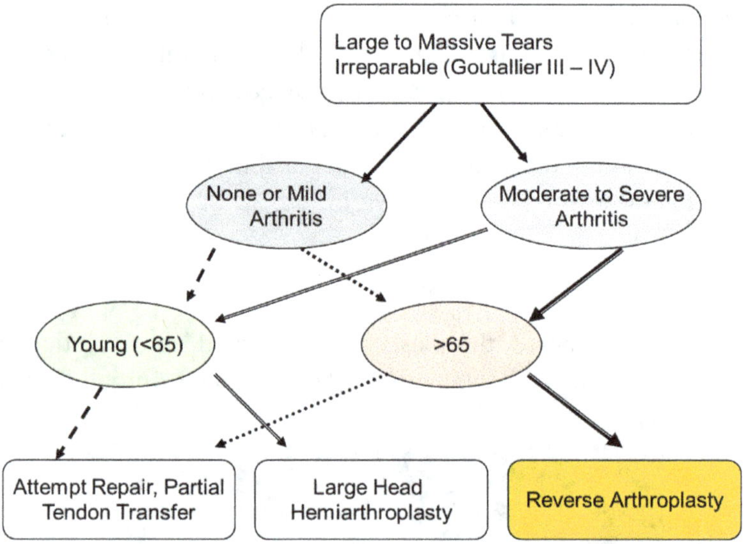

Fig. 3: Algorithm of treatment options in irreparable cuff tears. If there is mild arthritis, a partial repair or tendon transfer can be attempted. Younger patients with arthritis and massive cuff tears may benefit from large head hemiarthroplasty. RSA is typically indicated in elderly patients with irreparable cuff tears and arthritis.

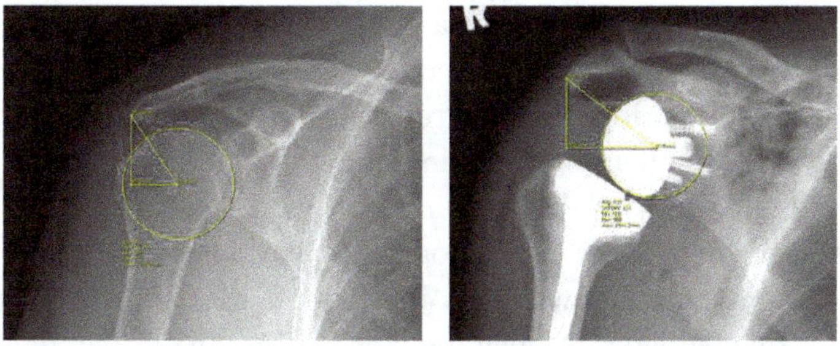

(a) (b)

Fig. 4: X-rays of RSA showing the Centre of Rotation (COR). The post-op COR (b) is medialised and distalised compared to the pre-op COR (a), giving the deltoid tension to make it an effective lever arm. This makes the RSA a stable prosthesis.

a high incidence of implant breakage and glenoid component loosening because of an underlying design flaw. Lateralisation of the shoulder's centre of rotation along with the highly constrained design of the prosthesis resulted in unacceptable forces at the bone-implant interface [10].

Paul Grammont's reverse prosthesis introduced in 1985 revolutionised shoulder arthroplasty with its novel design. This system utilised four key principles:

a. A fixed centre of rotation, distal and medial to the level of the glenoid surface (Fig. 4).
b. An inherently stable prosthesis.
c. Utilising effective lever arm of the deltoid from the start of movement.
d. A large glenosphere with small humeral cup to create a semi-constrained articulation.

5. Surgical Techniques

5.1 *Incision and Approach*

(a) **Delto-pectoral approach**

- The patient is positioned in a beach chair, inclined at about 30°. It is important that the affected humerus is allowed to hang vertically at the side of the table. The arm can be supported on a Mayo table or freely mobilised as the need arises.

- **Surface marking** is made, from the coracoid tip to the insertion of the deltoid, hence approximating the anterior contour of the deltoid.
- A **skin incision** is made along this marking; from the tip of the coracoid extend downwards for about 7–10 cm. The incision can be extended later. Deepen the incision into the fascia. Identify the cephalic vein (Fig. 5(a)).
- Develop the plane between the anterior deltoid and the pectoralis major, in which the cephalic vein sits. Mobilise the vein laterally with the deltoid, cauterising and tying the medial branches of the vein. **Tip: a guide to this plane is that the vein is accompanied and surrounded by a fatty plane.** Then lift the deltoid using a broad retractor.
- The upper third of the pectoralis insertion into the humeral shaft can be detached. This will help with manoeuvring during surgery.
- Identify the biceps tendon, if still present. Cut it as it emerges from the groove, and tag it with Ethibond 2/0 sutures.
- Medial to the biceps is the subscapularis tendon, detach it from the insertion at the lesser tuberosity, preserving as much tendon as

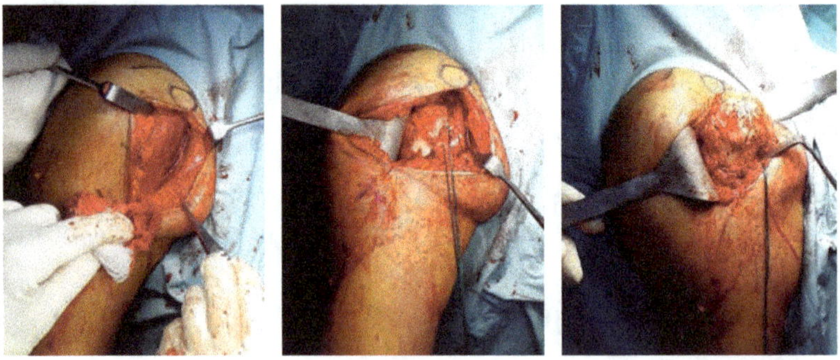

(a) (b) (c)

Fig. 5: Delto-pectoral approach. After the skin incision is made and fascia cleared, the delto-pectoral interval is identified and developed, as shown in (a). The subscapularis is identified, tagged and taken down, as shown in (b). The biceps tendon, if present, is tenodesed. The humeral head can then be subluxed superiorly, as shown in (c).

possible (Fig. 5(b)). At the inferior border of the subscapularis are the circumflex humeral vessels, these can be cauterised and need not be preserved.

- Detach the capsule from the anterior to the inferior humeral head, detach completely using a diathermy probe. **Tip: sometimes it is difficult to dislocate the humeral head, often it is due to adherent inferior capsule. Detaching this would free the head.**
- The supraspinatus tendon, if still present, can be cut. Then dislocate the humeral head by bringing the arm to external rotation and levering the head out (Fig. 5(c)).

(b) **Lateral approach**

- **Surface marking:** from the anterior clavicle, extend a line laterally along the deltoids, for a distance of about 10 cm (Fig. 6(a)).
- A **skin incision** is made along this line, the incision is deepened into the fascia. Develop the plane in the anterior deltoid raphe, seen by a fatty layer separating the muscle fibres. Separate the muscles by blunt dissection.
- Once the joint space is entered, clear the subacromial space of the bursa and any adhesions. Follow the capsule laterally and inferiorly to its infolding (Fig. 6(b)). **Tip: do not breach the infolding of the capsule lateral to the humerus, the axillary nerve runs**

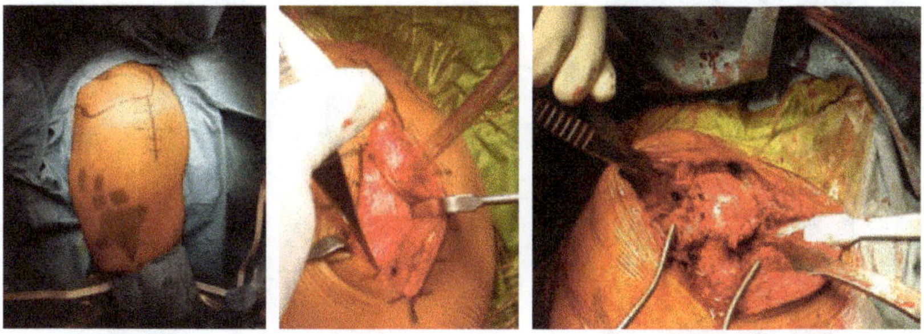

(a) (b) (c)

Fig. 6: Lateral approach. The skin markings of the approach are shown in (a). Incision is made along the anterior raphe of the deltoid muscle, this is along the extension of the anterior border of the acromion. The muscle layers are separated, taking care not to breach the capsule, shown in (b). If the supraspinatus tendon is already torn, then the humeral head can be subluxed easily, as shown in (c).

close to it. As long as the capsular fold is intact, the nerve remains safe.

- The supraspinatus, if still present, can be cut and removed.
- The biceps tendon is similarly tenodesed above the groove. It is difficult to properly access the subscapularis in this approach, and thus it is left alone.
- The humeral head can now be subluxed by pushing the arm from the elbow upwards, and levering the head out (Fig. 6(c)).

5.2 *Humeral Preparation*

- Mark a position at the confluence of the bicipital groove with the footprint of the supraspinatus, and perforate the humeral head with the awl (Fig. 7).
- Insert the intramedullary rod with the humeral head cutting guide. There is an anterior humeral head guide for the delto-pectoral approach and a lateral cutting guide for the lateral approach. The recommendation is to keep the guide in the "green" zone. However, in the smaller Asian humeral head, **the tip is to cut less of the humeral head, that is, leave the cutting guide slightly higher.** It is safer to cut less first

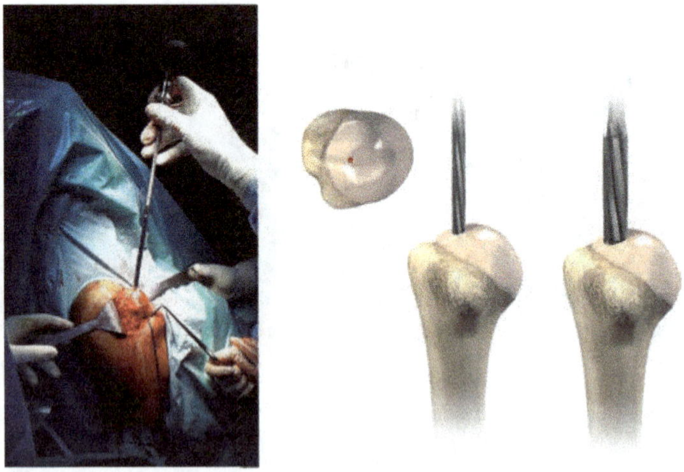

Fig. 7: Entry point of the humeral head. This point is at the intersection of the biceps tendon with the footprint. The humeral shaft is then reamed to size.

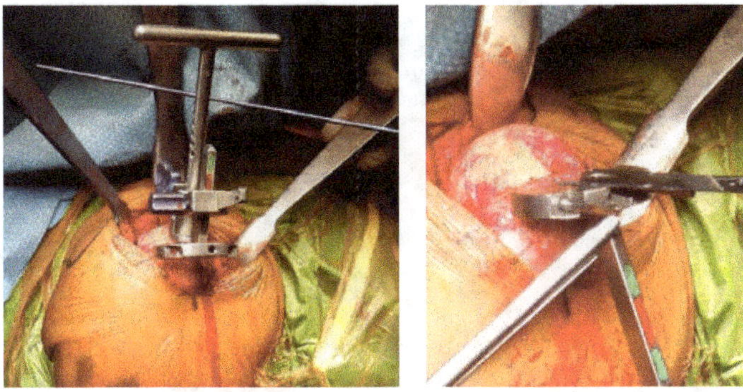

(a) (b)

Fig. 8: Cutting the humeral head. (a) The humeral cutting guide in position, it is best to follow the anatomical version. (b) The humeral head being cut at 155° inclination. It is best to cut less first.

and cut again later, rather than lose stability by cutting too much at this stage (Fig. 8(a)). Pin the cutting guide, which should be in the plane of the humeral neck. Then invert the cutting guide to enable sawing the humeral head off (Fig. 8(b)).

- It would be useful to review the anatomic variables in the humeral head cut:
  - **Neck-shaft angle:** This is unique to each system. In the Delta Extend system, this angle is 155°. (The Exachtech system uses a 135° cut).
  - **Version of the humeral head:** It is recommended to cut with a version of 0°–20° retroversion. In the author's experience, it is better to follow the natural anatomical version of the humeral head. Rather than imposing a fixed angle, study the morphology of the humeral head, then pin the cutting guide at the anterior face of the humeral head. Only then does one measure the version with reference to the direction of the arm. In our experience the version of the humeral head in the typical Asian is 20°–30° **retroversion**.
  - **Height of humeral head cut:** There have been reports of keeping the humeral head cut about 4 cm above the pectoralis major insertion but this in our opinion is NOT practical. An easier way is to assess the height of the greater tuberosity (GT) after cutting the

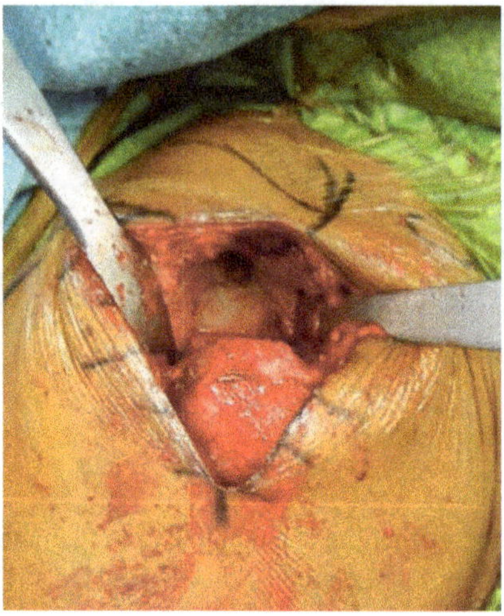

Fig. 9: Adequacy of the humeral head cut. With the muscles relaxed and exposed, the cut end of the humeral head should be at the level of the centre of the glenoid. If the glenoid is blocked, then more humeral head needs resection. If the whole glenoid is already seen easily, then too much of the humeral head has been resected.

head. With the arm relaxed by the side, the GT should be at the level of the centre of the glenoid (Fig. 9). Looking from the lateral view, the upper half of the glenoid should be visible, with the GT at the centre of the glenoid.

- Saw off the humeral head in its anatomical plane with the anatomical version, and assess adequacy of the cut. Re-do the cuts if needed.
- The cemented monobloc humeral implant shown in this technique has stem diameter ranging from 8 to 14 mm. The most common stem used is 10 mm in diameter.
- A trial stem is then inserted, over which the humeral cup reamer is used to create the cavity in the humeral head. Ensure the rim of the reamer sits at the bony rim of the humeral head. Failure to do this or inadequate reaming will result in the poor fitting of the humeral cup. Ream to Epiphysis size 1 or 2 (Fig. 10(a)). The assembled trial stem is then inserted (Fig. 10(b)).
- Then insert the humeral head cover (optional).

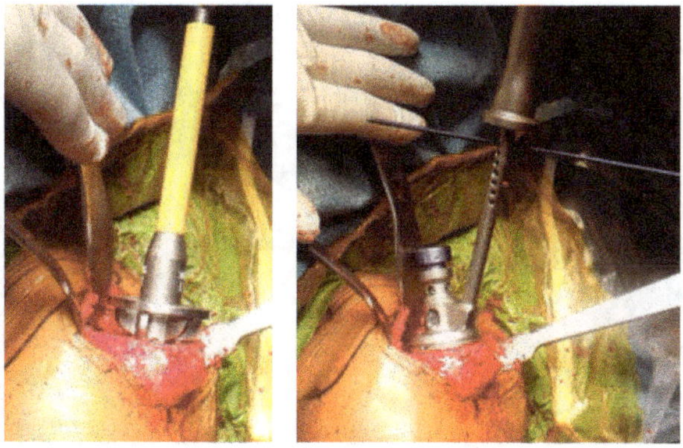

(a) (b)

Fig. 10: Humeral head preparation. (a) The humeral head being reamed, and a trial stem of size is fitted in, as shown in (b).

5.3 *Glenoid Preparation and Metaglene Fixation*

- The humerus is retracted postero-medially and kept out of the way using a two-pronged retractor. A sharp Hohmann retractor is positioned at the postero-superior corner of the glenoid to retract the bulk of the deltoid muscle, and another retractor placed anteriorly to keep subscapularis and pectoralis major out of the way. Thus a 3-point retraction is adequate to give a working view of the glenoid (Fig. 11(a)).
- Using a long diathermy probe, clear the labrum from the glenoid completely. Detach the labrum from the glenoid surface as well as the sides of the glenoid, peeling off the labrum and recessing it posteriorly, re-creating an ALPSA lesion.
- With the glenoid in full view, using the diathermy probe, mark the north-south vertical axis and perpendicular to it, the horizontal equator. Mark the centre of these lines to drill the central peg, it is not necessary to shift the intended position more inferior or posterior (Fig. 11(b)). **Tip: in the Asian glenoid, keeping the central wire in the geographic centre of the glenoid does not result in significant inferior glenoid notching.**

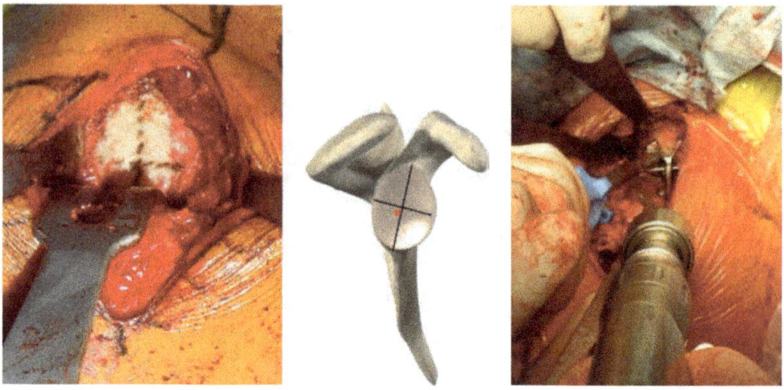

(a) (b) (c)

Fig. 11: Glenoid exposure and drilling. A dual prong and 2 Hohmann's retractors are used to expose the glenoid, shown in (a). (b) Shows the position to drill the wire at the red dot, just posterior and inferior to the anatomic centre of the glenoid. (c) Shows a guide to centre the drilling of the wire.

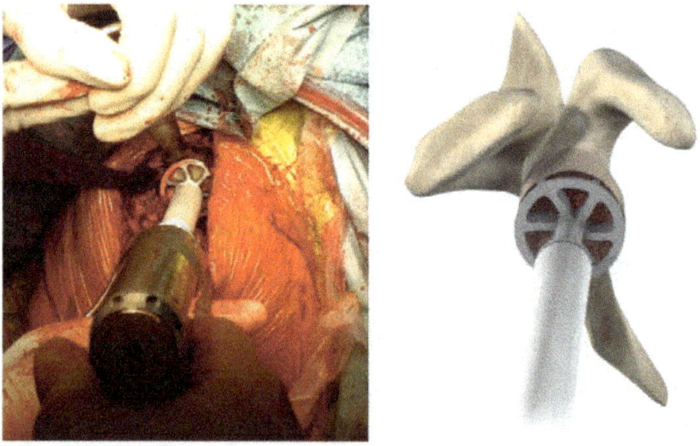

Fig. 12: Glenoid reaming. The glenoid cartilage is then reamed and the bone decorticated till cancellous bone is seen.

- Drill a wire to the central location; orientate the wire such that it is perpendicular to the surface of the glenoid in both the transverse and coronal planes (Fig. 11(c)).
- A cannulated reamer is inserted over the wire to clear the glenoid of cartilage and to decorticate it, leaving punctate bleeding when cancellous bone is revealed (Fig. 12). It is common that the inferior half of

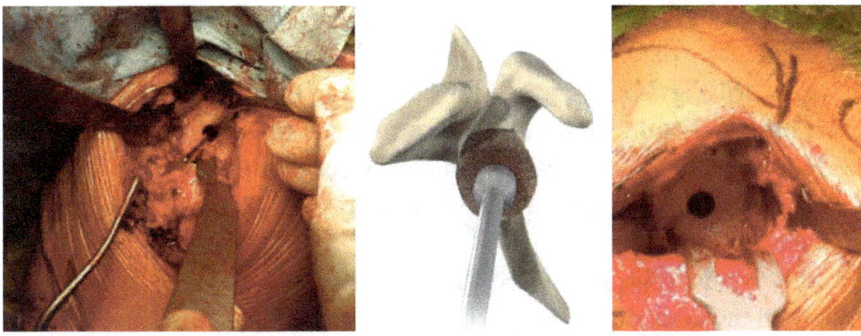

(a) (b) (c)

Fig. 13: Creating the central core. A large drill is used over the wire to create the central core, as shown in (a) and (b). The central core is shown in (c).

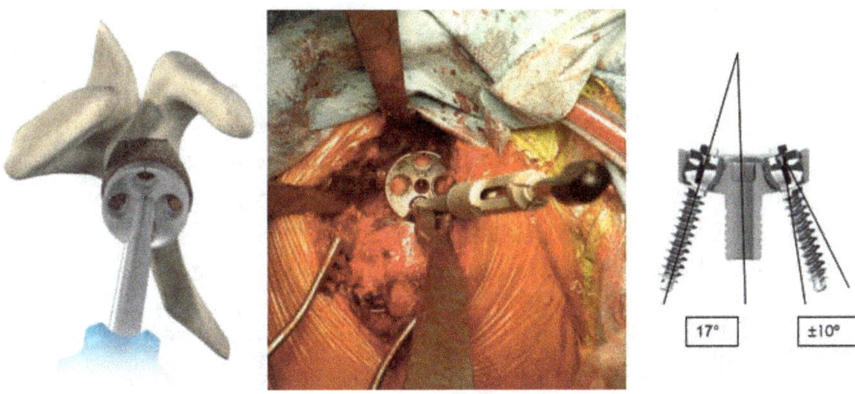

(a) (b) (c)

Fig. 14: Inserting and fixing the Metaglene. (a) shows the metaglene being inserted, the central peg being inserted into the core. The superior and inferior screws (b) are locked. The anterior and posterior screws diverge 17 deg from the peg, with 10° variation (c).

the glenoid is more decorticated, as the scapula is inclined slightly upwards laterally, leaving a smiley face on the glenoid. A (top-hat) reamer is often used to clear the superior part of the glenoid.

- Over-drill the wire with a peg reamer to create space for the central peg (Figs. 13(a), 13(b) and 13(c)).
- The metaglene is then inserted, keeping the same north-south orientation as that marked on the glenoid (Fig. 14(a)). Mallet the metaglene

slowly as the peg is slightly larger than the hole created. Ensure the metaglene is flat on the glenoid surface.

- Begin drilling the inferior screw hole (Fig. 14(b)). **Tip: tilt the drill bit inferiorly and slightly anterior, to catch the inferior vault of the glenoid where it merges with the scapula blade**. The locking screw required usually ranges about 35–42 mm long. Tighten the screw till finger tight.
- Similarly drill the superior drill hole tilting it superiorly to catch the base of the coracoid process. The superior locking screw usually measures 24–36 mm long.
- The anterior and posterior screws are non-locking and are less critical. Drill these holes directly or slightly convergent to catch more bone (Fig. 14(c)). Remember the base and vault of the glenoid narrows sharply, hence it is easy to miss bone if the screws are divergent. The non-locking screws required are usually 18–24 mm long. Tighten these screws definitively. **Tip: remember to keep the screws of differing lengths, if all screws are of about the same length, it creates a fault-line, a plane of potential fracture.** This is due to the higher elastic moduli of the screw-bone region, dropping sharply in the region of the cancellous bone without screws.
- Finally, tighten and lock the superior and inferior screws.

5.4 *Glenosphere: Smooth Entry*

- Before inserting the glenosphere (size is either 38 or 42 mm in diameter, the latter being more common), ensure the entire rim of the metaglene is free of any soft tissues. Also ensure the metaglene sits flat on the glenoid, without any lift-off or any osteophyte blocking the glenosphere (Fig. 15(a)).
- Adjust the retraction at this stage. The sharp Hohmann retractors should remain at the postero-superior and anterior aspect of the glenoid (Fig. 15(b)). The two-prong retractor is useful to keep the humeral head away but tends to block the passage of the glenosphere. In the author's experience it is better to use a bone hook or a Langenbach retractor to retract the humeral head away as the glenosphere is

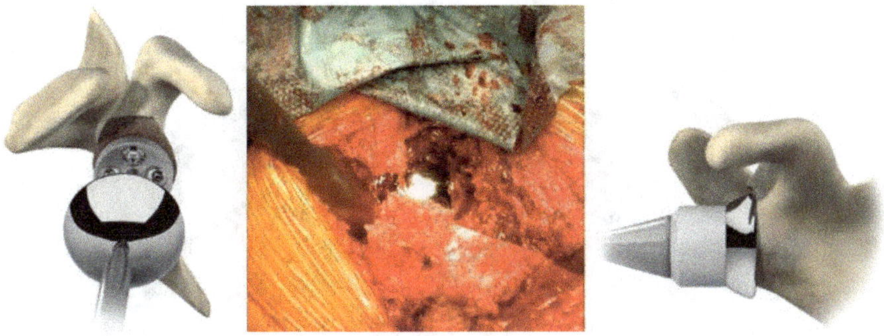

(a) (b) (c)

Fig. 15: Fitting the Glenosphere. The glenosphere is fitted using an inserter as shown in (a), with careful negotiation of the humeral head and retraction of the muscles, shown in (b). (c) is a schematic diagram showing the glenosphere in position.

inserted. Further, the cavity of the humeral head gives extra room for the glenosphere in a tight working space.

- A long wire is used to guide the glenosphere in its insertion. There is a snug feel as the glenoid sits on the metaglene. If it does not fit snugly, **a tip would be to look for the posterior bony rim of the humeral head/cup, which often gets trapped at the postero-inferior part of the glenosphere, not easily seen**. Retract the humeral head/cup away and toggle the glenosphere again to achieve the snug fit (Fig. 15(c)). Ensure no soft tissues are trapped between the glenosphere and metaglene before committing the screw (Fig. 16(a)).
- Reverse turn the screw in anti-clockwise direction first to ensure the glenoshere is well seated before turning it clock-wise. The threads are long, so it takes some time before the squeaks of the tightening screw are heard. If it happens early, the screw is cutting out of its threads. Stop immediately, re-adjust the glenosphere before resuming the screw fastening. Tighten the screw definitively (Fig. 16(b)).

5.5 *Humeral Cup: Size Matters*

- Dislocate the humeral head out, and insert a trial stem of appropriate size, maintaining the anatomical version established earlier. Then fit a

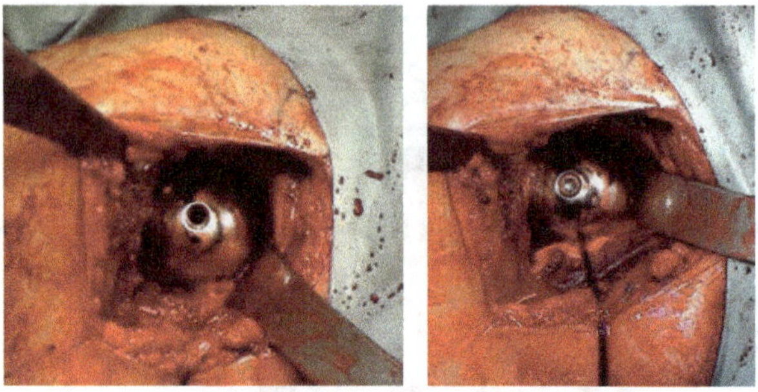

(a) (b)

Fig. 16: The Glenosphere. (a) Shows the glenosphere in position and (b) with the locking screw in place.

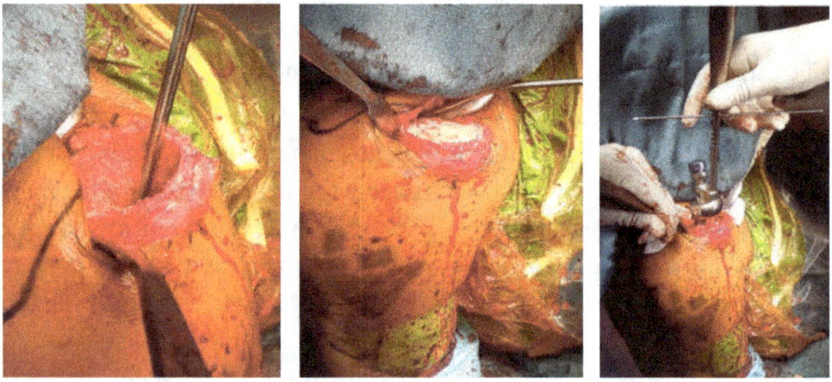

(a) (b) (c)

Fig. 17: Cementing and Inserting the Humeral Stem. Cementing the humeral stem is optional. (a) Shows the humerus prepared and (b) shows the cement ready. The Humeral stem is inserted, shown in (c).

humeral cup (size 38 or 42 mm diameter) and reduce the humeral head.

- Reduction of the humeral head is achieved by first applying a downward traction on the humerus at the elbow, then while maintaining an axial traction, bring the arm to abduction in the scapular plane (that is, about 45° mid-way between flexion and lateral abduction). Apply pressure on the humeral head as the arm is abducted, till the cup snaps into the glenoshere.

- Then assess for stability by these tests:
  (1) Passively bring the humerus to maximum flexion, abduction while internally and externally rotating the arm. The humeral cup must exhibit no or minimal lift-off as it is brought through its range of motion (Fig. 18(a)).
  (2) Apply an axial traction on the arm, the humeral cup must not be easily lifted off the articulation (Fig. 18(b)).

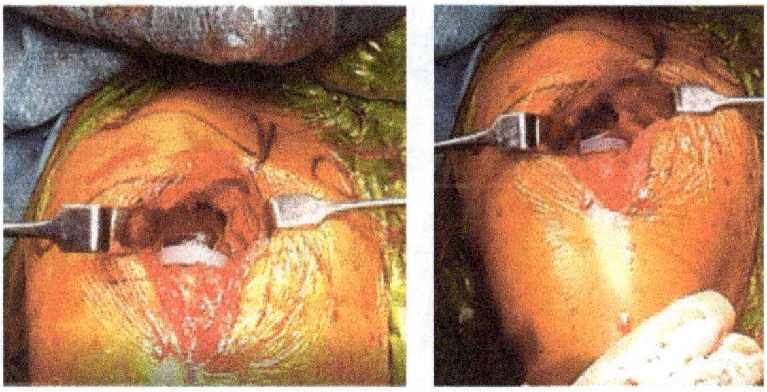

(a) (b)

Fig. 18: Testing the stability after reduction. The humeral cup is fixed and the humerus reduced. The shoulder is then brought to the range of motion in all directions. In particular, the arm is internally and externally rotated (a), to ensure there is no lift-off of the cup. As the arm is moved, anterior and posterior translation is tested, as shown in (b), to ensure there is no instability and the humeral cup remains enlocated.

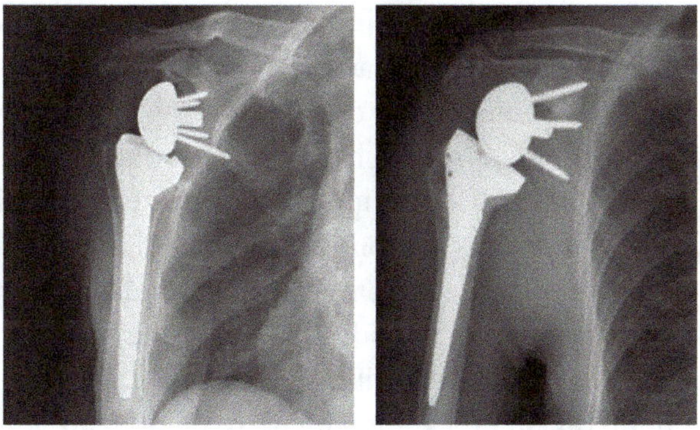

(a) (b)

Fig. 19: Post-op X-rays. (a) and (b) show X-rays after Depuy Delta Reverse Shoulder Arthroplasty have been performed.

(3) Finally, as the arm is internally and externally rotated, apply a translating force anteriorly and posteriorly on the humeral cup articulation. If it subluxes easily, it is not stable enough and a thicker humeral cup is required.

- <u>Dislocating the humeral cup: apply an axial traction force, bring the arm to abduction in the scapular plane, then insert a blunt retractor in the humeral cup/glenosphere articulation to lever the humeral cup out</u>. A considerable force may be required. If the humeral cup dislocates too easily, a thicker cup is required. If too much force is required, consider lowering the cut of the humeral cup, or sinking the humeral cup slightly deeper.
- Variables of the humeral cup:
  (1) **Size and Thickness:** Size is either 38 or 42 mm in diameter to correspond to the glenosphere. Thickness of the humeral cup spacer is +3, +6 and +9 mm.
  (2) **Eccentric dialling — not available in the Delta RSA**
  (3) **Deeper/more concave Retentive Cup (+6 mm) is available for improved stability**

5.6 *Humeral Stem Implantation*

- The humeral stem of appropriate length, size; humeral cup size and thickness is then selected.
- The option to cement exists in the current Delta Extend system (Fig. 17(a)). In general, for cuff arthropathy our practice is to leave the stem uncemented. Cementing is done only for post-fracture RSA. The cement is prepared and inserted, hand-packed (Fig. 17(b)). The stem is inserted slowly so as to maintain the cement mantle integrity (Fig. 17(c)). The version is anatomical and height as determined earlier for cuff arthropathy. In fracture cases, the humeral head version we use is 20° retroversion and the intended height of the humeral stem determined earlier, is maintained during cementing.
- Once the humeral stem is implanted, humeral cup locked in, the humerus is reduced and stability checked once again. The joint is then washed with diluted iodine, and closed in layers.

5.7 *Reverse Shoulder Arthroplasty in Trauma Cases*

Performing an RSA has been advocated in elderly, osteoporotic, displaced 3- and 4-part fractures of the proximal humerus. This would allow for earlier mobilisation, easier post-operative rehabilitation, and generally reliable outcomes which would not depend on tuberosity healing or rotator cuff status. Performed well, it would have a lower chance of requiring a revision than an internal fixation or hemiarthroplasty in this population [15].

The steps are generally the same, but the following points must be kept in mind:

- **Pre-op imaging:** A CT scan is necessary to assess the fracture configuration, and to assess the bone stock in the proximal humerus/ glenoid vault. If the greater and lesser tuberosities (and the surrounding rotator cuff) were still attached to each other, an osteotomy would be required along the bicipital groove to "open up" these two fragments and allow access to the glenoid. If the fracture extended distally beyond the metaphyseal region, one would need to plan to cement the stem slightly proud to compensate for any bone loss. The alternative would be to use thicker polyethylene liner, or an implant which uses onlay systems with thicker humeral trays.
- Have the complete prosthesis portfolio available: In certain situations, there may be a need to convert the procedure from a RSA to a hemiarthroplasty with a CTA head; having a platform system with all the necessary modular components at hand would easily allow for this intra-op, or even in the future if necessary.
- **Skin incision:** A Delto-pectoral approach is recommended, for good exposure and access. Can be safely extended to expose more of the humerus shaft if required.
- **Anatomy:** In trauma scenarios, the anatomy is severely distorted by haematoma formation and displacement of the fragments and their soft tissue attachments. Spend a little more time initially to identify your landmarks and get control of the major fragments

  Tag the lesser tuberosity through the subscapularis tendon with strong stay sutures anteriorly.

Tag the greater tuberosity through the supraspinatus and infraspinatus tendons with strong stay sutures placed superiorly and posteriorly, respectively.

Retrieve the inferiorly displaced humeral head fragment carefully, ensuring that any metaphyseal neck spike does not inadvertently harm the axillary artery or nerve.

Once the lesser and greater tuberosities are in control with stay sutures, and the humeral head has been removed, with clear access to the glenoid, one can proceed with the usual RSA steps for glenoid preparation/ implantation.

- **Humerus preparation:** Here one will be using cemented fracture stems, instead of regular uncemented stems. The native humeral version cannot be judged in a fracture scenario, one would have to rely on the system's version rod to dial in the amount of version for the stem. Generally, more retroversion gives more clinical external rotation; most surgeons prefer 20–30 degrees of retroversion.

  The fracture stems have fins with suture apertures to aid in attaching the tuberosities back to the stem and the shaft, similar to that of a fracture hemiarthroplasty scenario (see Chapter 21). It is also recommended that one takes small block fragments of cancellous bone from the excised humeral head for bone grafting between the tuberosities and the stem. This results in better union of tuberosities with better clinical ROM outcomes and patient satisfaction [16].

6. Post-op Management and Rehabilitation

Immediate goals postoperatively are to maintain integrity of the replaced joint while gradually restoring passive range of motion (Fig. 19). In our institution, the shoulder is usually immobilised in a 30° abduction type sling for the first 4 weeks. During this time active and active assisted elbow, wrist and hand activity is encouraged. Beyond 4 weeks, the patient's passive range of motion is gradually increased in the scapular plane. Gradual transition to active range of motion with incremental increase is started after 6 weeks of surgery. Moderate strengthening is attempted after obtaining adequate active range in the shoulder joint, usually after 12 weeks.

7. Outcomes

Numerous outcome studies have demonstrated reproducible improvement in pain, active elevation, overhead function and improvement of objective outcome scores. In our study, patients achieved 53° improvement from preoperative forward flexion and 51° in improvement from preoperative abduction after undergoing RSA. There is significant pain reduction as measured on the visual analogue scale of approximately four points with significant improvement in Constant-Murley shoulder score, UCLA shoulder score and Oxford shoulder scores [11,12].

Evidence in literature [13,14] reports greater than 90% satisfaction rate with an average postoperative active forward flexion of approximately 135°–150° alongside significant improvement in 5 year American Shoulder and Elbow Society (ASES) scores (from 31 to 77).

Acknowledgements

The schematic illustrations in Figures 7, 11(b), 12, 13(b), 14(a), 14(c), 15(a) and 15(c) were taken from Depuy DELTA XTEND Surgical Technique manual and have been used with permission.

References

1. Smith CD, Guyver P, Bunker TD. Indications for reverse shoulder replacement: a systematic review. *J Bone Joint Surg Br* 2012;94:577–583.
2. Neer CS, Craig EV, Fukuda H. Cuff-tear arthropathy. *J Bone Joint Surg Am* 1983;65:1232–1244.
3. Halverson PB, Cheung HS, McCarty DJ, Garancis J, Mandel N. "Milwaukee shoulder" — association of microspheroids containing hydroxyapatite crystals, active collagenase, and neutral protease with rotator cuff defects. II. Synovial fluid studies. *Arthritis Rheum* 1981;24:474–483.
4. Jensen KL, Williams GR Jr, Russell IJ, Rockwood CA Jr. Rotator cuff tear arthropathy. *J Bone Joint Surg Am* 1999;81:1312–1324.
5. Zeman CA, Arcand MA, Cantrell JS, Skedros JG, Burkhead WZ Jr. The rotator cuff-deficient arthritic shoulder: diagnosis and surgical management. *J Am Acad Orthop Surg* 1998;6:337–348.

6. Lippitt S, Matsen F. Mechanisms of glenohumeral joint stability. *Clin Orthop Relat Res* 1993;(291):20–28. PMID: 8504601.
7. Aydin N, Tok O, Gorgun B. Rotator cuff tear arthropathy: pathophysiology, diagnosis and treatment. *Orthopedic Muscul Syst* 2014;3:159. doi: 10.4172/2161-0533-3-1000159.
8. Ecklund KJ, Lee TQ, Tibone J, Gupta R. Rotator cuff tear arthropathy. *J Am Acad Orthop Surg* 2007;15:340–349.
9. McFarland EG, Sanguanjit P, Tasaki A, Keyurapan E, Fishman EK, *et al*. The reverse shoulder prosthesis: a review of imaging features and complications. *Skeletal Radiol* 2006;35:488–496.
10. Boileau P, Watkinson D, Hatzidakis AM, Hovorka I. Neer Award 2005: The Grammont reverse shoulder prosthesis: results in cuff tear arthritis, fracture sequelae, and revision arthroplasty. *J Shoulder Elbow Surg* 2006;15: 527–540.
11. Chay-You Ang, Kah-Weng Lai, Denny Lie Tjiauw Tjoen, Paul Chang Chee Cheng. Reverse shoulder arthroplasty: The Singapore General Hospital experience and a simple method of measuring change in the center-of-rotation. *J Orthop* 2014;12(2). doi:10.1016/j.jor.2014.04.019.
12. Mak Wai Keong, Tan Yeow Boon, Hao Ying, Denny TT Lie. Acromial greater trochanteric distance as a predictor of outcomes post reverse shoulder arthroplasty. *submitted to JOS.*
13. Wall B, O'connor DP, Edwards TB, Nové-Josserand L, Walch G. Reverse total shoulder arthroplasty: a review of results according to etiology. *JBJS* 2007;89(7):1476–1485.
14. Valenti P, Boutens D, Nerot C, Walch G, Boileau P, Molé D. Delta 3 reversed prosthesis for osteoarthritis with massive rotator cuff tear: long term results. In: Walch G, Boileau P, Molé D (eds.), 2000, pp. 253–259.
15. Du S, Ye J, Chen H, Li X, Lin Q. Interventions for Treating 3- or 4-part proximal humeral fractures in elderly patient: a network meta-analysis of randomised controlled trials. *Int J Surg* 2017;48:240–246.
16. Pascal Boileau, Tjarco D. Alta, Lauryl Decroocq, François Sirveaux, Philippe Clavert, Luc Favard, Mikaël Chelli. Reverse shoulder arthroplasty for acute fractures in the elderly: is it worth reattaching the tuberosities? *J Shoulder Elbow Surg* 2019;28:437–444.

https://doi.org/10.1142/9789811249846_bmatter

Index

www.ingramcontent.com/pod-product-compliance
Lightning Source LLC
LaVergne TN
LVHW010329220926
848484LV00004BB/863
* 9 7 8 9 8 1 1 2 4 9 8 3 9 *